Second Edition

Management of Pediatric Practice

Author: Committee on Practice and Ambulatory Medicine
American Academy of Pediatrics

Leonard A. Kutnik, MD, Editor
Edward J. Saltzman, MD, Associate Editor
Daniel W. Shea, MD, Associate Editor
Lisa S. Honigfeld, PhD, Staff Editor
Karen S. Palchick, Staff Editor

American Academy of Pediatrics
141 Northwest Point Blvd
Elk Grove Village, Illinois 60007

Library of Congress Catalog No 85-071788   ISBN No 0-910761-31-0

Quantity prices on request. Address all inquiries to:
American Academy of Pediatrics, PO Box 927,
141 Northwest Point Blvd, Elk Grove Village, IL 60009-0927

The recommendations in this publication do not indicate an exclusive course of treatment or serve as a standard of medical care. Variations, taking into account individual circumstances, may be appropriate.

Committee on Practice and Ambulatory Medicine
1988 – 1991

Leonard A. Kutnik, MD, *Chairman, 1988 – 1990*
Roger F. Suchyta, MD, *Chairman, 1990 –*

Guillermo A. Balfour, MD
Michael D. Dickens, MD
John L. Green, MD
James V. Lustig, MD
Kenneth E. Matthews, MD
Bruce P. Meyer, MD
Peter D. Rappo, MD
Thomas F. Tonniges, MD

Liaison Representatives

Jay Berkelhamer, MD, *Ambulatory Pediatric Association*
Maurice Bouchard, MD, *Canadian Paediatric Society*
Jay E. Noffsinger, MD, *AAP Section on Military Pediatrics*
Robert E. Sayers, MD, *AAP Section on Military Pediatrics*

Acknowledgements

Members of the Committee on Practice and Ambulatory Medicine wish to express their gratitude to all the Academy staff members who worked tirelessly on behalf of this book. The Committee also wishes to thank Mariann M. Stephens, Chicago, Illinois, for her invaluable editorial assistance through the various editorial and production phases of this book.

The Committee wishes to express its appreciation for the assistance of the following individuals, who contributed to the preparation of this book.

Ms Julie K. Ake, Elk Grove Village, Illinois
Sophie Julia Balk, MD, Bronx, New York
Donald P. Barich, MD, Parma, Ohio
Lee W. Bass, MD, Pittsburgh, Pennsylvania
John T. Benjamin, MD, Charlottesville, Virginia
Donald M. Berwick, MD, Brookline, Massachusetts
Richard R. Brookman, MD, Richmond, Virginia
Daniel D. Chapman, MD, Zeeb, Michigan
Philip E. Clemente, CLU, MSFS, Hollywood, Florida
Bradford P. Cohn, MD, San Francisco, California
William A. Daniel, MD, Montgomery, Alabama
Robert H. Drachman, MD, Baltimore, Maryland
Robert Grayson, MD, Surfside, Florida
L. W. Greenberg, MD, Washington, DC
Anthony T. Hirsch, MD, Los Angeles, California
Albert D. Jacobson, MD, Phoenix, Arizona
Leslie S. Jewett, PhD, Washington, DC
Harvey P. Katz, MD, Braintree, Massachusetts
Alan E. Kohrt, MD, Tafton, Pennsylvania
Ms Carolyn Kolbaba, Elk Grove Village, Illinois
Ivan R. Koota, MD, Great Neck, New York
Arthur Maron, MD, West Orange, New Jersey
Thomas M. McCutchen, Jr, MD, Fayetteville, North Carolina
Donald B. Moore, MD, Boulder, Colorado
John C. Moore, Jr, MD, Omaha, Nebraska
Lucy Osborn, MD, Salt Lake City, Utah
Stanley Pappelbaum, MD, Del Mar, California
Kay C. Pinckard, MD, Phoenix, Arizona
William O. Robertson, MD, Seattle, Washington
Penny Rutledge, JD, Washington, DC
James E. Strain, MD, Elk Grove Village, Illinois
Ms Beth Yudkowsky, Elk Grove Village, Illinois

Table of Contents

Illustrations

The health and well-being of children is the major goal of the American Academy of Pediatrics and its Committee on Practice and Ambulatory Medicine. To meet this goal successfully, pediatricians must also establish and meet a second goal – a well-run, efficiently operating practice. Management aspects of a pediatric practice should be a major concern for all pediatricians.

Pediatrics enters the 1990s in a climate best described by paraphrasing the famous opening lines from *A Tale of Two Cities* by Charles Dickens: "It is the best of times; it is the worst of times." For each change in the style of pediatric practice today, there has been something lost and something gained.

Technical advances in the field of medicine enable today's children to enjoy physically more healthy lives than their forebears. As a result, pediatricians spend less time in illness care, and are free to devote additional emphasis on the health supervision of children. Psychosocial and developmental guidance is enhanced as a result, and with it, the potential to improve the quality of patients' lives. Unfortunately, the financial realities of ambulatory practice necessitate high patient volume and shorter visits. Innovative strategies are needed to respond to these conflicting responsibilities. Good practice management techniques can enhance practice efficiency, and maximize the effectiveness of the pediatrician's time.

Pediatricians strive to provide the highest quality medical care for their patients. This requires continuous availability, 24 hours a day, 7 days a week, 52 weeks a year. Years ago, when most pediatricians were solo practitioners, this required constant "on call" status. The pediatrician enjoyed few vacations and often little sleep. While the pediatrician was often revered by patients as their special physician, the hectic schedule interfered with family life.

Today we practice in an era of large single specialty or multispecialty groups, fully salaried staff model practice arrangements or smaller practices with shared coverage arrangements. Careful attention to communication with patients and covering colleagues, accompanied by efficient, thorough practice operation, enable continuity of high quality care for children. While some closeness to our patients has by necessity been lost, the change in practice style allows the modern pediatrician additional time for family or other personal life activities.

Advances in medicine continue to unfold at a staggering pace, offering the opportunity to diagnose and cure diseases, such as leukemia and neuroblastoma, which were not amenable to treatment in the past. New antibiotics and other pharmacologic agents have dramatically enhanced the pediatrician's armamentarium in fighting disease; improved knowledge allows previously untreatable premature infants a good chance of survival. These opportunities to provide improved care greatly enhance a pediatrician's self-esteem and ability to take pleasure from practice. Regrettably, in today's litigious society, this success has so raised patient expectations that any adverse outcome is no longer considered acceptable. Patients also expect to be more involved in decision making regarding care, and many question the pediatrician's judgment and therapeutic approach. These factors add new stresses to the art of providing pediatric care.

Pediatricians are learning to cope with these changing expectations by utilizing the improved communication and educational opportunities now available. Computers and telephonic advances, including facsimile (FAX) machines, provide ready access to medical library information or distant experts for consultation on complex medical problems. Continuing medical education programs and risk management programs conducted constantly in all areas of the US enable all pediatricians, including those in the most remote locations, to hear and learn the latest ideas and approaches.

Preface

Leonard A. Kutnik, MD

The financial realities of pediatric practice have also changed. No longer can a high quality physician hang up a shingle and be guaranteed a successful practice. Today's patients often choose their insurance payment system first, usually through their employer. Rather than select a physician through traditional referrals, they select a physician from the specific provider panel, and assume that this guarantees competency.

Payment mechanisms in these managed care systems have complex requirements for billing, referrals, and hospitalization. Today's pediatric office must employ effective and flexible management systems for optimal patient care and financial reimbursement. These changes have complicated the management of a small medical practice, but those who can successfully adapt to this changing environment enjoy assured reimbursements for services (reducing the amount of delinquent accounts and bad debts) and the promise of additional patients to help a practice grow through health plan marketing programs.

Those pediatricians who find that these changes detract from the appeal of ambulatory private practice may select from a proliferation of alternate career choices, ranging from academic or administrative medicine to retraining in a pediatric subspecialty or joining an HMO. This variety can enable a pediatrician to switch career directions and develop a more satisfactory practice arrangement. All pediatricians, regardless of practice form, must always continue to exercise excellent practice management skills.

Teaching programs produce superb pediatric trainees who are well informed academically. The success of the American Board of Pediatrics in documenting the high level of training is a tribute to the integrity of the teaching and assessment systems in use today. Unfortunately, the realities of practicing ambulatory pediatrics, and the practical techniques needed for developing effective office systems and running an organized pediatric office, have been, to a large degree, neglected. Little time has been devoted to such aspects of practice as appointment books, personnel problems, separating and aging of accounts receivable, and collection of overdue accounts. The equally important psychological aspects of practice, such as the emotional trauma created by viewing jammed reception areas and the stress of dealing with irate parents, have also been underemphasized. The result has been that well trained pediatricians entering practice have been ill prepared for the nonmedical rigors of practice.

This second edition of *Management of Pediatric Practice* has been written to serve as a guide to help pediatricians steer their professional lives and practices through these changing times. It has been designed to facilitate the pediatrician's ability to be productive professionally through the exercise of sound business practice. The chapters in this book have been arranged to assist pediatricians in the development of an effective organization of their office systems. They progress from basic concepts in pediatric technique to specifics in the management of key areas of practice to suggestions and aids for areas of practice which require some understanding of special issues. A checklist at the end of most chapters and editorial comments in the form of counterpoints are intended to either reinforce the contents of the chapters (to emphasize the pitfalls and rigors of a practice situation) or to indicate alternate methods of problem solving.

Management of Pediatric Practice is designed for pediatric practice and the pediatrician, rather than general office management. It attempts to assist the pediatrician in reviewing various aspects of practice in a candid manner based on the personal experiences of professionals who have achieved expertise and the respect of their peers. The Academy's Committee on Practice and Ambulatory Medicine has striven for the concrete and practical, which may inadvertently give the impression that there is but a single solution to each problem. The reader should realize that there are many "correct" ways to approach a problem effectively, depending on the personality and style of the pediatrician. The didactic writing technique was used only to avoid vague generalities.

In the few short years since the publication of the first edition of this manual, the changes in the medical and pediatric world have been astounding. Almost every aspect of pediatric practice covered in the first edition has required some revision and updating. In addition, the rapidly changing environment, described earlier, has resulted in the creation of entirely new areas requiring identification and emphasis. Thus the second edition has added new chapters in order to help the pediatrician in keeping abreast of this rapidly changing medical practice landscape.

Residents today often enter practice by joining large established groups, single or multispecialty, or HMOs. Many are debating decisions regarding the issues of part-time or shared practice. The chapter on practice payment systems has been greatly expanded and new chapters dealing with the issues of contracting and alternate practice styles have been added to assist pediatricians in their deliberations.

The complexity of ongoing practice has increased exponentially over the last 5 years, stimulating the development of new chapters on charging for services and risk management. The need to evaluate continually the quality of one's practice has become the issue of the 1990s and the subject of a new chapter on continuing practice analysis. The multitude of demands on pediatricians in practice are causing increased stress and affecting the pediatrician's life satisfaction and life-style. A new chapter on stress management provides suggestions and coping techniques. Finally, for those who have served the needs of children for many years and are now ready to move on to new endeavors, we have included a chapter on retirement.

If additional technical advice is needed after reading this book, pediatricians can obtain guidance through published works or consultants. The AAP Division of Pediatric Practice also is available for further assistance.

Pediatricians will continue to experience ever-increasing technical improvements, patient life-style changes, demands on time and changes in practice emphasis from specific illness care to health supervision. All of these call for innovative strategies to provide efficient management of a pediatric practice. The quality of a practice and thus the ultimate career satisfaction of the pediatrician will depend on a combination of the pediatrician's professional skills and an understanding of the "how to's" of practice. The Academy's Committee on Practice and Ambulatory Medicine believes that a more efficiently managed practice will result in much greater satisfaction for both pediatricians and their patients. Additionally, an effective practice operation frees the pediatrician to pursue new subject areas as they become an important part of contemporary pediatric practice, and/or to enjoy additional hours with their families.

The pediatrician should look on this book as an offer of help. Just as you would make a selection of food from a buffet table, take from this book what you want and need. Even if no real changes are necessary, strengthen your current office techniques. Maintain standards of quality (superb pediatric care), yet reserve time to reflect, understand, and compete in the present. Take time to enjoy your chosen career.

This second, updated edition of the AAP manual, *Management of Pediatric Practice,* could well be alternatively titled: *Everything You Ever Wanted to Know About Managing a Pediatric Practice But Never Got Around to Asking.* It clearly represents the most useful, practical, and authoritative publication available, not only for the nascent pediatrician planning his or her future in practice, but also for anyone seeking useful suggestions to improve the "patient-friendliness," efficiency in provision of pediatric services, and economics of a pediatric practice, be it solo or group.

This manual was written by the Committee on Practice and Ambulatory Medicine of the American Academy of Pediatrics (AAP) with input from pediatricians across the US, and edited by three former chairmen of the Committee, all of whom are respected and successful practicing pediatricians. It covers all aspects of pediatric practice, from the choice of type and place of practice, to how to prevent embezzlement in the office; from keeping one's spouse content, to telephone manners when calling another physician.

All of this is done in a readable, nonredundant style which includes not only samples of standard forms for use in the pediatric office, but also specific references as to sources of such forms. The manual contains up-to-date references for those who want to go into more detail about any of the subjects covered, and provides handy checklists which cover a full spectrum of practice-related issues.

In short, this is a "must" book for anyone contemplating entering pediatric practice, and for anyone who wants to review his or her practice for whatever reason.

Foreword

Robert J. McKay, Jr, MD
Burlington, Vermont

I was greatly honored to have been asked by the practicing pediatricians who have assembled the Management of Pediatric Practice to write the Foreword. I say honored because pediatricians in practice generally have a degree of mistrust for full-time academic pediatricians, among whom I am theoretically numbered. The request meant to me that practicing pediatricians view me as a friend, not a foe; and this gives me distinct pleasure.

The Foreword is not meant to provide me with autobiographical space, but I cannot resist the opportunity to explain exactly why I have always taken the side of the practicing pediatrician in any debate or controversy and have developed a true feeling for his/her problems and points of view. When I completed my 4 years of military service in World War II, I returned to Boston only because I had gone there to college and medical school. Having enjoyed receiving a living wage while in the army, I had decided that practice rather than full-time academic work would allow me to live in the style I had become accustomed to as a first lieutenant, and I joined the office of Dr Warren Sisson, one of the first qualified pediatricians in the Boston area. Lacking a source of the wisdom contained in the present manual, I fell in with his custom of accepting patients from any part of Boston and its suburbs. One Sunday while I was on call, and with a blizzard raging, I made a home visit to a physician's child at one end of greater Boston. After 3 hours of digging out of drifts, a call to the answering service sent me 17 miles in the opposite direction. I reached home 8 hours after I left, having made two visits, one without charge. Picturing a short future with me lying dead from a myocardial infarct alongside my snow shovel, I resigned from private practice and accepted the position which had previously been offered me as Chief of Ambulatory Services at Children's Hospital. Academic salaries were such that I was allowed three afternoons a week of private practice, and I limited my patients to families living on either side of my route from home to hospital. Since my private practice experience, I feel utmost sympathy and understanding for the practitioner, despite the fact that home visits are a thing of the past.

I enjoyed reading this manual. Careful attention to its details will spare the young resident much time and anguish in looking for a place to settle. The various sections have been written by pediatricians who know exactly what is involved in giving superior service to children while simultaneously feeding, housing, and rearing a family. The pitfalls to be avoided are carefully spelled out. If a private practice is thoughtfully established, the joy of watching and helping young men and women develop and grow from the newborn state is one that cannot be matched by any other branch of medicine.

If at all possible, the young resident at the completion of training should start in a group practice made up of members who are not too far apart in years. They should have similar goals and levels of excellence, plus dispositions that allow them to relate warmly and happily to one another. I have always urged that, in such a group, each member by reading and by attending clinics develop expertise in one of the subspecialty areas so there may be referrals of problem patients for consultation within the group. It adds greatly to the pleasure of practice to have one's peers turn to you for advice and help in a special area of pediatrics. In the ideal group, if there is such a thing, the spouses also will be warm and understanding, have a good sense of humor, and have a minimum of jealousy. Solo practice, however, is preferable to a group split by discord.

To those of you who read and benefit by this manual, we wish you a happy and rewarding career. I take the privileged position of Foreword-writer to urge that you tell us of experiences which will correct any deficiencies in the manual and will assist it in keeping up with these rapidly changing times. To your good health!

Foreword to First Edition

Sydney Gellis, MD
Boston, Massachusetts

Section I

Getting Started

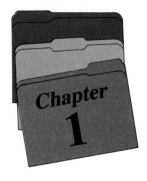

Basics of Practice

This chapter offers an introduction to basic concepts of pediatric practice management, including:
- **the pediatrician as practitioner**
- **pediatric career options**
- **communication and confidentiality issues**
- **office and personnel management**
- **the place for technology**
- **managing stress**

> "Children are our most enduring and vulnerable legacy. For nations as well as for individual families, they represent the link between past and future, experience and promise. The nurturing of future generations is a basic and most important activity."
>
> **Preamble to the Constitution of the American Academy of Pediatrics**

The role of the pediatrician has changed dramatically since the inception of the American Academy of Pediatrics (AAP). We no longer spend the majority of our time treating infectious diseases, but must address more comprehensive issues. The American Board of Pediatrics considers the primary focus of the pediatrician to be the developing child; the discipline of pediatrics seeks to maximize that development by treating disease, minimizing the deleterious effect of chronic conditions, and preventing social and medical conditions which may inhibit development.

Today's pediatrician is able to address the comprehensive biological and emotional needs of children. He or she acts as a practitioner, a counselor, and a teacher.

A pediatrician is the captain of the child's medical home. The physician should discuss the concept of a "medical home" for the child at the first visit. It is important for the parent to understand that the pediatrician is there to provide ongoing comprehensive care, and is available to assist the parent in the care of the child whenever the need arises. The pediatrician should serve as team leader for psychosocial disorders,

learning problems, and subspecialty referral care. This ongoing relationship is satisfying to the pediatrician and family and ensures the best possible medical care for the child.

Finally, today's pediatrician should serve as an advocate for children. Pediatricians have been instrumental in changing public behaviors with respect to such issues as seatbelt usage, and car seats for small children. Pediatricians are presently addressing the need for access to health care for all children.

Career options

The many facets of pediatric practice enable pediatricians to enjoy a wide variety of professional life-styles. Options abound in terms of practice style and location. While many still enjoy the independence of solo practice, more and more pediatricians are opting for group practice or institutionally based practice. The significant influx of women into pediatrics has paralleled an interest in job-sharing or part-time practice options for those who wish to balance work and family responsibilities.

The explosive development of subspecialties in pediatrics has afforded us a wide expanse of new choices. While pediatrics is traditionally considered a cognitive specialty, procedurally oriented pediatricians can enjoy careers in such subspecialties as intensive care, gastroenterology or pulmonary medicine.

Solo practice

Traditionally, solo practice has been said to afford a pediatrician the ability to make all practice decisions independently. Policies regarding office management, staffing, scheduling,

after-hour coverage and charges, may all be made at the discretion of the solo pediatrician. The pediatrician can determine how much time to spend with each patient, which services to offer in the office, and how to develop new services as time goes on.

However, all pediatricians need to provide care for their patients 24 hours a day. While solo practitioners enjoy the greatest ability to mold their practice to their wants and needs, they also have the greatest burdens in terms of arranging coverage and office management.

Pediatricians in solo practice often join together to establish "cooperative solo practices" in which independent practitioners agree to cover the others at night and on weekends on a rotational basis. This arrangement can provide for coverage during vacations, time away for continuing education or other mutually acceptable activities.

Partnership or group practice

The past decade has seen increasing numbers of pediatricians choose to give up their personal freedom and join a group practice or larger multispecialty group. In these situations, physicians band together to share the tasks of practice management, to develop new services for the practice, and to jointly determine such things as personnel policies, the format of the medical record, and policies for after-hours coverage, continuing medical education and vacation time. These arrangements allow pediatricians to profit from shared objectives and enhanced professional interaction. In today's highly competitive environment, with competition from family physicians and the advent of discounted managed medical care, many believe group practice offers a measure of security which solo practice may not enjoy.

Practice employment contracts

Structure in a group practice prevents ambiguities about policies. It is advisable to have a specific written agreement among all physicians in the group concerning the conduct of the practice.

The first step in formulating an agreement is to review the aims and goals of the group pertaining to matters of mutual concern, such as practice hours, coverage, academic needs, income and benefits, and time out of the office. Agreements should be reached in an atmosphere of mutual trust. All items discussed and agreed upon should be documented in writing and a copy given to those involved.

Members of a partnership or group practice must have a defined income distribution plan. The practice must have an identifiable management structure with specified accountabilities and consistent standards of care, which are agreed upon by the partners.

Pediatricians may choose to practice in a Health Maintenance Organization (HMO) which contracts to provide comprehensive health care services to a defined population of enrolled members on a prepaid per capita basis. There are two types of HMOs: the staff model and the group/IPA model. Staff model HMOs are usually limited to a single or finite group of locations and employ salaried physicians. The group/IPA model enlists a number of either single specialty or multispecialty professional practices that receive separate capitation payments from the HMO corporation. Physicians in this model may be either salaried or receive per capita payments plus a share of the group's/IPA's net income.

A pediatrician may also enter into an agreement with a PPO (Preferred Provider Organization) in which he or she agrees to provide services on a discounted fee-for-service basis for a defined group of patients.

Additional career options

Pediatricians choose from a myriad of models in developing a practice. Today's pediatrician weighs an increased prevalence of group practice, rapid growth in HMOs, greater proportion of women in pediatrics and an increased number of dual career families. As life-style becomes more of an issue for pediatricians, varying professional styles, including part-time practice, shared practice positions and other coverage arrangements, continue to evolve.

As there are differences between solo and group practice there are also differences between urban and rural practice. In an urban setting one is more likely to have rapid access to subspecialty consultation and pediatric-oriented intensive care settings. The rural pediatrician is more likely to act as a consultant to family practitioners in the area and to use intensive care stabilization skills.

General considerations

The majority of a pediatrician's professional time is spent in the office. Patients are seen for preventive health care, treatment of acute and chronic illnesses, injuries, psychosocial problems, developmental assessment, school problems, and anticipatory guidance.

General pediatrics is an ambulatory cognitive specialty. By caring for a group of patients over a period of time, the pediatrician is able to help maximize their potential while minimizing the morbidity attendant with any acute and/or chronic health problems. The "Guidelines for Health Supervision II"[1] developed by the American Academy of Pediatrics help focus the practitioner and result in the delivery of appropriate services for children. Health supervision visits include the elucidation of appropriate history, a complete physical exam, administration of appropriate immunizations, and administration of screening tests. In addition, anticipatory guidance is crucial in enabling parents to deal with problems which will occur as the child progresses developmentally. Following the guidelines enables the pediatrician to develop a comprehensive pediatric data base for each child in the practice. As new problems develop, they can be interdigitated into the pediatric data base, facilitating provision of appropriate services and treatments.

These considerations bring to mind the importance of planning. All pediatricians need to employ practice analysis to ensure that their practice and patient base are evolving in accord with professional goals. It is crucial to analyze and document your professional experience and to stay in touch with your personal interests. The current edition of this manual speaks to improving the quality of an office practice.

Office visits

If the initial visit is for health assessment, a complete history should be taken with special attention given to previous illnesses and hospitalizations and any family history of genetic disorders or chronic illnesses. A release of medical information form should be signed by the parent to allow the pediatrician to request a summary of the medical record from physicians treating the patient in the past. A thorough physical examination should be included in the visit. It may be necessary to do certain screening laboratory procedures, eg, hematocrit, urinalysis, sickle cell preparation, lead level and/or free erythrocyte protoporphyrin test. A developmental screening test may be appropriate, depending upon the age of the child, and screening for visual and auditory defects should be a part of the assessment. An immunization history should be obtained and immunizations given when appropriate. It may be necessary to delay immunization until records are obtained from former physicians.

If the initial visit is for treatment of an acute illness or injury, only the necessary procedures and pertinent past history need be performed. An appointment may be made for a comprehensive health assessment at a later date.

Hospital care

A newborn should be examined soon after birth if the obstetrician or nursery nurse expresses any concern about the baby. In any event, examination should be performed within 24 hours of delivery. A mother is anxious to know as much as possible about the care of her baby, and a daily visit by the pediatrician can give her much needed confidence in dealing with the problems she is likely to encounter at home. This is a time of "bonding" between parents and pediatrician which can help to establish a trusting and lasting relationship. Absent medical problems in mother or baby, mothers are now being discharged from the hospital on the first or second post delivery day. These mothers especially must be given the necessary information and thorough instructions to care for their babies at home.

Patient brochures are useful adjuncts to discussions with the mother. (See Patient Education Materials, Chapter 26.) They can include information about the care of the newborn infant, feeding schedules, use of the car seat and the need to observe for jaundice. If possible the handout should include the height and weight of the infant and any other vital information specific to the baby.

Time with the mother in the hospital is well spent, and usually results in fewer telephone calls after discharge. A mother who is confident in her ability to care for her baby is less likely to become anxious and concerned or overly dependent upon the advice of the pediatrician.

If the family is new to the practice, it may be wise to delay giving the patient extensive information about office policies until the first office visit. The mother should be given instructions for the first office visit as well as telephone availability whenever the need exists.

When illness occurs in the nursery or an infant is transferred to an intensive care nursery, it is extremely important for the pediatrician to keep the parents informed of the infant's condition. If neonatologists are involved, it is essential that they keep the pediatrician informed of the baby's progress. In addition, sharing the information with the obstetrician strengthens the interprofessional relationship.

Hospital newborn data should be affixed to the office chart to ensure that accurate information about the baby's birth, vital statistics and any nursery event are available at the time of the first office visit. It should be possible for the newborn records in the nursery to be multiple copy forms so that a legible copy may be taken by the pediatrician for the office record.

Hospital rounds

Hospital rounds should be made at least daily and more often if necessary. The pediatrician may be the admitting physician or serve as a consultant for a child admitted by a family practitioner or for a subspecialist who admitted a

child for tertiary care. In some communities, hospital-based pediatricians assume much of the responsibility for the inpatient care requested by the community pediatrician. Upon discharge, the community pediatrician resumes responsibility for the child's care. When planning for hospital rounds, time should be allowed for chart review, consultation with nurses, patient examination and discussions with parents.

Extended conversations with parents of children with serious illnesses, complicated problems or other conditions requiring explanation or reassurance may be carried out in the office or in a quiet room in the hospital. A meeting should be scheduled when both parents can be present. In addition, financial matters about the child's care: hospital fees, initial examination and daily rates, including the day of discharge, and fees for special procedures, are discussed more comfortably in the office setting. These should be carefully explained so that any future billing statement is understood by the parents as well as third party payers.

Emergency room

Emergency care is an important part of pediatric practice. As part of anticipatory guidance, parents should be encouraged to contact their pediatrician before going to the emergency room, although this is not always possible. Parents should know where to take their child in the event of a serious injury or life threatening illness. When such an event requires the skills of a critical care physician, the pediatrician can be supportive of the family and keep them informed of the child's condition.

Some patients will use the emergency room for after-hours primary care. This practice can be discouraged by making it clear that parents should make every attempt to reach the pediatrician *first* in after-hours emergencies.

Consultations

A pediatrician may be asked by another physician to consult on a child. This may occur in the hospital or in an ambulatory setting. The pediatrician must be certain the family has agreed to the consultation before it takes place. It is upsetting to parents to first learn of a potentially serious problem only after the consultant appears. The

consultation should be delayed, except in an emergency, until the family is informed and permission granted.

Occasionally a pediatrician may be asked by a parent to consult on a child. The family should be directed to discuss the consultation with the attending physician. The family should understand that a consultation should only take place if the request comes from the child's physician.

A consultation should consist of a complete history obtained from one or both parents. It should not be assumed that all essential medical information is included on the chart. A physical examination should be performed and the laboratory data reviewed before a conclusion is reached. The results of the consultation should be legibly recorded in the chart and discussed with the referring physician as soon as possible.

A pediatrician may seek the advice of another physician if a child's diagnosis or treatment is unclear or if skills beyond those of a pediatrician are required. The need for consultation and the names of possible consultants should be discussed with the parents, since the family may have a consultant in mind. If the physician requested by the family is not acceptable, there should be a careful explanation of why another consultant would be more appropriate.

Once the consultant is agreed upon, the pediatrician should contact the physician personally to give him the necessary background information needed to render an opinion. A written report of the consultation should be requested for inclusion in the child's office record. Exceptions may be made in the case of psychiatrists, whose information often must remain confidential.

Occasionally, a family will request a consultation because of lack of progress or dissatisfaction with some aspects of the treatment. An astute pediatrician can often discern this dissatisfaction before the request is made and will suggest a consultation to reassure the family.

When a consultation is suggested by a pediatrician in the office, the patient/parent should schedule the visit with the consulting physician. This allows the patient flexibility in scheduling an appointment and affirms the family's desire for a consultation. This is particularly important in referrals to psychiatrists or psychologists.

In an emergency situation, it may be important for the referring pediatrician to make the appropriate arrangements. It is often desirable to have one or both parents present when those arrangements are made. It is important for the pediatrician to continue to provide supportive care until the child is seen by the consultant.

The use of a consultant is a means of assuring the optimal care of a child with a complex and/or serious illness. Parents view this not as a deficiency in the medical knowledge of the attending pediatrician, but as an assurance of the pediatrician's desire to provide the best possible care for the child.

Communication

Communication between parents and pediatrician or adolescent and pediatrician is an important aspect of pediatric care. This means listening to the patient's concerns and responding appropriately. Physicians are often criticized for failing to address the specific complaints of the patient. Listening to patients takes time, but it is essential for a good patient-doctor relationship and for good medical care.

A pediatrician can create a relaxed atmosphere by extending a warm greeting and introduction to the parents, child or adolescent. Direct eye to eye contact when speaking is important. The pediatrician should share thoughts, opinions and concerns with patients whenever possible and be open in discussing illnesses that are not easily diagnosed. Illnesses in children often require continued observation before a definitive diagnosis can be made. Since most children's diseases are self-limited or respond rapidly to treatment, the pediatrician can usually be reassuring about the prognosis. On the other hand, if the disease is serious or life threatening, the pediatrician must be direct in explaining the nature of the illness and the probable outcome.

The use of medical jargon is confusing to laymen. Explanations should be given in a way that is easily understood by the parents. Language should be used to inform, not to impress. Care should be taken in the use of terms to describe a child's illness. Whenever possible, descriptive phrases that reassure rather than frighten patients should be used.

There may be times when a parent complains about office personnel or procedures. This may be justified, especially in a busy office practice or in group practices where large numbers of patients are being seen. The pediatrician should listen attentively to the complaint and make whatever changes are necessary if the complaint is valid. If a staff member is abrupt or abrasive, if a telephone call is not returned, if a billing error has occurred or if there is a prolonged delay in seeing a patient with a scheduled appointment, discussing the situation in a friendly manner will often resolve the problem.

When the patient or pediatrician elects to terminate their relationship, it is desirable for the pediatrician to communicate with the patient to share feelings and concerns. This also provides an opportunity to reassure the family that medical records will be promptly transferred to the "new physician."

The parents should also be assured that they will not be abandoned and that the pediatrician will remain in charge until another physician assumes responsibility for the care.

Confidentiality

Information obtained from a patient or parent should remain confidential unless permission is given to release it. This applies to the exchange of information between physicians when a consult is requested or when a patient transfers from one physician to another. A release of medical information form should be signed by the patient or parent when a transfer of records is requested.

For ethical and legal reasons, patient information should be shared with the immediate family only (parents, siblings). Divulging confidential information to anyone can have serious consequences for the physician and/or members of the community.

Adolescents especially need to be assured that information obtained in confidence will not be shared with their parents without their permission. An exception can be made in the case of an incompetent adolescent, and should be made if one shows signs of self-destructive behavior. The pediatrician should review state statutes regarding confidentiality and age of emancipation.

Sharing medical information with the school can also pose an ethical dilemma. In general, if the information would assist school authorities in dealing with a child's illness in school, it is appropriate to include it on the school health record. However, before the information is released to the school it should be discussed with the parent.

Medical liability

Medical liability was not a major concern in pediatrics until recently. However with the increasing number of suits involving DTP reactions, delay in diagnosing conditions such as meningitis and acute abdominal conditions, and prescribing errors, this is no longer the case.

A good patient-doctor relationship and good records will reduce the risk of a medical liability suit, but there are no guarantees. Another fallacy is that only "bad doctors" are sued. Conscientious, knowledgeable pediatricians have been involved in medical liability litigation, and the vulnerability of every pediatrician should be recognized.

Office location and design

The choice of an office location depends on the type of anticipated pediatric practice. For those establishing a new solo practice or forming a new group, the selection of a practice site becomes extremely important. Access to inpatient and outpatient hospital services and the availability of subspecialists and other professionals are important considerations. It is desirable to locate in an area where there are other medical and nonmedical professionals. Sharing experiences with those with similar interests can serve to enrich the lives of a pediatrician and his family. The cost of office space and decor provided by the landlord is an important consideration in many areas. Ease of access, parking, and access for handicapped persons should also be considered. A pediatrician and his/her family must be comfortable with the community's school system, social life, shopping, and entertainment.

To facilitate an efficient practice, office design has become more and more important. A clean, bright, well-run office encourages patients to feel secure and more relaxed. The office itself contributes mightily to the mutual satisfaction of the patient and pediatrician at each visit. It is important to remember that the way in which patients flow through an office during a visit significantly alters function of the office. The design also impacts on the manner in which personnel are able to function and influences the number of personnel required.

For those in established practices who wish to expand their catchment area, satellite offices may be useful. The development of a successful satellite office requires a major commitment on the part of the entire practice staff as well as careful preparation and planning to ensure the ability to attract patients to the satellite office. Some practices have even developed satellite offices to enable the provision of specialized services (eg, adolescent or subspecialty care).

Office emergencies

All offices must be properly prepared for treatment of emergencies. Emergency plans should be reviewed periodically and all emergency equipment should be checked regularly. Office personnel should be familiar with resuscitation procedures and emergency care. Manuals are available to provide specific information on emergency procedures and equipment.

All offices must be built and equipped to provide maximum safety for patients, parents and other visitors. Attention to safety details will avoid problems later.

It is important to carry liability insurance that covers injuries incurred in or about the office premises. Toys should be kept out of the traffic path of the reception area. Electrical outlets should be plugged or covered. Drugs and instruments should be kept out of the reach of children and children should not be left unattended on the examining table. (See bibliography at the end of this chapter.)

Personnel/personnel policies

As practices grow, the number of people employed by the practice may increase dramatically. This requires that pediatricians become competent

managers, and that a pediatrician always maintains final authority in matters of office personnel policy. The office must be organized so that employees understand the structure of the office, their relationship to other employees and those tasks for which they are responsible. Organization within the office must promote cooperation, team work, and direction to maximize efficient patient care.

Written job descriptions establish authority and responsibility while defining the duties of each position within the office. As job descriptions are developed, standards of performance should also be identified to evaluate and reward performance. Attention needs to be given to training personnel so that all members of the team perform efficiently and well. Pediatricians should also have a policy manual to outline those things which personnel are expected to do in a given situation. Regardless of the size of the practice, one pediatrician must take responsibility for personnel matters.

Reimbursement

To assure proper reimbursement, pediatricians must first document carefully what services they have performed and the outcome of those services. There should also be recognition and documentation of time spent in treating a patient's problems. Careful attention must be given to designing billing forms such as a superbill, using appropriate codes, and reviewing billings on a regular basis. The fee schedule should be clearly understood by office personnel, who should advise patients in advance of the cost of services. Office policy should encourage payment for services at the time of the visit.

With the development of alternative health care systems such as HMOs and PPOs, it is important to know the type of payment (reduced fee-for-service or capitation); the specific limits of coverage, such as whether the plan will cover health supervision visits; whether the system withholds a part of the payment; and if it places the pediatrician at risk. Careful attention must be paid to all of these issues to enable a pediatrician to deal with health care payment systems.

Office laboratory and other services

Many pediatricians have developed an office laboratory to provide their patients with efficient, cost-effective services. Developing such a laboratory requires careful planning, ongoing quality control and careful documentation of results so that patients are well served. At the present time, developing technology allows pediatricians to offer many more services for their patients than have been available previously. The Clinical Laboratory Improvement Amendments (CLIA) of 1988 will regulate all laboratories and may significantly alter the rules for office lab tests. Therefore, pediatricians contemplating developing a clinical laboratory should first check on the status of the CLIA legislation as well as any local or state regulations. The AAP Division of Pediatric Practice can inform you of the status of the CLIA legislation. Other services which may be offered in the office include dispensing medication and x-ray diagnostic services. These require special preparation and the ability to deliver consistently high quality services, and should be carefully evaluated by each individual practice.

Technology

Increased demands on a pediatrician's time have resulted in more and more dependence on technology. The chapters dealing with the telephone time conservation and computer systems help to address some specific issues with respect to some of these technologies.

The telephone is our most frequently employed technology and is critical to the development of a practice. Everyone who answers the telephone must understand that they are representing the practice. Telephone calls must be answered promptly and professionally. The content of all telephone calls regarding patient care issues must be documented, and the documentation made part of the patient's medical record. The office should have specific telephone policies and protocols, which are reviewed regularly by the pediatrician.

Pediatricians often find it advantageous to set aside specific time for telephone consultations. Others will return calls between patient visits during office hours. Calls from physicians or emergency calls from parents should be taken immediately. It may be desirable to delegate some of the responsibility for answering telephone queries to an experienced nurse or aide. This allows more time to see patients in the office and avoids a delay in returning calls. Parents must feel free to call the pediatrician, but many parents feel more comfortable in calling the office if they don't feel they are imposing on the physician's time. After an office assessment the pediatrician may want to follow a child with an acute illness by telephone.

As a matter of telephone etiquette, the pediatrician should place his own calls if possible, especially when trying to reach another professional. When a receptionist places a call and holds the party on the line until the physician is called to the telephone, that person has the impression that the physician's time is thought to be more valuable than his or her own. The pediatrician must make arrangements for telephone calls to be taken at home. It may be necessary to have two lines to accommodate both professional and personal calls. Pediatricians on call should be near a telephone and available.

Computer systems were at one time heralded as revolutionary breakthroughs; at present, most pediatricians have not yet exploited this technology. When considering a computer system, all procedures in the office should be audited to determine whether a true practice need exists. A specific computer system can then be obtained to fit the office requirements. Provisions must be made to introduce the computer into the office and train all personnel who will use the system. At least one physician in the office must understand and be able to operate the entire computer system.

Pharmaceutical representatives

The best source of information about new treatment modalities or indications for drug use is from university or professional society CME meetings and from the medical literature. A pharmaceutical representative can give the physician information about new products and new dispensing forms but the basis for their use should come from impartial scientific studies. Pharmaceutical representatives will often distribute useful patient information material and leave "starter samples" that can be used in an emergency.

A pediatrician will often find it difficult to see a pharmaceutical representative in the middle of a busy schedule. It may be desirable to schedule the visit over the noon hour or in late afternoon when it doesn't conflict with patient care.

Life-styles

Optimal performance is a professional obligation. A poorly rested, distracted pediatrician is ill-prepared to exercise his best cognitive skills. Proper attention to personal health, family, recreation, intellectual stimulation, and participation in the professional community provides a necessary counterbalance to the pressures of professional life. Almost by definition, pediatricians are subject to stress. Pediatricians must continually ask what it is they truly wish to do, which skills they bring to bear on their goals, and how they can modify preconceived goals to enhance success. The process of efficient time management can be enhanced by carefully structuring the day so that the office staff knows precisely what needs to be done during each period of the day. Interruptions must be kept to a minimum. Schedules must be followed.

It is important to emphasize that time spent with family and time away from the office for personal pursuits is important to the well-being of the pediatrician. Those who are not adept at time management are well advised to seek courses to facilitate development of this skill, as effective time management can significantly enhance professional satisfaction.

Continuing medical education

Only by constant education and integration of new knowledge can our practices remain productive and our lives fulfilled. Continuing medical education by reading, listening to or viewing audiovisual materials, and attending grand rounds or CME courses is essential if the pediatrician is to keep "up-to-date" in his medical knowledge.

The Academy's PREP materials (Pediatrics Review and Education Program), CompuPREP (its computerized version), and *Pediatrics in Review* journal serve as excellent sources for continuing medical education (CME) credits. Articles in peer reviewed journals also provide a pediatrician with current information on advances in pediatrics. Review journals often focus on the educational objectives to be used in the recertification process and are the best source of information on the "state-of-the-art" pediatrics. Audiotapes can be used in the tape deck of an automobile while videotapes require the pediatrician's undivided attention. Computerized disks are useful in reviewing the pediatric literature. CD-ROM is now capable of storing up to 7 years of *Pediatrics* on one disk with easy retrieval of information by title, author or key words.

Summary

Pediatrics remains an evolving, exciting specialty affording its practitioners many ways to enjoy a rich, full professional life. It offers the potential for lifelong stimulation and fulfillment, provided that we take the steps to nurture and protect the delicate balance of personal and professional goals and responsibilities.

Reference

1. American Academy of Pediatrics, Committee on Psychosocial Aspects of Child and Family Health. *Guidelines for Health Supervision II*. Elk Grove Village, IL: American Academy of Pediatrics; 1988.

Bibliography

Fuchs S, Jaffe DM, Christoffel KK. Pediatric Emergencies in Office Practices: Prevalence and Office Preparedness. *Pediatrics*. 1989;83:931-939

Hodge D. Pediatric Emergency Office Equipment. *Pediatric Emergency Care*. 1988;4:212-214

Lubitz DS, Seidel JS, Chameides L, et al. A Rapid Method for Estimating Weight and Resuscitation Drug Dosages from Length in the Pediatric Age Group. *Annals of Emergency Medicine*. 1988;17:576-580

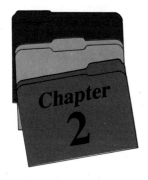

Chapter 2

Practice Location

Practice location is a major concern for all pediatricians. The issue is associated with the first years of practice, but can emerge again if relocation becomes necessary, practice mode becomes less satisfactory or a satellite office is contemplated. In making this decision the pediatrician should focus at three levels – life-style issues, professional and business considerations, and the specific site.

Pediatricians face increasing competition from a variety of sources, including other specialists, hospitals, and free standing urgent care centers. As competition increases, careful business decisions become more important. Location in a service-oriented profession is a critical ingredient for success, particularly when services are provided at the business site. As our society becomes more convenience-oriented, patients are less and less willing to travel or wait for medical care. Quality care must be provided to the patient in an accessible way.

Increased competition also restricts a pediatrician's ability to start over in a second location if the first one fails. Other desirable locales may be saturated with physicians. New neighborhoods and suburban developments quickly attract younger physicians. The opportunities for relocation are more limited than they were a generation ago. For all of these reasons, proper location of the office is of vital concern from a business standpoint.

Pediatricians and other medical specialists are also seeking improved lifestyles with better hours, less stress, and more family time. Practice location choice may rest as much on its promise of a better life-style as its likelihood of financial success.

Whether one is looking for a first practice site, a satellite or a relocation, it is best to approach the choice in a systematic manner.

The general perspective

In selecting a general area of the country in which to practice, the pediatrician should concentrate primarily on life-style issues. Any large geographic area (a specific state or contiguous states) offers any number of specific practice opportunities. The pediatrician should compare different areas in terms of their desirability as a place to live as opposed to work. Factors to consider would include climate, recreational opportunities, regional cultural opportunities, topography and transportation, family ties, and cost of living. At this level of decision-making, close cooperation with one's spouse or other family members is critical. By paying attention to personal life-style choices first, the pediatrician is consciously ordering his or her priorities in a manner most conducive to long-term success in private practice.

Specific perspective

In narrowing the focus, the elements of life-style preferences previously discussed are still important. However, at this stage the pediatrician must begin to give equal weight to professional and business considerations.

One early consideration involves whether the pediatrician desires a rural, suburban, or urban practice. Urban areas offer more opportunity to specialize. The pediatrician may be paid through contracts with health service organizations such as HMOs and PPOs, or deal with the federal government's Medicaid program. Also, the time spent traveling from home to work may be greater than in other settings. Pediatricians working in a suburban setting will probably practice as members of a larger group (either single or multispecialty), live near the office, deal with managed care programs and fee-for-service patients, and divide hospital duties among the group members. Pediatricians practicing in rural areas will tend to have smaller practices, may practice as solo doctors, may not be able to easily reach specialists unless they bring the specialists in on a contracted basis, usually have primarily fee-for-service patients, and may have less distance to travel between office, home and hospital.

Professional considerations should include type of practice (solo/partnership/staff model clinic), desire to have hospital facilities necessary to practice subspecialty pediatric care (including Level II or III nursery care), importance of working in a fee-for-service, managed care, community health clinic or other environment, availability of consultants and tertiary care medical centers and availability of adequate trained office staff.

For example, a physician who has decided for life-style reasons to settle in a warmer, seaside area of the country, might for professional reasons pick a number of possible specific sites within that region. The selection might be based on the desire to practice within a large group model that offers the opportunity for a part-time subspecialty practice. Another physician who has chosen the same general region might narrow the list of specific possible sites to a different set of communities based on different professional priorities.

To some extent, one's choice of a specific area based on professional considerations is also tempered by the desire of the physician to either start a new practice or join an existing one. Each pediatrician has to decide early on whether or not to reach for complete independence.

Having picked a small number of specific areas (cities, towns, or rural centers) that meet the individual's professional criteria, the pediatrician should review this shorter list again in terms of life-style priorities. This will further narrow the possibilities. In the example above, the pediatrician who wishes to practice in a warm, seaside area and has found several towns with group practices and hospital facilities compatible with pursuit of a subspecialty practice, might then pick one town over another because it is closer to the ocean.

Specific location

The choice of a specific location within a specific area (city, town, suburb) is primarily based on business and professional considerations. The major personal consideration in selecting a specific location is the travel time from home to office and hospital. While travel time obviously has professional and business implications, its major impact is on personal life-style – time at home with the family or available for personal activities.

The choice of a specific site location should be prefaced by gathering certain information critical to making that choice.[1] Figure 2-1 provides a location scorecard for comparing practice sites.

The first piece of information needed involves the ability of a specific site to demographically support another pediatrician. Local hospitals or chambers of commerce may be willing to supply further information on migration patterns, population trends, and breakdowns of age-groups within their given areas. Construction of new homes, schools, and hospitals is a good indication of a viable area for medical practice. Demographic profiles of specific communities are available from several sources including the American Medical Association.

Equally important is the number of providers of pediatric care in the region. This should include the number of family practitioners (the usual rule of thumb is that four family practitioners will have the same competitive impact as one full-time pediatrician), health clinics and urgent care centers in the area. It may be difficult to convert the competitive impact of an urgent care center into a defined number of pediatrician equivalents, but the longer the hours of care provided at the urgent care center and the greater the amount of advertising it does, the greater its competitive impact will be.

The pediatrician should also endeavor to find out the trends in the local OB community. Are there new obstetricians just setting up in practice who haven't established referral patterns yet? Is there a shortage of OB care in the area? How many family practitioners are delivering infants? Where are their babies being delivered?

One recent issue requiring evaluation has been generated by the increasing role of HMOs and other managed care programs. If a location has one or two large employers who provide the majority of the job opportunities in that area, it is important to determine if these employers are self-insured, have exclusive contracts, or are only contracting with a limited number of HMOs or PPOs. If you are not able to sign up as a provider for certain specific HMOs or PPOs, a large segment of the population in that region may not have access to your pediatric services, and may be excluded from your care.

The next question of critical importance is where these children and adolescents live. It has been said that patients will generally only drive 20 minutes one way to see a specific doctor. A drive longer than 20 minutes will cause most people to seek care closer to home, even if they find that source of care less desirable. Convenience is critical, and may work to help or hinder a new practice.

A new practice located in a new suburb may draw patients from a successful, established practice located some distance away simply because of convenience. On the other hand, a new practice is located more than 20 minutes from the target population group has a distinctly lower probability of success. The site location must be a compromise between convenience for the patient and convenience for the physician.

The 20 minute rule may be less relevant in rural localities if there are few competitors. Even so, the pediatrician who begins practice in a small rural town, counting on drawing patients from miles around, may be surprised to find that patients may not drive very far if some other provider of care, such as a general practitioner, is closer at hand.

Comparing a map of population centers in the proposed practice area with established practice sites in that area may give important clues as to opportunities for site location based on the 20 minute convenience rule.

In a similar vein, road and traffic patterns are also critical. Patients may be more willing to travel a longer distance if the roads to the office are generally not crowded and are easily negotiated. Similarly, being located near or on a good road allows quicker access to the hospital. Therefore the best location may not be on Main Street in the business section of town, but near the intersection of a major access road or nearby interstate highway.

The next step is to consider visibility of the practice site to the public. A practice located in a building plainly visible to passing motorists enjoys free continuous advertising. A small office in an office park is less noticeable than a free standing office building. A building near the street is more noticeable than one set back. Certain architectural styles are more readily noticed and identified as medical offices. The concept of physical visibility is important.

One should consult a knowledgeable commercial realtor to find available office space or land on which to build. The local hospital administrator may be a good source. Locating very close to an active obstetrical practice is always desirable for a pediatrician, and the hospital administrator should be able to tell you which OB practices are the most active.

Other factors to consider in site selection include its closeness to neighborhood schools and available pharmacies. Practices located near schools, in visible locations, should receive a great deal of free advertising as parents drive past on the way to and from the school. Asking young families in the area about their perceived health needs and interests is another good way to measure the medical needs of the community. A pharmacy located near the office is very convenient for patients who need to have a prescription filled after leaving your office.

Finally, the availability of adequate parking cannot be overemphasized. A practice in a charmingly restored older house with only street parking is not nearly as likely to succeed as a practice in a nondescript medical building with ample free parking. Primary care physicians should have enough parking spaces for the staff plus 6–12 additional spaces per physician for patients. (See Design of the Office, Chapter 6.)

Satellite offices

A satellite office is an extra office (or offices) in a nearby location to be serviced by the major office. The concept

Location Decision Scorecard

I. Rate a prospective location 10 ways

Fill out one column for each area visited. Score 5 for Yes,
3 for Doubtful, 0 for No.

	Communities		
	A	B	C
1. I'm convinced a need is here			
2. The medical society was encouraging			
3. Local doctors didn't dash my hopes			
4. I can get hospital privileges			
5. Coverage would be no problem			
6. Consultation facilities are adequate			
7. Postgraduate education is accessible			
8. I can get suitable office space			
9. Skilled office help is available			
10. Key citizens think there's room for me			
Totals			

II. The rate your economic prospects this way

Fill out one column for each area visited. Score 5 for Yes,
3 for Doubtful, 0 for No.

	Communities		
	A	B	C
1. Population growing			
2. Diversified industry			
3. Good employment level			
4. New firms moving in			
5. Local bank debits rising			
6. High wages			
7. Low welfare rolls			
8. Consumer credit good			
9. Health insurance is popular			
10. Going health-care rates are acceptable			
Totals			

III. Now rate the residential prospects this way

Fill out one column for each area visited. Score 5 for Yes,
3 for Doubtful, 0 for No.

	Communities		
	A	B	C
1. Spouse likes the place			
2. Attractive residential section			
3. Zoning laws guard property values			
4. House prices within reach			
5. Reasonable local taxes			
6. Adequate public services			
7. Plentiful shopping facilities			
8. Good public school system			
9. Adequate churches and cultural facilities			
10. Adequate recreation facilities			
Totals			

IV. Finally, compare the towns' total scores

	Communities		
	A	B	C
Professional prospects			
Economic prospects			
Residential prospects			
Totals			

*Figure 2-1: Location Scorecard. This scorecard can be used
to rate and compare the professional, economic, and
residential characteristics of potential practice sites.*

of an additional facility, accessible to physicians and staff alike, has been developed in response to specific pediatric practice needs.

The placement of a satellite office is almost purely a business decision based on the desire to attract a new patient population. All of the demographic, road, visibility and parking considerations apply as before, but are complicated by the need to carefully consider the interaction of two offices. What is the travel time between offices? Will patients need to get to both offices or just one? Are both offices within reasonable distance of the hospital? Will records need to be transported between offices?

Great care should be taken to ensure that the financial viability of the practice is not compromised by the satellite operation. The satellite office should be successful on its own merits. If it simply draws patients from one office of your practice to the other for convenience, it will not be independently successful. The demographics of the community should support another pediatrician in that specific location before a satellite is opened. Staffing patterns should also be considered: without a consistent physician at the satellite office it is not likely to be a success.

If the extra office is to succeed it must be close enough for all of the users yet far enough from the "main" office to provide its own professional identity and the perception of a "full and complete" office.

The need for a satellite office

An additional office location may fulfill a need to expand the "draw" or "catchment" area of your pediatric population. Because new communities of young families develop so rapidly and easily in our mobile society, many pediatric practices in established locations experience the loss of large numbers of patients or a significant decrease in the new patient potential when residential patterns change.

Convenience and accessability can fill a new practitioner's office in a new area or a satellite office for an established practice. The decision to open a satellite will be specific to each practice and will require planning and foresight.

The development of a new community that builds schools and/or a new hospital should especially signal the presence of practice opportunities. A critical self-evaluation that reveals a decline in office visits, relatively little practice growth despite population growth, or changing patient zip-code clusters, may point to the necessity of change. If traditional real estate values in your present practice area are no longer affordable for young "growth" families, or there is a need to develop a greater practice base to facilitate addition of new pediatricians within the established practice, or simply an interest in increased practice earnings, a satellite office may have potential.

In marketing your practice, the dictum to "identify patient needs and fulfill them" should be critical. If you choose to open a satellite office, patients must be assured of the same efficient quality that the main office provides. Additionally, once the family perceives convenience as an option, they may be eager to make a change to a closer office, so it behooves the satellite office sponsors to provide for the proper blend of quality and completeness from the outset.

Preliminary planning

This must include site selection and purchase or rental land and building, with affordable financing. Always keep in mind that a common mistake in planning is to underestimate the amount of square footage and equipment which the new office requires, as well as the total financial commitment this entails.

Other factors in site selection include ease of staff travel between the offices, parking, accessibility to the patients, and the previously mentioned hospital and school development.

Developing a satellite office

Once an executive decision has been made to open a satellite office, a combined meeting for physicians and staff should be arranged.

At this meeting, specific reasons for the new venture, anticipated realistic goals, and practice concerns that led to the decision should be shared with everyone present. This eliminates counterproductive rumors, and threats of practice or job security.

Once the attendees have a fair opportunity to express their feelings, an expression of agreement and commitment should be obtained. Details of the venture, planning, and specific assignments for task completion are the next consideration.

Prior to opening a satellite office, identify current patients who would best be served at the new location. Notify them regarding the new office and offer the opportunity to shift to the new location. Make it clear that they can change back to the parent office any time they wish.

The main medical record should be kept in the office of patient preference. If a patient is seen at a facility which does not have his medical record because of an emergency, because of pediatrician preference, or for an evening or weekend visit, the record of the visit should be transferred to the main record as soon as possible to assure chronological entries in the chart/flow chart. Practices which use a number system for medical records should code the chart to clearly identify the patient's primary office. Electronic facsimile (Fax) transmission is a godsend for the interoffice transfer of needed information.

Office staff should be hired and assigned to one office during traditional hours. Patients relate to staff personalities. If the staff is consistent, they frequently can overlook occasional encounters with different pediatricians. There should be one billing for the entire practice. A notation on the statement should indicate where the services were performed.

For efficiency in purchasing, all business, office, and medical supplies can be centrally ordered. Ideally, this should be done by one or two individuals at most.

Physician assignments and schedules should be made out far enough in advance so the staff assignments can be coordinated efficiently. Schedules should be posted in both offices and include vacations and days off.

Daily communication between pediatricians in the two offices assures good continuity and updates associates about patient and practice problems. This can be by telephone, speaker phones, or direct interoffice lines. Plans for the satellite office must include a communication system. All personnel meetings, whether business or nursing-care oriented, should include staff members from both offices to aid the development of a total practice concept.

It is wise to be aware of potential problems in any new endeavor, and creation of a satellite is no exception. Areas of concern fall into six generic categories.

If you are planning to create a satellite, here is a brief list of some of the potential problems that might develop.

Pitfalls in satellite office

1. Lack of time commitment by pediatricians as required for travel and ongoing marketing of the practice/satellite office.
2. Lack of commitment by pediatricians to fully equip the office.
3. Lack of careful financial planning so that expenses of the new office will not be a burden during the developmental phase.
4. Lack of regular, ongoing communication between offices – paperwork, doctor to doctor, staff to staff, and doctor to staff.
5. Lack of understanding by pediatricians that the needs of the satellite office may be different in the new community, (eg, hours, basic skills, etc).
6. Lack of appreciation of the need to cultivate referral sources in the satellite region.

Miscellaneous considerations

There are several factors which are of less importance than those mentioned earlier, but still worthy of consideration by anyone considering where to locate their practice.

The medical environment of the area should be assessed to determine if it is "specialty oriented" or "family practice" oriented. In a strong family practice area, for example, a pediatrician may plan to establish a primarily consultative practice as opposed to a direct primary care practice.

Ensure that the local hospitals meet your professional standards. If the new office or satellite is in a different state, review that state's licensing requirements.

Availability of business support services in a community, such as medical supply houses, accounting firms, etc, should also be assessed.

Finally, in the initial planning process, the pediatrician should consider the possibility that the first location choice may not work out. If so, consider the other alternatives available in the community which is being selected. Moving a practice to a different location in the same community is far easier than moving one's entire family to another area to relocate the practice.

References

1. Cotton H. *Medical Practice Management*. 3rd ed. Oradell, NJ: Medical Economics Company, Inc;1985

Checklist

✓ Have you picked the general area based on a careful consideration of family and personal life-style preferences?
✓ Have you picked a specific locale that you feel you have had adequate time to investigate in terms of demographics, economic trends, and the quality of health care being delivered in the area?
✓ Have you checked with physicians who have left the area recently for their reasons for leaving?
✓ Have you looked at several locales in the general area to obtain comparisons?
✓ Have you spoken with a competent, experienced realtor?

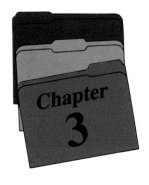

Chapter 3

Rural Practice

Pediatricians and their expertise are sorely needed in rural America. Rural practice is very rewarding, and the establishment of a fulfilling practice is both financially viable and emotionally satisfying.[1] That sentiment remains true today. As you read this chapter, remember these four points:

- **there is a definite need for pediatricians in the rural areas of our country**
- **successful rural pediatric practices have been developed in many communities**
- **the professional, personal, and family rewards to a rural lifestyle are significant**
- **rural practice allows you to be a complete pediatrician, using all of the education and skills that you learned in medical school and in residency**

Practicing pediatrics in small town/rural America is not only possible, it is stimulating, rewarding and fun. The rural pediatrician can affect the health status of children not only in the office and the hospital, but also in child care centers, schools, public health networks, and community organizations. The rural pediatrician is a source of health care and information for patients, their families, and the entire community. In a smaller community, a greater knowledge and understanding of patients and their families is more easily attained. However, deciding on a rural practice requires that the pediatrician and his family make sometimes difficult choices about life-style, goals and values.

Why rural?

Why do pediatricians choose to practice in small town, rural America? The most important factors are:

1. The pediatrician and his or her family want a *rural life-style*.
2. The pediatrician wants to use most of the skills and knowledge received during pediatric education.
3. The pediatrician wants to practice where there is a definite need, where he or she can have a direct impact on the children and where the families are appreciative.

Definition of rural

Images of rural life in America include the apple orchards of the Northeast, the wooded hills of Appalachia, the white-washed homes of the Midwest, the wheatfields of the plains and the expansive ranches of the West. Just as these visions are diverse, so are the definitions of what "rural" means. There are geographic, population and sociological definitions. The federal government divides the country into metropolitan (>50,000 people) and nonmetropolitan areas.[2] Other definitions include towns of less than 25,000 population or located more than 30 minutes from a population center of greater than 50,000.[1] For the pediatrician, practicing in a community more than 1 hour from a major pediatric hospital could be seen as "rural."

Economically, rural is no longer defined as only farming communities or "backwoods" areas of America. As transportation and communication technologies have advanced and more individuals and families have become concerned about the quality of their lives, there has been a move by small businesses and light industry to small towns and rural areas.

Rural life-style

Most importantly, rural is defined by the community and the life-style of the residents of that community. What is a "rural life-style?" Just as every urban and suburban community differs from the next, so do rural communities. However, there is a common ground of rural living that can be found in most small towns. Some families will describe it as a sense of community, others as a life with less hassle and still others as a more natural mode of living. In rural practice the patients and their families are also your friends and your children's friends; you attend church, community and school activities together. There is a general loss of anonymity and a sense of common purpose and concern for one's neighbors. Small towns provide a sense of belonging, but they also ask for participation in the community's activities.

Rural residents have fewer problems with congested transportation systems, crime and pollution; they enjoy a less harried pace in life. Living in the country also provides the entire family with easily accessible outdoor activities, including camping, hiking, hunting, fishing, biking, skiing, and sailing. One can plant a garden, have a tree farm or an orchard, raise livestock, or just enjoy the mountains or the wide open spaces.

However, there are the choices and the priorities. The family and the pediatrician have to decide whether easy access to cultural activities, professional sporting events, and shopping is important to them. While these activities may be relatively close, they still require extra effort, extra planning and extra time.

Rural practice

Is there really a difference between rural practice and urban/suburban practice? The major difference is the proximity to a pediatric training center or children's hospital. Most small towns and rural communities cannot support a large medical complex with its teaching faculty and residents. This has significant effects.

Pediatricians in rural private practice have to maintain their procedural skills – resuscitation, intubation and LPs. They also have to be available for emergency C-sections and acutely ill children. Rural pediatricians often have to stabilize and care for critically ill children. They also have to provide care and coordination of services for the chronically ill or disabled child. There may be state or tertiary center outreach clinics nearby, but children's centers and subspecialists are seldom readily available. In some urban/suburban communities the pediatricians feel medical/legal or parental pressure to refer every critically or chronically ill child to a subspecialist. In rural areas, the pediatrician can still transfer and refer the critically or chronically ill, (albeit with some difficulty) but is more likely to be the general pediatric specialist and the families' link with the health care system.

Solo versus group

In the past, many rural pediatricians were solo practitioners. Solo practice can be very rewarding for some, especially those who adjust well to the major complaints of professional isolation and lack of adequate coverage. More and more small groups are being formed in rural areas as pediatricians are insisting on an acceptable life-style for their personal, family, and professional lives. Some groups are centered in the middle of a large drawing area while others prefer to reach out through satellite offices to serve a wider area.

Rural need

Is there a need for pediatricians in the rural areas? The answer is an unequivocal YES. There are 21 million children living in the nonmetropolitan areas of the United States: approximately 20% of the total population below age 19.[3] One third or 7.4 million children live in the over 1400 counties that do not have a pediatrician.[4] While family practitioners have moved into over 96% of the communities with populations of 5-10,000, only 35% have an obstetrician

and only 25% have a pediatrician.[5] In rural communities there are over 700,000 children with significant chronic illness and another 300,000 with some limitation of daily activities.[6]

The need exists not only for the development of new practices, but also for new partners and colleagues to join existing practices looking for a second, third, or fourth pediatrician.

Deciding rural

Goals

How do you decide if a rural area is where you would like to live and practice? First, examine your own personal, professional and family goals and needs. If you are married, both partners must examine their own goals and those of the family. In addition, consider any special needs that you or your family may have. Consider all aspects of rural living, from the level of pediatric care you will have to provide to the quality of the schools to the availability of cultural events. If you have been raised or lived previously in a rural area, you may have a good idea of what rural life is like. If you have not had previous experience and you are a resident, it might be worthwhile to consider a second or third year elective in a rural practice to try it out.

Community assessment

After you have examined your goals, and assuming that the community can otherwise meet your needs, how do you decide if the community can support a pediatrician (or another pediatrician if you are joining a group)? Several factors[1] should be considered in your analysis:
1. *Population demographics,* including size, age breakdown, birth rate trends, and projected influx of families.
2. The *economic status* and future projections for the area, including the unemployment rate, number of new jobs, average annual income, and percentage of the population on medical assistance.
3. *The number and type of health care providers* and the current health service referral patterns.

The county planning office, child care centers and the school district should be able to give you accurate population information, birth rates,

and an idea of the number of families moving into and out of the area.

The planning office and the county social service agencies should be able to provide the economic information. Rural families pay a greater share of their health care with "out of pocket" money. Fewer have health insurance and even less have preventive services and immunizations paid by a third party.[6] Therefore, economic trends will have a significant effect on the families' ability to pay.

The local hospital administrator and the state medical society should know the number and type of local health care providers. You should also examine the total catchment area population and the present patient referral patterns. If the entire county of 40-50,000 uses the local hospital and its physician staff, a positive effect is anticipated. If most of the population uses hospitals and physicians outside of the county, it may be very difficult to develop a practice, as rural referral patterns are often slow to change.

Other child health providers

While the overall population of the area is important, it has to be examined in relation to the number of child health providers and the percent of the population below 20 years of age. Small towns of 5,000-10,000 may be able to support a pediatrician if at least 30% of the population is children and there is not an oversupply of other child health providers.[1] It is also important to know how many obstetricians deliver at the local hospital and how many births are reported annually. If there is no obstetrician, it may be very difficult to develop a practice, as family practitioners will care for the babies they deliver.

Most family practitioners spend approximately 25% of their time on pediatrics, so four family practice specialists generally see as many children as one primary care pediatrician.[7] It is important to determine if the local FPs deliver babies and provide well child care. Ask who may be retiring, and whether the established practices use Family Nurse Practitioners (FNPs) or Pediatric Nurse Practitioners (PNPs). Do they see you as a specialist to whom they can refer patients and/or a provider of primary care? If you are seen as only a specialist for referrals, you may require a much larger population base.

Community agencies

Community agencies may be a source of competition or a source of income. Most rural communities have a public health clinic. Does it provide quality, AAP-recommended well child care, or is it only an immunization clinic? Remember to consider not only how the clinic sees itself, but also how the families in the community see it. How many children come here for their health maintenance visits and immunizations? Who manages the clinic? Would your participation be mutually beneficial?

Look at the school system, preschool, and child care. Who does the child care, school, and athletic physicals? At what ages are the physicals mandated? Could you participate? If a school nurse practitioner handles these physicals, who supervises him/her? What are the opportunities for consultation roles, paid or voluntary? Will they refer patients to you? Some of this information could be obtained from the private and public school systems or the State Department of Education.

Consider the voluntary agencies – will they only refer patients to the subspecialist, will they communicate with you? Are they interested in your involvement?

Overall impression

As you consider the community, seek to develop a feeling for the area, a gestalt, an ambience. Does the community welcome you? Were the schools, the child abuse team, the public health nurses excited that you might be moving to their area? Does the medical community welcome you as a source of help or only see you as competition? How hard you have to work to develop a practice may depend on these more subtle factors.

Hospital and other health care providers

HOSPITAL – The rural community hospital has to be evaluated to determine what level of care can be delivered and what areas need to be improved to be able to provide quality pediatric care. This may be one of the easiest areas to evaluate and one of the hardest to change. It is important to assess the level of interest among hospital administration, nursing, and medical staffs. Some rural hospitals are willing to provide income guarantees, rental space, or other financial incentives to encourage a pediatrician to practice in their community.

FAMILY PRACTITIONERS – In small towns and rural areas, the relationship between pediatricians and family practitioners is unique. This can be a very positive, cooperative relationship where the pediatrician's expertise is sought by the family practitioner (FP), where the pediatrician conveys a sense of respect for the FP and assures that patients will return to the FP after the consultations, and where the competition is healthy and beneficial for all, especially the patient. The pediatrician has to set the tone for this relationship.

SURGICAL AND MEDICAL SPECIALISTS – The community also has to be evaluated to see what specialists are available for orthopedics, ENT, ophthalmology, neurosurgery, and general surgery. Of particular concern is the quality of anesthesia practice in the rural hospital. How much experience have the local surgeons and anesthesiologists or nurse anesthetists had with pediatric patients? Are they comfortable with children or do they always refer them to the distant medical center? Usually there are no pediatric subspecialists in rural areas, but there may be adult cardiologists and neurologists. Do they see children and have they had any pediatric training?

PEDIATRIC SUBSPECIALISTS AND REFERRAL – How are patients who require consultation and referral handled in the community? If your training program is relatively close, you may not need to decide where you will send patients. However, if you are not familiar with the region, it is important to look at a few areas. How far away is the nearest neonatal ICU and Pediatric ICU? Are they responsive to transfers? How do they transfer patients? In terms of consultations and referrals, who has a reputation for good communication and quality care?

Community relationships

The rural pediatrician needs to work with the community agencies and organizations. The schools, child care centers, public health clinics, county welfare, and child and youth programs can be a source of education, referral, and occasionally, extra income. It is important to develop good communication so that one may learn more about the services these agencies provide and the overall health status of children and families in the community.

Practice management and finances

The rural pediatric practice should be managed in the same manner as a suburban or urban practice. In recent years, it has been shown that rural practice costs as a percentage of gross income are just as high, if not higher, than those in the urban areas.[8] However, incomes can also be close to those of the urban/suburban peers.[9,10]

Continuing medical education and time off

The need for continuing medical education is no different than that of your urban/suburban counterpart. Every effort should be made to become involved in teaching, with special emphasis on residents and medical students visiting your practice.

Time off is important no matter where you practice. In a rural practice, especially if you are solo, it is important to have time for your family and for yourself. You should provide for coverage by a neighboring pediatrician or family practitioner with whom you are comfortable. In rural group practice, coverage is not a problem and many groups take 4 weeks of vacation and CME time.

Summary

While rural pediatric practice will be a challenge, it can be rewarding personally, professionally, financially, and emotionally. It can also be part of an overall life-style that reflects the rural environment. Rural pediatric practice is not for everyone. If you are interested and would like to speak to someone about rural practice, please do not hesitate to call your state pediatric society or the Division of Community Health Services, American Academy of Pediatrics (800/433-9016).

References

1. American Academy of Pediatrics, Committee on Community Health Services. *Rural Health Notebook*. Elk Grove Village, IL: American Academy of Pediatrics; 1986
2. Moss A, Parsons V. Current Estimates from the National Health Interview Survey, 1985. *Vital and Health Statistics*. 1988:10(160); DHHS pub no (PHS) 86-1588
3. American Academy of Pediatrics, Task Force on the Future Role of the Pediatrician in the Delivery of Health Care. The Report on the Future Role of the Pediatrician in the Delivery of Health Care. *Pediatrics*. 1991;87:401
4. Nadler HL, Evans WJ. The Future of Pediatrics. *AJDC*. 1987;141:21
5. Budetti P, Kletke PR, Connelley JP. Current Distribution and Trends in the Location of Practice of Pediatricians, Family Physicians and General Practitioners 1976-1979. *Pediatrics*. 1982;70:780-789
6. McManus PA, Newacheck PW. Rural Maternal, Child and Adolescent Health. Presented at the Rural Health Research Agenda Conference; February 1988; San Diego, CA
7. Budetti PP, Frey JJ, McManus PA. Pediatricians and Family Physicians: Future Competition for Child Patients? *Journal of Family Practice*. 1982;15:89-96
8. Holoweiko M. Practice Expenses Take the Leap of the Decade. *Med Econ*. 1990;67:82
9. Physician Payment Review Commission. *Annual Report to Congress*. Appendix C. Summary of the Commission's Hearing on Rural Practice Costs. Washington, DC: 1990
10. Owens A. Earnings Make a Huge Breakthrough. *Med Econ*. 1990;67:90

Checklist

✓ Have you explored the pros and cons of rural living with your family?
✓ Are you comfortable with the professional limitations rural practice might impose?
✓ Have you assessed demographic characteristics for areas of practice being considered?
✓ Do you have a structured approach to establishing and maintaining a rural practice?

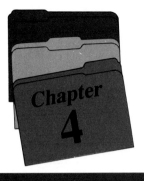

Chapter 4

Joining a Practice

The pediatrician joining a practice may wish to review the following topics included in this chapter.
- **contracts**
- **compensation**
- **practice responsibilities**
- **interviewing**

Contracts

The difficult process of selecting a type of practice is the first step of a complex decision tree.

It is said that physicians are not good business people. This may or not be true, but no level of personal competence can replace appropriate advisors in areas of business and law when starting a new practice or joining a pre-existing one. Any pediatrician joining a practice should be represented by his or her own attorney. It may cost some money when you feel you can least afford it, but the investment could save many times the money (and much heartache) if professional relationships subsequently dissolve. (See Professional Advisors, Chapter 17.)

Contracts are written to protect both parties. They should be fairly negotiated and satisfy all concerned. It is important that the parties have an honest and forthright discussion in an atmosphere of mutual respect among equals. If any of the parties are dissatisfied before the relationship even begins, there will be trouble. Everything controversial and difficult to discuss should be placed on the table for consideration. Resolution of any problems should be agreeable to both parties.

One may join a practice with expectations of eventual equal ownership, partial ownership, or to remain a salaried employee. Whatever the goal, each requires a contract that covers certain important areas of mutual concern. Contract duration merits serious consideration from the outset. Ideally, the contract should not only address the initial year of employment, but additionally describe the future expectations and rights of each party if the relationship continues. All parties should have a sense of the practice's long-term viability and patient base.

Compensation

If one is joining the practice as an employee, the specific salary should be identified. Incremental increases can be based on longevity, performance or both, and should be so stated. The actual dollar amount of the increase may be difficult to place in the contract but the intent for increase should be clearly stated. Contracts may even stipulate a threshold for productivity bonuses.

If the goal is eventual partnership and ownership, the original salary should be identified and the terms leading to the partnership stated clearly. This may be achieved incrementally over a 2- or 3-year period by adding a percentage of practice profit to the starting salary each year until parity with the original partner(s) is achieved. For example, if one is joining a three doctor practice, the ultimate goal is 25% ownership. If the agreement stipulates parity at 3 years, for example, the first year salary might be 18%, the second 21%, and the third 25%.

Also to be considered is the possibility of an additional amount of compensation for expertise in subspecialty areas or for administrative responsibilities.

Buy-in

The buy-in is perhaps one of the most complicated, least understood, and most important areas of any practice contract. It must be perfectly clear what is being bought. Items for purchase include accounts receivable, physical assets of the practice (capital equipment), medical records, leaseholds, and the nebulous goodwill factor. It is important to know the realistic collectability of the accounts receivable being purchased. The dollar amount on the books may not take into

account bad debt, amounts which will not be reimbursed by third-party payors, especially Medicaid, or funds owed by people who have left the community. As a general rule accounts under 60 days are assumed to be 100% collectible. The amount assumed to be collectible decreases rapidly over time, to as little as 20% for accounts more than 120 days past due.

It is also important to know which portions of the purchase price are deductible and which portions are not. This will have important short-term tax ramifications and impact the dissolution of the agreement should that need arise.

One alternative to a buy-in is to close the books of the pre-existing practice and start anew. This eliminates the need for the accounts receivable portion of the buy-in while allowing for a lower purchase price on office equipment and other items and retaining the goal of parity.

Benefits

Agreements should clearly state which expenses are the responsibility of the joining physician and which are the responsibility of the existing physician or group. Who will pay the costs for malpractice insurance? Who is responsible for the tail coverage if the relationship is severed? Who will pay for health, dental, life, and disability insurance premiums? Is the entire family or just the physician covered for these benefits? Is any allowance provided for relocation costs?

Is the benefit of a retirement plan available to the joining physician? Does he/she have responsibility for the employee costs related to that plan?

Will the practice offer reimbursement for continuing medical education meetings, dues to professional organizations such as the AAP, or dues for hospital staff privileges? Are your telephone costs, pager costs, and periodicals covered? These may seem like minor points, but such issues, when they become an argument of principle, can lead to great disagreement.

Practice expenses

Does the joining physician have any responsibility for practice expenses? If salaried, these are usually borne by the existing party, but this should be clearly stated.

Practice responsibilities

Will the duties of the new member of the practice be the same as those of the established pediatricians and, if not, how will they differ? Often times, the new physician may be given additional night call and the senior partners less. If this is to be the case, it should be clearly stated in the contract. Are house calls required of the physician? Will there be different hospital assignments or responsibilities for the new physician?

Does the joining physician have any teaching responsibilities? If they are not part of the existing groups' pattern but the joining physician wishes to teach, this should be stated in the contract. In addition, whose time is taxed for the teaching? Is the time spent teaching a cost to be borne by the entire practice or reconciled apart from the teaching pediatrician's other time commitments?

Time away from the practice

It is important to clearly identify the amount of time allotted for vacation, continuing medical education (CME), and sick leave. Is there a time when vacation cannot be taken, such as periods of high volume or periods when pre-camp and pre-school physicals are done? Another crucial area for clarification involves provisions for maternity or paternity leave. If maternity leave is provided, is it compensated and to what degree? How many weeks or months are permitted? Is there a provision to return to work part-time if desired?

How does this affect the participation in any practice bonus arrangement?

Counterpoint

With the increasing number of female pediatricians the maternity leave issue will be a crucial one for many practices to address. All aspects of the issue should be evaluated, including the emotional needs of the pediatrician mother-to-be and her baby as well as the hardships which this unpredictable change in the office routine and coverage will create for her pediatric partners. The capacity to discuss and come to terms over this issue may be a good indication of the ability of the group to work together as a team.

Dissolution

It is hard to enter into a new agreement by discussing what happens to all parties if things do not work out. Unfortunately, this is a reality of life for which both parties must prepare. Things to consider are the terms and duration of the payments for a "buy-out." Be sure to include the items purchased during the buy-in period.

Is there an escape clause that allows either party to terminate a contract after a specified waiting period? What is that period to be? It is very hard to continue to work in an environment of acrimony once an individual has announced plans to leave. It truly is the medical equivalent of a divorce, and 60-90 days is not an unreasonable period of time for either party to give notice, especially if the decision is made at a time of year when there is a good opportunity for the parties to find a new position or a new associate as their needs indicate.

One of the most valuable assets of the practice is the telephone number of the practice. Agreements should clearly state who has rights to that number.

Restrictive covenants may be legal in some states if they are deemed reasonable by the courts. These can prohibit the leaving physician from practicing in a 5-10 mile radius of the office for a period of time considered reasonable, such as 2 years.

In summary, approach a contract to join an existing practice with optimism. It is a necessary evil of our business world. If properly executed, it can alleviate many problems should the misfortune of a dissolution occur.

Contracting with alternate delivery systems

The pediatrician in practice who makes a business decision to become a provider for an alternate delivery system and contracts with an HMO or PPO faces a different series of choices. Alternative delivery systems take many forms. Chapter 15, Practice Payment Systems, provides an overview of some typical considerations.

A word about interviewing

The interview process and its inherent skills are often foreign to newly trained physicians. This can provoke surprising anxiety in one so competent in life-threatening emergencies. Despite perhaps a dozen years beyond high school in college, medical school, residency, and perhaps, fellowship, this may be the first critical "job interview." You may feel somewhat unprepared or uncertain. This section is designed to help mitigate these anxieties and increase the probability of an optimal outcome.

The interview is a learning process for both parties. You will need to discover as much as possible about the particular characteristics of the practice and the physicians. At the same time, you will want to communicate clearly your desires, needs, personal attributes, and skills. Many corporations offering practice management consulting services have developed programs on a variety of issues, such as interviewing.

Some general points to remember include the following. Dress in a professional manner, consistent with the position you are seeking. Project confidence and self-assurance – remember to smile and make good eye contact. Get the interviewer to talk about him/ herself and to give you a description of the position. Remember, you also want to interview the practice. It is helpful to be attuned to the interviewer's signals and to anticipate questions.

Formulate questions in advance in such areas as office hours, on-call schedules and coverage, salary, benefits, vacation and CME allowances, parental leave and other special needs, licensure, cost of buy-in, partnership requirements, dissolution buy-out or restrictive clauses. Above all, satisfy the interviewer that you do or do not have the specific qualifications they need. Have a curriculum vitae (CV) prepared for interviewers to use during the interview, and leave a copy of your CV with them. (See "Sample CV.") A follow-up thank-you letter, emphasizing your interest in the position is very effective.

In brief, be on time, be prepared, keep the opening statement brief, relax, stick to the agenda, develop interest in you, and be positive and complimentary!

Checklist

✓ Do you realize your right and need to independently review your contract?
✓ Have you reviewed your responsibilities?
✓ Does the office provide time away from practice?
✓ Have you considered the pros and cons in contracting with an alternate delivery system? Have you reviewed Chapter 15, Practice Payment Systems?
✓ Have you had your own attorney review your contract?

Sample Curriculum Vitae

A curriculum vitae is the equivalent of the business resume in the medical world. It confers information of both a personal and professional nature and should be brief and succinct. The sections on services, and publications and lectures can be more lengthy, depending on one's activity in these areas. A general format with possible options follows:

CURRICULUM VITAE

Name:	
Office Address and Telephone:	
Date of Birth:	
Place of Birth:	
Marital Status:	*(status): spouse's name, date*
Children:	
Education:	*Undergraduate: university, degree, date* *Graduate: medical school, address, dates*
Internship:	*Internship hospital, program, address, dates*
Residency:	*Residency hospital, program, address, dates*
Fellowship:	*Program, address, specialty, dates*
State Licensure:	*State, date, number*
Board Certification:	*Diplomate (or eligible), board, date*
Membership in Professional Societies:	
Awards and Honors:	
Academic Appointments:	
Hospital Privileges:	
Other Memberships & Services:	*(Committees, church activities, etc)*
Presentations, Lectures, and Publications:	
Other topics listed may include:	*Major Research Interests, Teaching Experience, Military Service, and Special Interests*

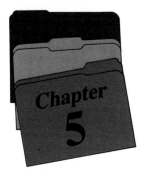

Practice Options

Today's pediatricians select from a menu of practice options that didn't exist just a generation ago. This chapter examines some of the reasons for this change, and the choices available today, including:
- **reasons for the development of alternate practice styles**
- **impact of the increasing role of women in pediatrics**
- **examples of practice variations**

Until recently, the predominant form of pediatric practice was the solo fee-for-service practice model. This has changed because of major trends, which include: 1) the increased prevalence of group practices; 2) the growth of alternative delivery systems (HMO, PPO, IPA, etc); 3) the increased proportion of women in pediatrics; and 4) the larger number of working mothers and dual career families.

The past decade has seen a steady rise in the number of group practices. According to the American Group Practice Association,[1] there were an estimated 300 such practices 20 years ago; now the estimate is 20,000. About 200,000, or 40% of all physicians, are involved in such practices; 20 years ago that number was 17%. The groups vary in size, location, organization, philosophy, and objectives.

Group practices have flourished, largely because of economic factors. These include the large financial outlays needed to start a new practice, the tremendous debt burden from training carried by many new physicians, today's accelerating constraints on health care costs, the increasing amount of paperwork requiring administrative support, and the growth of new health care delivery systems in managed care. The number of separate, qualified HMOs more than doubled from 243 in 1981 to 595 in 1986.[2] And according to Interstudy, there were approximately 33.6 million enrollees in HMO plans by mid-1990.[3]

One of the most dramatic changes for medicine in general and for pediatrics in particular has been the upward trend in the number of women in pediatrics.[4,5] Women pediatricians tend to have different needs and responsibilities, usually related to the care of their own children. More often, they choose

practice styles which enable them to balance several responsibilities.

> ### Some recent facts[4,5]
> - In 40 years the number of female medical students has quadrupled.
> - Over half of all pediatric residents are women.
> - Women comprise 35% of all pediatricians.
> - If the trends continue, over half of all pediatricians will be women by the year 2000.

Several publications have addressed issues of women in pediatrics, including the Report of the Task Force for Women in Pediatrics[6] and a more recent survey of 3000 pediatricians undertaken by the American Academy of Pediatrics.[7] They assessed issues related to women pediatricians and requested information on postgraduate training, family life, and professional activities. The Academy's findings were in agreement with findings from previous studies.[8]

The AAP survey showed that women practice significantly fewer hours per week and fewer weeks per year than do men pediatricians.[7]

Women in this survey earned less. Income differences were related to several factors, including women's younger age, their fewer years in practice, greater tendency to be in salaried positions, and working fewer hours.

Why do women pediatricians practice fewer hours? This is related to childbearing and childrearing. Most women physicians are married, and about two thirds have children at some point. According to the AAP survey, 50% of women pediatricians are married to a physician. In fact, other studies have shown that 80% are married to

another professional, which may lead to a more pressured home life.

About 90% of married women pediatricians have a spouse who works full-time outside the home. One third of male pediatricians have spouses working part-time and one third have spouses *not* employed outside the home. Whereas men are much more likely to rely on spouses for the care of their children under age 6, women rely on help inside the home, or help outside the home such as day care or home day care providers.

In summary, there are many more women in medicine now, and particularly in pediatrics. These women practice differently than do men; for many women this is because of child care and household responsibilities. Having both a career and a family is a difficult undertaking and a suitable practice style helps to alleviate the conflicts which arise when balancing many responsibilities. There are many pediatricians, both women and men, who have developed innovative ways of practicing. Several hybrids of practice variations are presented to demonstrate some of these innovative styles.

A shared position within a group

Drs B and C, who are husband and wife, both practice general pediatrics. After their residencies, he did a neonatology fellowship, while she worked full-time at a child development center. During this time, he decided against a career in academics and chose to practice general pediatrics. He and his wife were also beginning to realize that they would want to spend time with their children. They decided to look for a group practice which would accept both of them for one position, each half-time. Although the idea of a woman working less than full-time was acceptable to physicians interviewing them, most who spoke with him opposed their plan, stating that "a man would not be fulfilled working only part-time." But he was determined not to work full-time.

They found a group practice in a geographic area which was attractive to them. Despite initial misgivings, the group was willing to offer the two of them one position on a trial basis.

They began over a decade ago; their practice has worked out very well for the two physicians and for the group. The two doctors are now partners in a four-position practice, sharing one full-time position. Each doctor works 2 full days a week: he works Mondays and Tuesdays and she works Thursdays and Fridays. Wednesdays are their day off. Night call is split between them – each works every eighth night and half of every fourth weekend.

This practice style affords numerous advantages to the entire practice as well as to both pediatricians:

- The practice has been broadened by the skills of two physicians rather than one. He has expertise in neonatology and sports medicine; she in adolescent gynecology and developmental pediatrics.
- Each of the two doctors is often available to patients even if not in the office. If he has a question about a patient of hers, he will call her, and vice versa.
- The practice gets "coverage insurance." When she was on maternity leave, he covered her full-time for 8 months; similarly when he broke his leg, she took over full-time until he was able to weight-bear.
- Because the two physicians are less tired and less stressed, they are more willing to make schedule changes with their partners.
- This practice affords the physicians involved more personal time. Both are involved with their childrens' schools and are frequent visitors there. He is on his community's school board. She works in the town's library and teaches downhill skiing to children in the winter. They also have time to spend with each other. In addition, every 3 or 4 years they spend their month's vacation providing medical care in Haiti.

Counterpoint

Part-timers serve an important function and there are major advantages to hiring women who work part-time. There are many well-trained women coming out of residencies now who want to spend more time with their families. Many observers believe that when these women work part-time, medicine gets the best of everything. The pediatricians are happy because they can be with their children and aren't stressed. The patients are happy because they are getting well-trained and empathetic people. The practice enjoys the services of physicians who are motivated to work hard at half a regular salary. For these reasons, many small to moderate-sized pediatric group practices are taking in part-timers as associates.

The main disadvantage to this practice style is that only one salary is generated; if a family needs more than one full-time income, this situation will not work. For these two pediatricians, however, the income of one full partner is sufficient to live in their area. In the future they may need to add a few sessions when they need money to pay for college tuition. For now, the arrangement "couldn't be better – we will probably do it forever."

A part-time position in an academic group practice

A pediatrician employed at a major medical center in upper Manhattan offers another perspective. She wanted to do a fellowship after her residency, but wasn't comfortable about leaving her children for long hours. She felt a need to be part of her children's lives when they were smaller. There had been multiple problems with babysitters when during residency, and she felt it would be a very pressured situation if both spouses were in high-powered jobs. The pressure, in part, was attributed to their family situation. She began looking around for a part-time position and found a clinic-based

group practice associated with a teaching hospital in upper Manhattan, in an area inhabited largely by a poor minority population.

There are 15 practitioners in the group. Some work full-time, and are scheduled for six or seven patient-care sessions, and three or four other sessions. Part-timers are usually scheduled for five or fewer patient-care sessions. Each physician has a panel of patients whom they follow for planned visits. The physician is also available to patients for unplanned or "walk-in" visits during regularly scheduled hours. And for one session a week, each physician is scheduled to be the "walk-in" doctor to see patients whose physicians are not there at the time.

At nights and on weekends, the physicians take turns covering each other's patients. Weekends on-call are scheduled about every 8 weeks; when on-call, physicians make daily rounds on hospitalized patients and are available by phone at all times to any of the group's patients. Patients who need to be seen at night or on a weekend are referred to the teaching hospital's emergency room. Although they are consulted by telephone, only rarely do the group doctors come in to see patients unless they are hospitalized.

The advantages to this situation include academic stimulation and ready access to subspecialists, who can sometimes see the patient the same day. There are regular teaching rounds, x-ray rounds and journal clubs in which the practitioners take turns presenting cases and papers. Camaraderie develops when colleagues engage in similar work. The teaching role encourages the physician to keep up on current pediatric practice.

A major reason this job works for her is because her colleagues support her, and are always able to switch around schedules if needed.

A full-time position in a "staff model" HMO group practice

Dr "E" practices in an HMO group practice. Originally, he was in academic medicine. Although he was teaching and doing some research, he derived his main satisfaction from patient care.

Five years ago he decided to change his career and accepted full-time employment with the HMO practice. He chose this situation because he did not want to risk beginning his own practice, where it might take 2-3 years for him to break even financially. He didn't want to join someone else's practice, because beginning salaries were too low and because of his concern about potential personality conflicts. He wanted more limited on-call responsibilities so that he could spend more time with his family and was interested in working for an organization where his salary and benefits, (including malpractice coverage, retirement, vacations and sick days) would be assured. This could have been provided by a large fee-for-service group practice, but at the time he was looking for a job, this opportunity was not available.

After the first few months, he knew that for him, leaving academics had been a good decision, because he enjoyed practicing pediatrics in the new situation, where he could establish ongoing relationships with families.

He works full-time in this practice and is scheduled for 33½ in-office patient care hours per week, and is expected to see 3-4 patients per hour. Because of his special training in behavioral pediatrics, he has been given one morning per week to do developmental assessments for children in his own practice and is referred children from others in the HMO as well. On-call is every fourth night and weekend. He is supported by an excellent community hospital which has a level two nursery and a neonatologist readily available.

Life in the office and after hours is made easier by the availability of a 24-hour nurse service whose job it is to give advice to parents and to arrange for children to be seen if needed. The nurses work from protocols and check with the doctor for questions. All calls are recorded on advice slips with copies going to the chart and to the patient's primary care physician, which allows for review of what was said.

The pediatrician enjoys working in a system where the medical care is prepaid, although he believes some people may take advantage of this system. The extra work generated by these patients is offset by knowing that

patients who do need frequent doctor visits will not put off the visit because of inability to pay.

As with anyone working in a large group practice, our pediatrician has lost some autonomy. He is accountable for his time and he does not have complete control over his working environment. Although his ultimate earning potential may be less than in some private practices, this is offset by the real advantages he finds in this situation.

A nighttime pediatric clinic

A board-certified emergency physician founded a pediatric clinic, to be open only in the evenings and on weekends. His determination to begin this clinic arose, in part, because he had always felt that the emergency department was not the proper milieu for a patient with a non-urgent illness. He enlisted the support of fifteen of the area's practicing pediatricians to be shareholders in a new corporation. The goal of this practice, modelled after the original night time pediatric practice in Salt Lake City, Utah,[9] was to provide a special setting for children outside of usual practice hours.

The success of a practice such as this might be predicted by the recent dramatic change in the nature of American families. In 1985, the latest year for which statistics are available, 62% of all mothers were employed outside the home, compared to 9% in 1940 and 49% in 1975.[10] The most startling increase occurred among mothers of preschool children. Mothers who have jobs during the day cannot take sick children to the doctor without missing work. These mothers would be likely to

use medical facilities operating during evenings and on weekends.

The intent of this nighttime practice is to complement the care given by primary pediatricians, not to substitute for it. Parents whose children need care outside of usual work hours call the child's pediatrician, who determines the nature of the problem. True emergencies are referred to the emergency room; non-emergent cases needing to be seen are referred to the clinic.

The practice is located in a shopping center. Its hours are 5:00 pm – 11:00 pm on weekdays, 12:00 noon – 11:00 pm on Saturdays and 9:00 am – 9:00 pm on Sundays. It is staffed by one of two pediatricians and a pediatric nurse at these times and specialists are available on-call.

For patients, the clinic has many advantages. They do not have to wait long hours to see a physician and charges are about one-half the ER fee. Lab tests entail additional charges, but generally there are fewer lab tests ordered than in an ER, where the doctor on-call may be unfamiliar with children.

All children are referred back to their primary care physicians, with written records sent the next day. On occasion, the primary pediatrician will be consulted by the clinic physician regarding treatment options. To ensure that the service is used only for episodic care, it offers no well-child visits, routine physicals, or immunizations.

There are disadvantages to this practice style. The main disadvantage to the physician is that he is unable to follow his own patients as he would in practice. There is no hospital work. He offers only episodic care. In addition, more traditional pediatricians sometimes resist participating in this practice, feeling that patients ought to be

Number of Hours Worked Per Week All Pediatricians[7]	
Male	
Board Certified	51.4
Non Board Certified	49.4
Female	
Board Certified	43.3
Non Board Certified	39.6
P<.01	
AAP, 1988	

Number of Weeks Worked All Pediatricians[7]		
	$\bar{x}$	± SD
Male		
Board Certified	48.1	2.9
Non Board Certified	47.5	6.3
Female		
Board Certified	46.0	7.8
Non Board Certified	44.5	10.5
P<.01		
AAP, 1988		

followed by their own pediatricians at all times.

For the pediatric practitioners who refer to the service, this situation works very well. Their patients see well-trained, known pediatricians. The primary pediatricians are relieved of the stress of seeing non-urgent patients after hours and of referring them to hospital/emergency rooms for fragmented crisis care.

Exploring alternatives

The issues of access and availability of care to various poorly served groups are leading some pediatricians to explore very innovative and challenging practice options. Some practices are being established in inner city locations or in conjunction with state or county programs. Others have explored mobile health delivery systems or established practices in more rural settings or for migrant children. Finally, practice opportunities to overseas locations or through various health organizations have allowed pediatricians to take their skills to other parts of the world.

One final alternative to the office based practice is a "practice sabbatical." Around the country, pediatricians are taking a leave of absence from their practice to either return to an academic center to take a "mini residency" in a specific area or to try something different in a new setting. These absences, usually for 6 or 12 months, serve to build up skills, learn new ones or to experience a whole new practice option. At the end of the sabbatical, the pediatrician returns to practice with renewed enthusiasm.

Conclusions

The practice options outlined represent just a few of many adaptations to changing needs. Pediatricians are developing practice situations which enable them to balance their professional and family lives. Because there are so many women in pediatrics today, their practice styles may have major impacts on the future of pediatrics.

It is safe to say that the demographics of our patients are changing as well. The influx of mothers into the work force has created a need for pediatric care outside of usual work hours. This, coupled with the increased demand for episodic care, has encouraged the development of nontraditional practice forms such as a nighttime pediatric clinic. In addition, this practice form suits the needs of pediatricians seeking to work well-defined hours.

Pediatric practitioners and educators will continue to develop new and innovative practice options. As these become more popular, pediatricians will continue to enjoy the many effective alternate ways to practice pediatrics.

References

1. Heyssel RM. Administrative Medicine. *JAMA*. 1990;263:2620
2. HMO balances up in '89 as membership growth slows. *American Medical News*. Chicago, IL: American Medical Assn.; June 8, 1990:11
3. Flexible HMOs show enrollment gains: Interstudy. *AHA News*. 1991;27:3
4. *Women in Medicine Statistics*. Washington, DC: Association of American Medical Colleges; February 1989
5. *In the Marketplace*. 2nd ed. Chicago, IL: American Medical Association; 1987
6. American Academy of Pediatrics, Task Force on Opportunities for Women. Report of the Task Force on Opportunities for Women in Pediatrics. *Pediatrics*. 1983;71(suppl): 679-714
7. LeBailley SA, Brotherton SE. Career Paths of Men and Women in Pediatrics: Descriptive findings from the Survey on Pediatric Careers. Working Paper #15. Elk Grove Village, IL: American Academy of Pediatrics; June 1988
8. Bowman M, Allen D. *Stress and Women Physicians*. New York, NY: Springer-Verlag; 1985
9. Pollary RA. These pediatricians work only at night. *Contemporary Pediatrics*. 1987;4:56
10. Balk SJ, Christoffel KK. Advising the working mother. *Contemporary Pediatrics*. 1988;9:56

Section II

Business Essentials

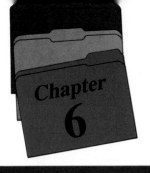

Chapter 6

Design of the Office

The design of a pediatric office sets the tone of the practice. Pediatricians should consider their needs, as well as those of staff and patients.

The design of the pediatric office plays a leading role in the efficiency of each patient visit. An office which is clean, bright, and decorated with attractive and cheerful colors encourages patients to feel comfortable, secure, and more relaxed. The professionals and staff in a well designed office are more likely to be effective and to enjoy their work. Mutual satisfaction with each visit is increased, leading to enhanced professional and economic success. This chapter will review some important points to consider in planning an office.

Sources of information

Acquire as much knowledge and experience as possible in planning a new office. Read, talk with others who have recently moved into a new office, visit other offices, and involve appropriate consultants. The process requires time and additional cost, but long-term savings and added satisfaction make it worthwhile.

The references cited throughout this chapter provide more in-depth information. *Perspectives in Medical Office Planning*[1] is a particularly helpful general reference. Sample floor plans for offices of different sizes are given, and the planning and building process is presented in detail.

Visiting other offices of similar size can offer much practical information. Be sure to walk through the buildings, check out the rooms for size and efficiency, and – most importantly – talk with those who work there. Ask what they like and what can be improved about the design.

Consider involving experienced consultants such as an architect, an office design expert, a building contractor, and an interior decorator who specializes in professional offices. Once a final decision is near, bring in a financial advisor, banker, and perhaps an attorney.

Ownership versus tenancy

An essential first step in planning an office is consideration of ownership versus tenancy. Ownership implies incorporating the land and office/building space into an investment program. This is generally preferable, and should be considered when adequate land is available in a good location and financial considerations approximate the same burden as "fair market" rental expenses.

An owner enjoys investment growth and tax benefits, and has total control of the physical environment of the practice. Ownership of proper facilities in a good location can have significant long-term benefits.

Financial planning

Realistic planning begins with assessment of all owned or available resources. This includes land, building, and financing. Is there enough land for an office, parking, and driveways,[2] or must more land be purchased? Must a new building be built, or can the existing building be renovated? Is an existing building amenable to change, or must the present floor plan be used? What amounts and methods of financing are available?

Building codes

The office must meet existing local and state regulations and building codes, and these will vary from one locale to another. Several considerations apply to all practices. There must be adequate access to the building and its rooms for handicapped patients,[3] fire safety must be considered, and exits must be well marked. Parking spaces must be provided and must comply with local codes. There may be restrictions on zoning setbacks and easement, preventing you from building on either side of the building.[1]

Size of the practice

The size of the practice is an important factor in determining the size of the building. A solo practice may require a building with a minimum of 1,000 sq ft[4] whereas 2,500 sq ft or more may be required for a three-physician practice.[5,6] The number of physicians will influence the number of examining rooms, private offices (or consultation rooms), administrative space (business office), storage requirements, and the size of the reception areas.

Careful thought should be given to this aspect of planning to ensure that the needs of the practice do not outstrip the physical facilities. Consider the ancillary services that will be provided and the necessary clinical and administrative supporting staff personnel. Examples are laboratory, x-ray, vision and hearing testing, tympanometry, psychological testing, patient education (reading material, cassettes, videos), and physician extenders. Consider the possibility of in-office medication dispensing, and allow space for it if this is a likely possibility. Take into account the future growth of the practice and allow a reasonable amount of space for additional patients, staff members, pediatricians, and allied health professionals.

Once these decisions have been made, prepare an estimate of total space requirements by combining the individual needs. Compare these figures with estimates from research, advice from consultants, and information from colleagues with similar practices.

Practice style

The style of practice should influence the basic interior design of the office. The office design should be a logical extension of the pediatrician's philosophy of practice, ie, "form follows function." Does a group practice consist of separate practices under one roof, or does it function as a shared practice with a team approach? Does each physician have a nurse, or do all nurses work with all physicians? A group practice functioning as separate practices usually shares laboratory and administrative functions and has one or two support personnel working with each physician, frequently in a separate portion of the office. The design of the office must reflect this style of practice, and attention must be focused on easy access for patients and personnel to the separate areas as well as to the shared services. However, a group practice functioning as a team in which all physicians may see all patients and all nurses may assist all physicians can function well within a more open office design. For example, the examining rooms, consultation rooms, lab and testing rooms can form a perimeter, while staff members move among the patients from a central or core area[6,7] which may be open.

Think through the design as a reflection of function. How closely can the conceptual goal of "form follows function" be achieved? What human and physical realities will be limiting factors?

A functional arrangement of space will allow you to move and service patients efficiently and in a way they "feel cared for – not manipulated."[1] It also enhances staff satisfaction. Develop a plan in which you arrange individual room space within the larger, total office space, working out appropriate functional relationships and traffic patterns.[1] Spend time with this, and continue to rearrange the spaces until you are satisfied.

Staff involvement

Now is the time to involve your staff in the planning process. Their suggestions and input can be invaluable, and their involvement certainly enhances their feelings of commitment to the practice and to the new office. Their early and continued involvement can prove practical and may prevent later design revisions.

Office emergencies

All offices must be properly prepared for treatment of emergencies. Emergency plans should be reviewed periodically and all emergency equipment should be checked regularly. Office personnel should be familiar with resuscitation procedures and emergency care.

All offices must be built and equipped to provide maximum safety for patients, parents and other visitors. Attention to safety details will avoid problems later.

It is important to carry liability insurance that covers injuries incurred in or about the office premise. Toys should be kept out of the traffic path of the reception area. Electric outlets should be plugged or covered. Drugs and instruments should be kept out of the reach of children and children should not be left unattended on the examining table.

Patient areas

Reception Area

A pleasant, easily accessible, and well marked main entrance should introduce patients to the reception area, the "living room" of the pediatrician's professional home. The reception area is the first impression patients have of the practice, and it should be spacious, inviting, and well maintained.[1]

If space allows, have separate waiting areas for well and sick children.[6-8] Although this may not always be effective in preventing transmission of contagious illness, most parents seem to appreciate it. If possible, a play area in a reception area designated for healthy patients will appeal to young children. A small table and chairs, books, and entertaining educational materials will keep children (and parents) happier while waiting.[1,9] A separate reception area, perhaps with its own entrance, is recommended for practices which cater to adolescents. If separate rooms or areas are not possible, partitions or room dividers can be used to achieve a similar effect.[10,11]

To estimate the amount of reception space required, figure the maximum number of patients scheduled during a peak hour, add 50% for relatives and friends, and multiply the total by 20 sq ft. The minimum size a reception area should be is 144 sq ft.[11,12] Moving patients promptly into examining rooms may compensate for a smaller reception area.

Separate seating is preferred to couch or sofa seating. Avoid intimidating "bus station" seating, where patients sit side by side around the room.[1] Make sure chairs selected are stable. Consider chair rails to protect walls. Provide coat racks or a closet to store coats. Low shelves for books and toys will be appreciated. Consider an area for a television or educational video equipment. (See Patient Education Materials, Chapter 26, for current information on AAP health education programs.) A bulletin board can be a center for patients' artwork and pictures.[1] Use another board for patient education articles or announcements.

Strive to arrange the reception window so patients can easily approach the receptionist upon entering the office.[7] Seating should be arranged so that the entire waiting room is in view of the receptionist.[7,13] A frosted glass reception window does not contribute to an inviting reception area. Patient flow to the interior of the office should be free and unobstructed. The exit route should lead patients by a signout window or counter, which should offer privacy from the general waiting room. This encourages a more confidential and unhurried atmosphere to discuss any necessary financial arrangements. Carefully designed, professional quality signs should direct patient flow.

An effective interior design should create an office environment that is an extension of the home – one that emphasizes a personal rather than institutional attitude.[1] Interior design is a complex issue and involves the thoughtful combination of colors, window treatments, light, furniture, wall and floor coverings, and decorative accessories.[1] By all means involve a professional decorator with expertise in interior office design.

For those who favor a different practice style, the "drive-in" pediatric office concept eliminates the usual reception area as it has a separate outside door for each examining room.[14,15]

Examining rooms

There should be a minimum of three, and preferably four, examining rooms for each pediatrician seeing patients. This allows time for undressing, dressing, and preparing of patients before and after they are seen, allowing the pediatrician to remain steadily at work. One room may routinely be left open for injections, procedures and emergencies.

The size of the examining room depends upon the furniture, equipment, and number of people in the room at one time. Usually, 80 to 120 sq ft is adequate.[1] A 8×10 ft room should be comfortable for infants and younger children, while a 12×12 ft room equipped with an adult examining table would be more appropriate for adolescents. The preferred method to determine the best room size for your style is to visit as many existing offices as possible to evaluate working spaces. An excellent method is to evaluate your present room size for comfort. Another way is to perform a dry run. Outline the exact size room chosen in an open area. After placing within this outline simulated or actual equipment, pretend you are performing different procedures and practice usual movements within this simulated space.[12,16] Check whether the "flow" of the room accommodates a right- or left-handed physician.

Ideally, each examining room should be designed to be flexible enough to accommodate all age-groups of patients from newborn to young adult. This will speed patient flow and minimize inconvenience to patients and staff.

Each room should have an examining table which can be free standing or built in. It can include a built-in infant scale, complete with paper roll and ruler for measuring length, and it should be at least 5½ feet long to accommodate older children. An infant scale is usually part of every room. A stand-up scale may be part of every room or centrally located, depending upon your budget and personal preferences. Handwashing facilities, a paper towel dispenser and a waste receptacle should be conveniently located in each examining room. Create as much useful storage space as possible, eg, underneath tables, in cabinets beneath the sink, and under the desk or writing table. A writing surface with space to store paper forms can be built into one corner or part of the sink cabinet, examining table or a free-standing desk. A chair rail around the room will help prevent damage to the walls from chair backs. Door stops should be toddler resistant. A bulletin board and information rack in each examining room can be dedicated to patient education. Coat hooks and a small wall-mounted mirror are appreciated by the patients and parents. A larger mirror behind the examining table can be a source of entertainment for young infants and toddlers, and also may

prove helpful during the examination. Make the examining area small enough to allow the pediatrician to reach all necessary equipment without moving. Lighting should be adequate[17] and should simulate natural daylight in spectral quality. This is best provided by a 4 foot long fluorescent fixture containing four "daylight" bulbs. This type of lighting allows the best evaluation of a patient's color. Windows, if present, should have adequate coverage to ensure privacy and block external light during eye examinations.

Each room should have a heating/air-conditioning duct and an adjustable vent for adequate fresh air. Non-connecting, insulated ducts will muffle noise transmission from one room to another.[4,18] The doors should be sturdy and soundproof, and the walls also should have ample insulation for soundproofing.[10,18-20] One specific room (usually the largest) should be identified as a treatment room which contains emergency equipment and supplies as well as a locked cabinet for emergency medicines.

The examining rooms should be easy for patients to find. It can be helpful to identify each room by a number, color of door, or a picture of an object or animal on the door.[8,21] Door knobs should be placed higher than usual to prevent small children from "escaping" while waiting for an exam. Pediatricians and other staff members should be able to reach the rooms quickly and easily.

Nurses' station

Many offices have a working space designated for use by nurses and other assistants. This is used for storage for medical supplies and other equipment utilized in diagnosis and treatment. Space should be allowed for a writing shelf or table and chairs which the nurses will utilize while performing telephone guidance, obtaining lab and x-ray results, and working on medical records. It should include at least one sink and a refrigerator to store appropriate medications, immunization and hyposensitization materials. Allow at least 70 to 100 sq ft for a station with one or two assistants, and add 20 sq ft for each additional assistant.[1] If in-office medication dispensing is planned, this may be an appropriate location for the medications and supplies.

Laboratory space

The amount of space dedicated for laboratory use depends upon the quantity and nature of the laboratory services provided. (See Office Laboratories and Other Services, Chapter 21.) When only simple screening tests are used, the laboratory and nurses' station often can be combined in the same area. More extensive testing which involves equipment and lab personnel requires dedicated laboratory space. The laboratory should be easily accessible to those using it from anywhere in the office. The space and facilities needed will vary with the services provided. Counters with built-in cabinets above and below should be planned to utilize all available space. A separate, free-standing counter may add more work and storage room. Adequate electrical outlets and at least one sink are essential.

Administrative space (business office)

Combining smooth patient flow and efficient administrative functions is indeed a real challenge, especially in a large and busy practice. Smooth patient flow is more likely when careful attention has been paid to the location of the sign-in, sign-out, and appointment windows. Influencing these decisions are factors such as method of financial record-keeping (pegboard, computer terminals, etc), number of personnel, need for privacy in sign-out functions, and existing design limitations such as available space and its arrangement. Pegboard or similar writing systems generally require that sign-in and sign-out functions are at the same or adjacent locations. Computer terminals usually can be at separate locations, and the printer for discharge forms can be located near the sign-out window. However, terminals must be accessible to the place at which office personnel are stationed. Ideally, the sign-in area should be readily accessible to the reception area, and the sign-out area should be located near a common exit path. Design the sign-out area to ensure privacy, and include an extra wide shelf or countertop for patients to securely place purses, infant carriers or other personal items.[1] Appointments are made by telephone as well as in the office. A busy office may function more efficiently if appointments are scheduled at a different area than signing in and signing out, assuming there are adequate personnel. Ask the office staff members for their suggestions and encourage them to perform "dry runs" of different designs. Visit other offices of similar size, talk with their personnel, and observe patient flow and satisfaction.

A one-employee office requires approximately 125 sq ft of space for the employee work. For each additional employee add 60 to 80 sq ft.[4,13,22,23] A larger practice may require a private office of 80 to 110 sq ft for a business manager or bookkeeper.[1] This should be located near the main reception area. Plan adequate space for all the necessary furniture and office equipment, as well as storage for office supplies and administrative records. Counters may be of different heights, and full use should be made of wall cabinets and under-the-counter space.

Include adequate space for a computer system. Even if one is not anticipated in the near future, present planning should allow room for eventual acquisition of a suitable system. A computer consultant can be helpful in suggesting the number, size, and location of the hardware modules, including the central processing unit, terminal display units with keyboards, and printers. Conduit placed during initial construction will facilitate later cable installation, and counters can be designed to accommodate display terminals and keyboards. Adequate numbers of electrical outlets, surge protectors, and isolation capacity wiring are essential. A centrally located wiring closet should be planned if anticipating eight or more hook-ups.

Plan adequate space for medical records. Records should be kept long enough to coincide with the statute of limitations for professional liability. Active medical charts should be filed in a location convenient to the reception area, the nurse providing telephone guidance and screening, the clinical work area, and if possible the appointment area.[6,24] Open-shelf vertical files against walls[25,26] or as free-standing, back-to-back structures[6] can save space and help make filing easier. Be sure to plan space for future growth and for storage space for inactive files.[27] Inactive files in a pediatric practice require considerable space unless microfilmed.

If at all possible plan at least an additional 100 to 120 sq ft for future growth as reflected in additional personnel, equipment, and storage.

Pediatrician's private office

The pediatrician's private office should transmit a message of confidence and trust.[1] The furniture, carpet, wall coverings, colors, lighting, and diplomas on the wall should convey a positive message of welcome and reassurance to patients. Family pictures and other personal objects, as well as growing green plants, add a personal and unique touch.[1]

The private office is often used as a consultation room. Some pediatricians prefer to combine the private office with the office library and use a separate, small room as a consultation room. Communication between physicians in a group can be enhanced while maintaining privacy if the physicians' offices are adjacent and have doorways between them.[6] Some group practices choose to have a large room with a desk for each physician instead of individual private offices.

While a comfortable private office can be as small as 80 to 100 sq ft, when it additionally is used for patient consultation it should be 100 to 140 sq ft.[1] It can contain built-in counters, cabinets, and bookshelves. As an added touch, some pediatricians opt for an adjacent lavatory with a shower.

Other services

Procedures such as vision and hearing screening, impedance audiometry, and psychological testing may require special space. If Snellen charts are to be used for vision testing, a 10 or 20 foot eye lane will be needed. However, a mechanical vision tester can be set up in any standard-sized room or mounted on a wheeled cart and brought in to the examining room. Rooms specifically planned for performance of ancillary services can be smaller than examining rooms and should be readily accessible to patients.

Staff lounge/ conference room

The office staff will appreciate a nice lounge area away from the main patient flow. Its size depends on number of staff, space availability, and its intended function.[1] If it is large and well furnished, it can double as a conference room and even as an office library. Counters and cabinets with a small refrigerator, microwave and possibly even a kitchen sink offer "at-home" convenience. Consider including built-in, lockable spaces for purses and other personal items. A staff lavatory should be adjacent to the lounge, and a separate staff entrance can be provided.

Rest rooms

There should be a minimum of two rest rooms – more in a multiple practice office. They should be readily accessible from both the reception area and the examining room/nursing station area. The walls and doors should be soundproofed, and each should have an exhaust fan. Built-in storage under the sink is a necessity. Restrooms should be large enough to accommodate a wheelchair and the door lock should be of the type that can easily be opened from the outside when necessary. Be sure local building codes are met. A countertop or secure shelf which parents can use as a changing table will be greatly appreciated.

Corridors

The hallways should be a minimum of 4 to 4½ ft wide if they are used by everyone, including patients.[10,28] This allows two people to walk around one another without crowding. Heavy traffic areas should be up to 5 feet wide.[1] Water fountains are a convenience but also are an attractive nuisance (chipped teeth and congestion of patient flow).

A private outside entrance for pediatricians and staff is recommended.[10] This entrance also can potentially be used by contagious patients.

Storage space

Plan storage areas for janitorial supplies, disposable items, inactive medical records, medical samples, and office supplies. Storage for some of these items can be combined, eg, putting janitorial and disposable supplies in one storage area. A maximum of 10% of the floor spaces should be considered for storage if inactive records and old equipment are stored elsewhere.[29] Replace nonload-bearing walls with enclosed shelves to create additional storage space.[30,31]

Parking

There are many factors to consider in planning the parking area. These include the number of physicians, the number of patients seen by each physician, the size of the staff, the amount and shape of available land, the number of exits, and any existing local zoning requirements. In addition to enough parking spaces for the staff, 6 to 12 additional spaces per pediatrician will be needed for patients.[32] One parking space per 200 sq ft of office space is recommended by some practice management consultants. Do your research, then agree upon a formula at the outset. Two driveways with angled parking is the easiest, but more cars can be accommodated with perpendicular parking.[1,4,32-34]

A carport adjacent to the office entrance is a nice feature, especially in inclement weather. However, be aware of the potential safety problems created by pedestrian flow patterns which require crossing a busy entrance or exit for cars.

Communication systems

The office which functions with quiet efficiency probably will be using systems which allow communication with a minimum of talking and confusion. These systems are primarily for staff use, but they also may involve patient communication. The communication systems available are telephone, intercom, voice paging, radio paging, fire alarm, smoke and heat detectors, security, examination room signal lights, dictation, computer hookup, closed-circuit television, and background music.[1,6,35,36] Together with an outside communication consultant and staff, evaluate each work area and enumerate the procedures that take

place there. The final system should reflect the needs of the practice style and office design.

Conclusion

The opportunity to design and build a pediatric office is indeed a unique challenge. A source of comfort and reassurance for the patient and a professional home for the pediatrician and staff, a well-designed office is an integral part of a satisfying pediatric practice.

References

1. Ross Planning Associates. *Perspectives in Medical Office Planning*. Columbus, OH: Ross Laboratories; 1987
2. How much land to buy for a medical building. *Med Econ.* 1975;52:56
3. Office design with easy wheelchair access in mind. *Med Econ.* 1978;55:41
4. American Medical Association. *Planning Guide for Physicians' Medical Facilities*. Chicago, IL: American Medical Association; 1979
5. Sparer CN. Organizing the physician's office. *Pediatr Clin North Am.* 1981;28:537
6. Baum AZ. An office that's efficient to the core. *Med Econ.* 1977;54:162
7. Three pediatricians with young ideas. *Med Econ.* 1971;48:85
8. A practice that runs like clockwork. *Med Econ.* 1967;44:98
9. Bass LW, Wolfson JH. *The Style and Management of a Pediatric Practice*. Pittsburgh, PA: University of Pittsburgh Press; 1977
10. Baum AZ. A shopping-center office that doesn't look like one. *Med Econ.* 1971;48:134
11. How big should your waiting room be? *Med Econ.* 1977;54:36
12. Cotton H. Sizing up your office setting. *Med Econ.* 1971;48:152
13. Whether to install a sliding glass receptionist's window. *Med Econ.* 1980;57:59
14. Shivers O, Garner RC. The drive-in pediatrics office. *Pediatr Clin North Am.* 1969;16:983
15. Johnson HW. 130 patients a day – and no waiting room! *Med Econ.* 1975;52:109
16. A method for deciding on exam-room size. *Med Econ.* 1975;52:57
17. Correcting deficiencies in office lighting. *Med Econ.* 1975;52:57
18. Gossett JW. Tips on how to dampen office noises. *Med Econ.* 1969;46:108
19. Griffin GC. Is your office a land of giants? *Pediatr Clin North Am.* 1969;16:977
20. If your walls are too thin for talking in privacy. *Med Econ.* 1975;52:55
21. Hirsch RL. Can your examining rooms pass this test? *Med Econ.* 1977;54:191
22. Space requirements for an efficient front office. *Med Econ.* 1977;54:55
23. How much space for your business office? *Med Econ.* 1969;46:49
24. How to find out if your office design thwarts efficiency. *Med Econ.* 1978;55:49
25. Office planning guide. *Med Econ.* 1969;46:107
26. A two-way wall makes it easier to get at charts. *Med Econ.* 1971;48:93
27. A way to utilize "free" office file space. *Med Econ.* 1980;57:57
28. The ground rules for hallway width in a busy office. *Med Econ.* 1971;48:75
29. Storage space requirements in a new office. *Med Econ.* 1977;54:56
30. Novel storage area: shelves within a wall. *Med Econ.* 1970;47:107
31. Saxl G. An office full of time-saving ideas. *Med Econ.* 1967;44:109
32. How many cars your office parking lot should accommodate. *Med Econ.* 1974;51:72
33. Office planning guide. *Med Econ.* 1969;46:87
34. Getting the most out of a parking lot. *Med Econ.* 1975;52:55
35. Wershing SM. Four office signal systems: Are you ready for one? *Med Econ.* 1976;53:177
36. Baum AZ. A step-saving office signal system. *Med Econ.* 1968;45:100
37. Fuchs S, Jaffe DM, Christoffel KK. Pediatric Emergencies in Office Practices: Prevalence and Office Preparedness. *Pediatrics.* 1989;83:931-939
38. Hodge D. Pediatric Emergency Office Equipment. *Pediatric Emergency Care.* 1988;4:212-214
39. Lubitz DS, Seidel JS, Chameides, L, et al. A Rapid Method for Estimating Weight and Resuscitation Drug Dosages From Length in the Pediatric Age Group. *Annals of Emergency Medicine.* 1988;17:576-580

Checklist

✓ Is there adequate room for storage of records?
✓ Does the floor plan provide for an adequate traffic flow?
✓ Is the laboratory accessible?
✓ Is the decor appropriate for the age varieties in your practice?
✓ Did you include the staff in planning?
✓ Can you afford the total "package," including equipment and furnishings?
✓ Are you proud of the look of your office?

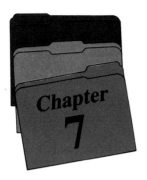

Appointments: Scheduling for Patient Care

Chapter 7

This chapter discusses the many factors that constitute a workable appointment schedule, including:
- **starting on time**
- **minimizing interruptions**
- **scheduling appointments for practice style and productivity**
- **teaching the staff the appointment policies**
- **using patient and staff feedback to assess effectiveness**

Appointment scheduling is critically important because the request to schedule an appointment represents a potential patient's initial contact with the pediatrician. This first contact presents a valuable opportunity to demonstrate that the pediatrician and staff are interested, concerned and caring. Unfortunately, there is an inherent danger that a negative perception of uncertainty, confusion, inefficiency, or disinterest may so alienate the patient that efforts to establish physician-patient rapport are frustrated at the onset. There is never a second chance to make a first impression. The family's first impression must be that the practice is well-organized, efficient, professional, and concerned about the needs of the patient.

The hallmark of a well managed practice is an appointment schedule that allows the precious time available to be utilized in the most efficient manner. Without a workable appointment schedule, the goals of the practice relative to quality pediatric care, financial success, and professional and patient satisfaction cannot be easily met.

The workable appointment schedule will be equitable, orderly, and predictable; it will take into account the frequently noted frustrations in pediatric practice:
1. Appointments are behind schedule and never seem to catch up.
2. Routine is always disrupted by patients without appointments.
3. Excessive congestion and confusion in the waiting room is disturbing to both the patients and the staff.

4. The disorganized staff and harried pediatrician lose the confidence of the patient.
5. Telephone interruptions.

The advantage of proper appointment scheduling may seem obvious, but pediatric practice involves many variables not encountered on a routine basis in other types of practice. Pediatric practices coordinate health supervision, illness care, school or camp physicals, anxious new parents, sick infants, acute injuries, parent and patient counseling. These variables influence scheduling and must be considered when planning a new appointment scheduling system or evaluating a current system. The system also must be assessed in light of how it affects the patient and family, the staff, and the pediatrician. The pediatrician and staff need to keep in mind that their punctuality is imperative regardless of the system used, and that any system must incorporate methods to minimize interruptions.

Designating and maintaining a specific time for an appointment demonstrates the pediatrician's commitment and underscores the importance of that visit. Additionally, educating the family to assume responsibility for making and keeping appointments encourages other parenting skills. It is well to remember that "routine" precamp, or preathletic physicals may seem "urgent" to the family, and patient accommodation and staff flexibility is a MUST at this time.

To devise the most workable and efficient system of appointments, a number of principles must be considered and put into practice. Efficient

allocation of time and office resources will ensure that the staff and facilities function at a steady, productive, and predictable pace. Patient charts should be pulled and prepared in advance of the visit, which will save valuable time later on a hectic day.

While it is important to recognize that different types of appointments will require varied time assignments, it is equally essential to understand that the practice styles of pediatricians do vary – and schedules must be adjusted accordingly. By assigning a specific amount of time to each type of service, the hourly flow of patients can be more accurately predicted. A written policy of assigning one unit of time (eg, 10 minutes) to an ear re-check, two units of time to a health maintenance visit and three units to a new patient will help facilitate appointment scheduling. This concept will allow, for example, six patients to be scheduled per hour for one-unit procedures, but only two patients for three-unit procedures. Appointments for such matters as weight checks, throat cultures, and allergy injections do not generally require a time-unit designation and can be listed in an accessory area of the daily appointment log.

It can also be helpful to differentiate appointments by category of patient. Scheduling appointments by category cannot be rigid, but overtime in the system tends to become automatic. Sick patients can be allocated different times from the well patients at the beginning or end of the morning or afternoon hours. Some larger practices give one pediatrician the responsibility for sick visits each office day. This may ease disruption of health supervision visits for the other pediatricians. The office schedule should be flexible enough to allow sick patients some priority over others. This will enhance patient satisfaction and allow for smoother patient flow.

Other possibilities include additional sick appointment time on the day after holidays, weekends, and vacations, (and possibly on school holidays) anticipating extra visits prior to vacations, and making allowances for pre-school, camp and similar physicals.

Adolescents often are the most adamant about not sharing the waiting room with "babies." School hours will allow a natural selection of young children early in the day and teens after school. With the increasing importance of adolescents in pediatric practice, however, serious consideration must be given to specific "adolescent hours" late in the day, or evenings, or Saturdays. Adolescent visits will be encouraged by a change in the waiting room magazines, appropriate audio accompaniment, and separation from parental figures.

Scheduling appointments by category also allows the innovation of "group dynamics" for specific age-groups, so that parents of toddlers might view a videocassette, nursing mothers (and their husbands) might attend a group lecture, and parents of college applicants might discuss their unique concerns. If appointments for infants are grouped during one time of day, the waiting mothers have an opportunity to share experiences and develop relationships.

Expanded office hours

The expansion of office hours beyond the traditional schedule assumes greater importance as more and more working parents request early morning, evening, and weekend office hours. With many mothers working outside of the home, and many children staying in day care settings, the convenience of expanded office hours is becoming more significant. Sometimes a simple reversal of hospital rounds with early morning office hours, or a hospital conference scheduled mid-day to permit late hours, will address the dilemma. With larger groups, evening office hours until 9 pm

by one associate which include several scheduled check-ups can assure some patient activity in addition to waiting for sick children.

The solo or small group practitioner can share expanded hours with other solo or small group practitioners. This assures limited but adequate availability for health supervision and follow-up care and consistent after-hours illness care. This can make after-hours call more manageable, as it limits the call responsibility and reduces some stress.

Office telephone hours

Telephone calls should be efficiently handled by the staff according to a system implemented by the pediatrician. (See Chapter 8, The Office Telephone: Triage, Training, and Technique.) Phone checks should be scheduled at regular intervals, perhaps every 15 minutes, to ensure that all necessary communications are accomplished. The pediatrician should not be interrupted for calls unless there are emergencies, family calls, or other physician calls.

A morning contact or "telephone hour" for either pediatricians or office assistants facilitates scheduling acute care appointments. Verbal contact with the pediatrician or a trained staff member will quickly allay a mother's anxiety after a long night of caring for a sick child. A telephone answering device with a recorded message cannot serve this function adequately. The early morning personal contact helps "set up the day" for the pediatrician. Other obligations (eg, rounds, lectures, or nursery visits) can be coordinated with the number of sick appointments added to the day's schedule.

Many practices offer a block of time during which a parent (or older patient) can call in to talk with the pediatrician. This time period provides an open door for parents to ask a question, initiate an evaluation or reaffirm the appropriateness of what they have been doing. The usual time for this "telephone access" is either first thing in the morning schedule, mid morning or at the end of the morning clinic. Physicians may take turns manning the phone line, or delegate routine calls. Some practices take messages and assign each pediatrician several blocks of time through-

out the day's schedule to return them. This system alleviates repeated interruptions and allows the staff to pull the patient's medical record.

Mechanics of appointment scheduling

When an appointment request is made by phone, the person receiving the call is responsible for determining the reason for the appointment, the urgency of the problem, and the number of time units required. The patient should be offered two firm, alternative times, eg, "Would you prefer Monday, April 2, at 10 am or Tuesday, April 3 at 1 pm?" When the appointment has been agreed upon, repeat the date and time (and in groups, identify the doctor involved) and gently suggest that the parent mark the calendar now.

The in-office return appointment is made after the pediatrician has advised the interval and plans for the next appointment. Saying something like "See you in 8 weeks" helps ensure that the patient returns on the most convenient day for them. The staff is most often alerted by a notation, on the superbill or routing sheet, or in the chart, and a written appointment card is given to the parent or patient.

After the appointment has been made and clearly confirmed (and appointment card given), the patient's name and telephone number should be entered in the daily appointment schedule or computer. Supplementary identification that is part of the practice routine, such as chart number or other code, also should be noted at this time. Soliciting and including on the appointment schedule a current working hours telephone number also can be extremely helpful. The current telephone number can then be verified against the chart, and will be readily available for a reminder call or appointment change.

Accurate appointment record maintenance during office hours can be enhanced by a number of methods. For example, the patient's name can be checked when the patient arrives, and missed appointments can be highlighted or underlined rather than erased. A missed appointment cannot be documented easily if the name was erased.

Chronic offenders can be pinpointed if the missed appointments are "flagged."

If several "no shows" are occurring in the office daily, a reminder phone call can be made on the day prior to the appointment. A review of the appointment system might identify the source of the problem and call for modification.

Periodic health examinations should be encouraged during the patient's birthday month because it is impossible to schedule every camp physical during May and every pre-school checkup during August. Most families will cooperate with this policy, particularly when it facilitates their appointments, and will respond to a mail or phone request to commemorate their child's birthday with a checkup.

A school or nursery form may ask that the examination be performed within a specified time, such as within the last 30 days. This requirement is unreasonable and inappropriate, especially if the patient has been seen in accordance with the Academy's "Guidelines for Health Supervision." (See The Health Supervision Visit, Chapter 20.) A statement attesting to the patient's good health will usually suffice.

As it is vital that the staff be aware of the pediatrician's availability, pediatrician and staff should review the appointment schedule format at regular intervals. The pediatrician must inform the staff of any changes in his or her personal schedule which will affect the office schedule (eg, medical meetings, vacation).

Enforcement of appointment scheduling

No scheduling system can work without support from the pediatrician, the office staff, and the patients. All must believe in the system and adhere to it. As team leader, the pediatrician must set the tone by starting on time and maintaining a pace. The team effort will be successful when each member understands his or her responsibility and function. The office staff must impress on the parents or patients the importance of appointment times and the need to adhere to them, barring emergencies and unforeseen circumstances. The person answering the phone should be prepared to accommo-

date sick children, some of whom should be told, "Come right now."

The pediatrician should not assume that the scheduling system is working and that he or she is always on time. Check with the office staff periodically about "backups" in the waiting room, complaints from patients who feel they have waited too long, and parents' response to a sick child seen before their own child. Occasionally ask patients how they feel the office appointment system is working.

Counterpoint

No one should debate the merits of a well controlled appointment schedule. However, patients must never feel you are too efficient or too organized to see them or their children in moments of need. You and your staff must understand the importance of allowing some available time for the immediate visit of an ill child and be noncombative when a patient feels a "walk-in" is justified. The pediatrician who understands these principles retains the loyalty of his or her practice without using an inordinate amount of time.

Any smooth-working system can be sabotaged by the "walk-in" patient. However, even the "walk-in" need not cause a major disruption to an efficient system. Emergencies (eg, lacerations, febrile convulsions) should be seen immediately. Other children who "walk-in" should be seen as soon as possible. At the most, the immediate problem should be managed, and an appointment should be made for a more comprehensive visit if necessary. The parent then should be advised that waiting times are shortest when appointments are made.

Unscheduled walk-in patients present an opportunity as well as a challenge. Inappropriate walk-ins provide the chance to build positive rapport when the pediatrician promptly cares for the child's problem and simultaneously educates parents about planning to seek proper care for their child. The challenge of patiently but firmly converting an inappropriate walk-in to a

later scheduled appointment will single out the exemplary receptionist.

Habitual or manipulative offenders will abuse any system, and firm management is essential. The alienation of an occasional patient will be far outweighed by the appreciation of the majority, who expect to be treated with efficiency, promptness, and fairness. The survival of the practice – even of the pediatrician – requires an appointment system that simultaneously fits individual requirements and firmly adheres to established principles.

Examples of appointment systems

Regardless of the system used, some practices request that the first patient of the morning or afternoon, as well as all new patients, arrive 10 to 15 minutes before actual appointment time. This period is required for patient registration and preparation. It allows the pediatrician to arrive and start office hours promptly. If the first patient is consistently not ready and waiting when the pediatrician arrives, the tendency will develop to arrive a few minutes late, and a destructive spiral may ensue wherein office hours are behind schedule from the first appointment.

Classic time-slot system

The rigid scheduling of appointments every 10 or 20 minutes throughout the day[1] (see Figure 7-1) may be satisfactory if the practice is a low-volume, consultative-type or if the patients are highly motivated and cooperative. Tardy patients and missed appointments are more disruptive to this type of scheduling than to other methods. Also, this system requires that sufficient staff are always on hand to prepare children for examination and process their records.

Basic wave system

Rather than scheduling patients in a regular, repetitive fashion, the basic wave system[1] allows several patients to arrive at the start of office hours and at regular intervals thereafter (eg, every half hour). This method assumes that the patients in each wave will arrive a few minutes apart, (some early, some late) average their time requirements, and be

Scheduling patients every 10 or 20 minutes requires sufficient staff on hand to prepare children and process records. This system is easily disrupted by tardy or missed appointments.

DATE _____

DOCTOR _____

9	:00	Lisa H.	RC
	:10	Diane J.	Sick
	:20	Beth E.	Seizures
	:30	Richard K.	PE
	:40	Michele S.	PE
	:50	Robert E.	Injury
10	:00	Peggy M.	Ingrown Toenail
	:10	Laura K.	RC
	:20	Mike H.	
	:30	1st PE	
	:40	Susan M.	NB
	:50	Amy P.	RC
	:00	Ashley D.	Sick

Figure 7-1: Classic time slot appointment scheduling. Each pediatrician has a separate appointment sheet for each day. The sheet is prepared from the appointment worksheet and is typed late in the prior work day; some appointments are written in later.

This modified wave system typically schedules three patient time units on the hour, one patient time unit at the quarter hour, two units at the half hour, and no units scheduled at the three-quarter hour. It allows catch-up time and flexibility for patient tardiness, walk-ins, and emergencies.

DATE _____

DOCTOR _____

9	:00	Lisa H.	RC
	:00	Diane J.	Sick
	:00	Beth E.	Seizures
	:15	Richard K.	PE
	:30	Michele S.	PE
	:30	Robert E.	Injury
10	:00	Peggy M.	Ingrown Toenail
	:00	Laura K.	RC
	:00	Mike H.	
	:15	1st PE	
	:30	Susan M.	NB
	:30	Amy P.	RC
	:00	Ashley D.	Sick

Figure 7-2: Modified wave appointment scheduling. Each pediatrician has a separate appointment sheet for each day. The sheet is prepared from the appointment worksheet and is typed late in the prior work day; some appointments are written in later.

seen in time for the next wave to arrive. This system is difficult to manage.

Modified wave system

The modified wave system[3] appears to provide for the best patient flow and continuity of office hours. A typical hour using this system would consist of: three patient time units scheduled on the hour, one patient time unit scheduled at the quarter hour, two patient units scheduled at the half hour and no patient units at the three-quarter hour. (See Figure 7-2.) This system allows catch-up time, recognizes the natural inclination of patients to be a few minutes early or late, and allows sufficient numbers of patients to be prepared (weight, measurement, interval history) prior to seeing the pediatrician. It also allows for some walk-in time, emergency time, etc.

Computer systems

Computer systems were at one time heralded as revolutionary breakthroughs; at present, most pediatricians have not yet exploited this technology. When considering a computer system, all procedures in the office should be audited to determine whether a true practice need exists. A specific computer system can then be obtained to fit the offices requirements. Provisions must be made to introduce the computer into the office and train all personnel who will use the system. At least one physician in the office must understand and be able to operate the entire computer system.

Conclusion

Scheduling for patient care is a complex balancing act requiring consistent vigilance. Effective scheduling sets a tone of calm and competence. A flexible, workable appointment system accomodates patients and eases day-to-day stress. The system should be selected on the basis of its suitability to the practice, and monitored carefully for patient and staff satisfaction.

Reference

1. Sparer CN. Organizing the physician's office. *Pediatr Clin North Am*. 1981;28:537

Checklist

✓ Are you ready to see your first patient on time?
✓ Is your staff punctual?
✓ Is your appointment system satisfactory to both you and your staff?
✓ Are interruptions kept to a minimum?
✓ Does your office staff prioritize patient sequence (eg, an acute visit before a health supervision visit)?
✓ Are there gaps in your schedule for walk-in's or work-in's?
✓ Do you advise staff of any personal schedule changes (eg, meetings, business appointments) that will alter your practice schedule?
✓ Do your staff and patients give feedback about the effectiveness of your scheduling?

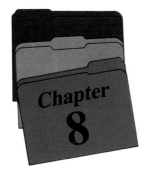

The Office Telephone: Triage, Training, and Technique

Chapter 8

The office telephone should be regarded as a practice builder and treated in an efficient, responsible manner. Telephone encounters set the stage for subsequent office encounters and may result in clinical decisions. Areas discussed in this chapter include:
- telephone and messaging equipment in and out of the office
- teaching telephone techniques to office personnel
- documenting the telephone encounter
- guidelines for using the telephone as a practice builder

While the office telephone system has become an integral part of medical practice, it has also become the number one source of patient complaints and a major cause of dissatisfaction among clinicians and medical support staff. All too often, the office telephone is neglected or left to chance. Repeated busy signals, reflex requests to "hold," delays in returning calls, unresolved health care questions, and worries not eased, all serve to undermine confidence in what otherwise may be high quality pediatric services.

The large volume of calls common to the typical pediatric practice mandates that the telephone system be as effective as possible. The dependence, trust, and confidence placed in the telephone system by patients' families are even more compelling reasons to ensure that the quality of telephone medicine is as excellent as any other component of the practice. Problems within telephone medicine segregate into seven general categories:[1]
1. Inadequate number of telephone lines, volume overload and access difficulties.
2. Outdated telephone technology.
3. Understaffing.
4. Failure to define what should be done via phone and who can perform these functions.
5. Lack of a well-defined telephone triage system.
6. Inadequate documentation of phone calls and the response to these calls.
7. The stress produced by non-emergency nighttime calls.

Managing the telephone represents one of the great challenges of ambulatory medical practice. Responsibility for managing the majority of calls should be appropriately delegated to someone other than the pediatrician. The flood of requests by telephone flowing into our practices may undermine our capacity to respond. Acutely ill patients calling for same-day appointments; camp and school physical exam forms due yesterday; emergency calls when least expected; questions about insurance coverage, immunizations, and the latest medical article's revelation in the local newspaper; routine and follow-up requests for medical advice and home treatment all become an unending, unpredictable current across the lines. The person answering the telephone has a critical role and becomes an extension of the physician, literally creating the image of our practice for our patients.

The purpose of this chapter is to discuss ways in which the office telephone system can work for the patients, the staff, and the physician in both the new and the expanding practice. It will deal with the following subjects:
- goals of an optimal telephone medicine system in the office
- basic equipment needs
- out-of-office needs
- elements of the telephone encounter
- training office staff
- organization and function of a telephone medicine system
- medical/legal issues and the telephone encounter record
- telephone personnel
- telephone quality of care checklist for evaluating how the telephone works in your office.

Goals of an optimal telephone medicine system in the office

For the patient and family
- getting through on the phone quickly and not being put on "hold"; (if the caller must be put on "hold," a custom-made background tape providing practice information can ease patient irritation);
- acquiring an appointment for the correct amount of time within an acceptable period of time;
- receiving efficient, effective service and problem solving when calling;
- knowing when to expect a call-back;
- interacting with staff who are pleasant, helpful, and considerate;
- understanding how phone calls fit into the care process and ground rules of the practice while having the health care needs well-planned and facilitated.

For the clinician
- finding adequate support to ensure that most direct clinical time can be spent providing hands-on care;
- having the ability to rely on the office staff to consistently perform defined tasks which support the care process for the patient and family;

- establishing an office triage and appointment system which provides the highest quality care, maximum efficiency and both patient and staff satisfaction.

For the office staff

- understanding the responsibilities of the medical telephone job and knowing the methods and procedures used to perform them effectively;
- having written job descriptions;
- having written protocols for triage and management;
- receiving recognition when the job has been performed well;
- enjoying opportunities for growth and development.

Our common goals are improved quality of care, service, and both patient and staff satisfaction. The quality of your telephone system can be estimated with the Telephone Quality of Care Checklist (see box).[2] Score one point for each YES. If your score is close to 12, hearty congratulations! If there is room for improvement, it would seem that the telephone should demand more time.

Telephone Quality of Care Checklist[2]

	YES	NO
1) Do you know how many phone calls your office receives daily and the top six reasons for calls?	YES	NO
2) Is the average duration of employment for your office telephone staff greater than 2 years?	YES	NO
3) Have you recruited the right person for the job?	YES	NO
4) Do you have a formal training of telephone management/triage in your office practice?	YES	NO
5) Do you have written protocols, specific guidelines, and office procedures for your staff?	YES	NO
6) Do you have written protocols for emergencies and for what to do when physicians are not in the office?	YES	NO
7) Do you document all medically significant phone calls?	YES	NO
8) Do you write smarter rather than longer?	YES	NO
9) Does your staff have a low threshold to bring patients in for an office visit?	YES	NO
10) Have you received no complaints from patients about the telephone or telephone staff in the last month?	YES	NO
11) Do you personally review telephone procedures regularly with your staff to be sure that only conditions that are appropriate for management by telephone are so managed?	YES	NO
12) Have you met with your staff in the last 2 months to talk about the telephone and to listen to their problems?	YES	NO

To evaluate your telephone system, above score one point for each "yes" answer and zero points for each "no" answer. If your score is less than 100%, you may want to examine each area where you have answered no.

Basic equipment considerations

It is wise to consult with the local telephone company and communications consultants about the needs of any individual practice. Needs will vary by setting, namely private practice, HMO, or hospital based, and the number of clinicians in the practice. A minimum of three telephone lines generally are required for solo pediatric practice. A telephone equipment company, such as NYNEX® or the Bell Operating Companies® and others, can provide information for a specific physical layout and blueprint. Placement of telephones within the office is determined by staff needs. A base unit in the appointment/reception area, an extension at the back office station, and a readily accessible, privately located telephone for the physician are minimum requirements. Telephones in examining rooms are a matter of personal taste but create confidentiality problems, as would an intercom or speaker phone equipment. Questions should be addressed to the telephone equipment company regarding location of phones, the number of

lines required for the number of incoming calls, the utility of state-of-the-art digital equipment, ACD (automatic call distribution) possibilities, voice messaging or the ability to self-direct calls, and the advantages and disadvantages of PBX® (private branch exchange) with an on-premise switch versus Centrex®, where the switch and responsibility for maintenance is owned by the telephone company. Whatever system is planned, particularly in an expanding practice, it is wise to anticipate growth to avoid more costly expansion in the future.

Out-of-office needs

Rapid on-call accessibility to the physician is a prime component of patient satisfaction. Telephone calls after hours or on weekends can be managed by call forwarding to an answering service or to a hospital switchboard if an answering service is not available. Either the answering service or switchboard will contact the physician on-call. A radio paging system or "beeper" should be considered a necessity. Two home telephone lines are desirable if personal

and family telephone needs might compromise on-call accessibility. An answering service increases accessibility for the physician and, when not on-call, forestalls unnecessary interruptions. All telephone answering services or systems should be monitored for efficiency and quality.

Cellular car phones provide freedom, mobility, and productivity enhancement with a personal touch. There are also problems, which include an increased risk of accidents, cost, and less freedom from the stress of the telephone. Telephone answering machines which only record messages are not appropriate for the physicians on-call and may cause patient dissatisfaction. However, an answering machine may be useful if the message provides an emergency number and is easily understood by even a distressed patient. For example, the message may say, "Office hours are 9 am to 5 pm, Monday through Friday. In case of an emergency, call _____." The use of the terminology, "in case of an emergency _____," defers non-urgent calls until office hours and enables a patient who has an emergency to obtain an immediate personal response.

A Four-Step Approach To Improved Telephone Service and Quality[2]

Step 1: Survey of Existing Telephone System

Objectives

1. To analyze the current telephone system in a detailed, descriptive fashion, including the number of phone calls by hour and day of week. There should be a particular focus on predicting the busiest hours, staffing levels during these hours, and what can be done to reduce volume and smooth out peaks wherever appropriate.
2. To evaluate the telephone behavior of staff and the current training program used to prepare personnel for telephone medicine responsibility.

Methods

1. Use a telephone encounter form to collect the important telephone data (number of calls for advice versus administrative or appointment information, total number of calls hourly and at peak times, number of referrals, and number of same-day appointments versus home management advice).
2. Personally listen to the way support staff are answering the telephone and talking to patients (with a double headset for simultaneous listening).
3. Call your office to evaluate the number of rings before the phone is answered, whether and how you were put on "hold," and how the support staff greet you.
4. Ask a representative from the telephone company to observe the telephone behavior of office personnel and the mechanics of your present system, and make recommendations for improvement. This service is usually free of charge.

Step 2: Study of Written Materials by Staff Under the Supervision of a Clinician

Objectives

1. After study of training materials, staff should be able to obtain a relevant medical history and distinguish between:
   a. a true emergency
   b. problems that can be safely managed at home
   c. problems that require an appointment
2. For problems that require an appointment, staff should be able to determine whether the appointment is needed:
   a. immediately
   b. same session
   c. same day
   d. future appointment
3. Staff should be able to present home management advice for specific symptoms accurately, safely, and efficiently.
4. Staff should be aware of how evaluations by telephone are different from face-to-face encounters, and how to avoid potential pitfalls and errors.
5. Staff should appreciate the importance of how the voice creates an image of the practice, and the value of professional telephone behavior.

Methods

1. Staff should study a manual on pediatric telephone management. (See bibliography.)

2. Mock telephone role playing should be incorporated into team meetings where one support staff plays the patient and the other plays the telephone assistant. The scenarios described in the training manual can be used in combination with those created by the staff from actual cases.
3. Lectures and discussions of specific disease entities and management techniques should be regular agenda items for office or team meetings.

Step 3: Direct Observation of Experienced Senior Staff

Objectives

1. To reinforce techniques in history-taking that improve the ability to differentiate between problems that need appointments and those that can be managed safely at home with home treatment advice.
2. To learn how to schedule appointments and keep pace with heavy volume.
3. To learn how to respond to acute emergency situations.
4. To learn how to manage upset or angry patients.
5. To become fully informed about the management of administrative matters, including:
   a. prescription refills
   b. requests for laboratory results
   c. referrals
   d. health education information, such as immunization schedules.

Method

1. All new staff should spend approximately 24 hours in direct observation of a senior staff member, divided over a 3-month period, listening to telephone conversations on a double headset adjusted for simultaneous listening only.

Step 4: Evaluation by Supervising Clinician

Objectives

1. To evaluate the telephone assistants' ability to distinguish between and manage emergency situations, problems that need appointments, and problems that can be safely managed at home with appropriate advice and follow-up.
2. To improve knowledge and skill by constructive dialogue.
3. To encourage outside reading and listening to tapes in areas recommended by the supervising clinician.

Methods

1. A 1-hour meeting should be made for the telephone assistant to meet with a key member of the health care team on a regular basis.
2. Topics (to be evaluated) should be divided among the health care team members and distributed in advance to the telephone assistant in preparation for the meeting.
3. Mock role playing should be incorporated into the evaluation.
4. Live tapes of actual telephone scenarios as well as video scripts can be used as springboards for discussion.
5. Strong points should be congratulated, and further study or tapes should be assigned for those areas needing improvement.

Figure 8-1: A Four-Step Approach to Improved Telephone Service and Quality.

Elements of the telephone encounter

As complicated as a face-to-face patient encounter may be, the telephone encounter is even more complex. There is less time, no body language, and few opportunities for second thoughts once the call has been completed and the staff member goes on to the next call. In the heat of a hectic day, we frequently lose sight of the complexity of the multiple variables which influence a single telephone encounter. These variables include:
- the patient
- the skill and preparation of the staff and the supports provided them
- the environment in which they work
- the nature of the call
- the medical/logical constraints within the system

The interplay of these multiple factors determine the outcome of every telephone encounter. Although training and preparation of support staff in telephone skills is only one process in the system, its importance surfaces in all categories.

Training office staff

Parents often ask "When should my sick child see the pediatrician?" There are no hard and fast rules, but a child should be seen whenever parents are worried about how the child is acting in response to an illness. These decisions usually are made independently at home. A mother instinctively decides her child is playful and not too ill, and a call to the pediatrician is unnecessary. In contrast, a child may appear so listless and irritable that medical attention should be sought immediately. Decisions in the grey zone, and sometimes even in the extremes, vary from parent to parent; and telephone advice may be extremely valuable in the triage process. An appropriate balance between benefits versus the risks of home management for a given medical situation and sound, informed judgment are required. Written telephone decision guidelines and policies should be available to help parents and staff decide when an office visit is indicated and what to observe while the child is being managed at home. Guidelines should also provide information about when it is important to see the pediatrician to help promote a more informed decision-making process, and how emergencies should be managed. A four-step training approach to improve telephone service and quality is presented (Figure 8-1).[2] The four-step process includes: (1) survey of existing telephone system; (2) a study of written materials by staff under the supervision of a clinician; (3) direct observation of experienced senior staff; and (4) evaluation. This approach is for those who wish to improve the performance of their staff in telephone care and to increase the knowledge of those answering the telephone in a pediatric office. This training requires the most careful physician supervision.

Organization and function of a telephone medicine system

It may be helpful to view the telephone care system in two parts. These are: (1) non-medical or administrative, including primarily future appointments; and (2) medical or problem care.

Approximately 60% if incoming calls are health care or problem related. Nearly half of these calls will require a same-day appointment; about one third require home management advice.[2] Regardless of the feelings about giving medical advice over the telephone, it is done all of the time by every practice. The person entrusted with responding to calls from parents must be carefully trained for this extremely important function. It is important to determine what background and training are appropriate for personnel answering telephone calls. How should their performance be evaluated? Should their function be limited to triage, or can office staff advise patients? Responsibilities delegated to non-physicians have been accepted by most parents, but it is the pediatrician's responsibility to be sure that telephone advice is appropriate and enhances care. A telephone care policy should be established consistent with the patient care philosophy of the individual practice. In order for the telephone to be used appropriately, it is also important that ground rules for the practice are communicated to those under our care.

Establishing a protocol for telephone screening

Staff members must know when a pediatrician should be called to consult with the parent immediately. Appropriate training will enable competent staff to make these decisions. Review of the phone chart at regular intervals, perhaps the quarter hour, ensures that other necessary communications are made promptly.

Many practices establish a morning or afternoon "telephone hour" when the pediatrician is available for immediate consultation. A morning telephone hour facilitates appointment scheduling and enables the pediatrician to speak directly with anxious parents whose children have been ill during the night. Parents who call during office hours for nonemergency consultation can be told when to expect a response.

Checking Your Telephone Courtesy Quotient

- ☐ Do you answer promptly and greet callers pleasantly?
- ☐ Do you put "good morning" and "thank you for calling" into your voice?
- ☐ Do you identify yourself properly and show that you will take responsibility for the call?
- ☐ Do you use the caller's name and give your full attention to the call?
- ☐ Do you take notes on an encounter form to avoid asking that your caller repeat information?
- ☐ If you are unable to help a caller, do you explain that you are leaving the line or transferring the call?
- ☐ Do you apologize for delays?
- ☐ All callers consider their call important (or he or she would not have made it). Do you handle each call this way – as if it were from a good friend or close relative?
- ☐ When you promise a call-back, do you follow through without delay?
- ☐ Do you place calls as courteously and efficiently as you like to receive them?
- ☐ Do you await the caller's approval before placing the call on "hold?"

It is important to establish a system which ensures appropriate communication without disrupting direct patient care. Inadequate telephone management can have a drastic impact on all aspects of daily practice; that subject is also discussed in Chapter 7, Appointments: Scheduling For Patient Care, under "Office telephone hours."

All staff should be trained when and where to schedule appointments relative to the presenting complaint: a true emergency, an immediate or same-day appointment, or an appointment in the future. (See box, "Appointment Decision Guidelines."[2]) The office staff member who receives a request for problem clarification needs to make one of three basic decisions:

- Schedule an appointment – same day or session versus future appointment;
- If no appointment indicated, advise patient in home management with follow-up advice; or
- Make a referral or other disposition after consultation with physician or under established protocol.

The management of emergency situations should be reviewed carefully so that each person answering the telephone knows in advance the exact procedure to follow if there is an indication of a life-threatening emergency, especially when the pediatrician is not immediately available.

Staff must be made constantly aware that other situations may arise which require direct referral to the pediatrician.
1. The parent has called before and the child's condition is worsening;
2. The caller may be very upset and the problem difficult to evaluate;
3. The medical problem appears to be complicated or the complaints are unusual;
4. The caller provides too little information or shows questionable competence (such as a babysitter or young child).

Registered nurses, licensed practical nurses, and on-the-job trained non-nursing pediatric personnel are all capable of telephone health care management if properly trained and supervised.

Appointment Decision Guidelines[2]

The following is one way to look at the need to schedule appointments using appointment groups with examples listed for each group. This is only one suggested approach, and should be evaluated carefully based upon the specific makeup and requirements of the individual pediatric practice and patient population.

Examples of Emergencies (life-threatening illness)

Respiratory difficulty
Epiglottitis
Convulsion
Overdose of medication
Diabetic reaction
Poisoning
Coma or unconsciousness
Behavior change following head trauma
Lethargy in small infant
Blood loss leading to shock

Examples of Situations Calling for Immediate Appointment

Acting extremely ill (extremely irritable or lethargic)
Sudden worsening in any condition or symptom
Difficulty breathing in known asthmatic
Possible fracture
Initial convulsion that has stopped and child now acting well
Severe abdominal pain or pain localized to the right lower abdomen
Acute allergic reactions without respiratory symptoms
Extremely anxious parent

Fall from a high place
Forceful and repetitive vomiting
Paralysis or weakness of a limb
Head trauma
Severe pain of any type
Stiff neck and ill appearance

Examples of Situations Calling for Same-day Appointment

Earache
Significant diarrhea
Stiff neck with muscle strain
Sore throat
Swollen glands
Skin infection
Pain or burning on urination
Abdominal pain

Examples of Situations Calling for Future Appointment

Emotional or behavior problems
School problems
Growth problems
Diagnostic problems with nonacute symptoms that have been present for a long time: headache, enuresis, abdominal pain
Other diagnostic problems and follow-ups as indicated according to the pediatricians' guidelines

Medical-legal issues and the telephone encounter record

Telephone medicine has become the newest medical-legal threat.[3] It is important that all medically-related telephone calls be documented. We should consult with risk management experts to learn how to write smarter, not longer. Written decision guidelines and procedures are essential and risk management issues should be discussed with all staff. There should always be a low threshold for giving appointments. *Supervision, as well as consultation, should always be available by the physician to staff.* Evaluation and review should be integrated into the system and well-documented.

The telephone encounter record

A record of the telephone encounter is important for continuity of care. Methods and formats of encounter systems differ widely.[2] Some offices use a Telephone Encounter Record (Figure 8-2);[2] others use a spiral notebook. Portable, pocket-sized pads adapt nicely for after-hours use (Figure 8-3). In-office dictation equipment can be easily extended to record after-hours telephone encounters.

The telephone encounter form may, at first glance, appear cumbersome; but as staff become familiar with the format, recording of the relevant information during the conversation becomes second nature. The encounter

Telephone Encounter Record

DATE _____ TIME _____ CALLER _____

PATIENT _____ AGE ____ MD _____

COMPLAINT _____

_____

_____

DISPOSITION _____

_____

_____

DATE _____ TIME _____ CALLER _____

PATIENT _____ AGE ____ MD _____

COMPLAINT _____

_____

_____

DISPOSITION _____

_____

_____

DATE _____ TIME _____ CALLER _____

PATIENT _____ AGE ____ MD _____

COMPLAINT _____

_____

_____

DISPOSITION _____

_____

_____

Figure 8-2: Sample Telephone Encounter Form.

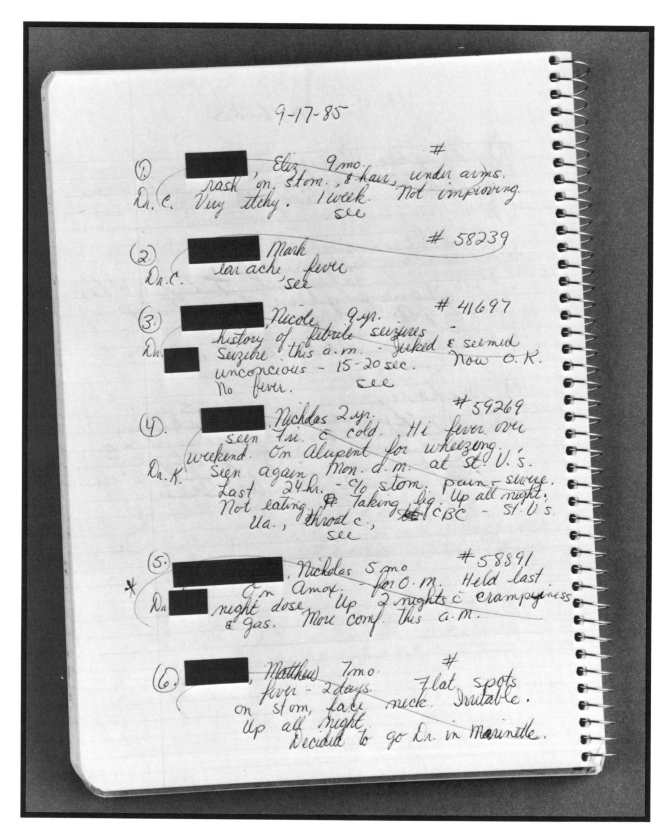

9-17-85

① ▮▮▮▮ Eliz, 9 mo. & hair, under arms.   #
Dr. C. rash on stom., 1 week. Not improving.
        Very itchy.
                see

② ▮▮▮▮ Mark   # 58239
Dr. C. ear ache, fever
                see

③ ▮▮▮▮ Nicole   9 yr.   # 41697
Dr. ▮▮ history of febrile seizures -
        seizure this a.m. - jerked & seemed
        unconcious - 15-20 sec.   Now O.K.
        No fever.   see

④ ▮▮▮▮ Nicholas 2 yr.   # 59269
        seen Fri. c̄ cold. Hi fever over
        weekend. On Alupent for wheezing.
Dr. K. seen again Mon. a.m.   at St. V.'s
        Last 24 hr. - c/o stom. pain - severe.
        Not eating # Taking liq. Up all night.
        Ua., throat c̄,   CBC - St. V.'s
                see

⑤ ▮▮▮▮ Nicholas 5 mo.   # 58891
*   Dr ▮▮   On Amox. for O.M. Held last
        night dose. Up 2 nights c̄ crampiness
        & gas. More comf. this a.m.

⑥ ▮▮▮▮ Matthew 7 mo.   #
        fever - 2 days.   flat spots
        on stom, face neck. Irritable.
        Up all night.
                Decided to go Dr. in Marinette.

*Figure 8-3: Telephone encounter entries when a spiral
notebook is used.*

Staff Summary Guide to Office Telephone Use

1. Be alert, wide awake, and always express interest in the caller.

2. Convey a friendly smile and greeting with your message.

3. Speak clearly, distinctly, and confidently.

4. At all times, be polite, warm, and businesslike.

5. Go out of the way to be helpful; put yourself in the patient's position.

6. Be expressive and put the punctuation into your voice – the ???
   and the !!!

7. Talk naturally. Use a normal tone of voice and a moderate rate of
   speech. Avoid slang, technical language, and irrelevant, personal
   chitchat. Other patients are waiting. Make every effort to be efficient
   and relevant so you can get to the other calls quickly.

8. Answer the telephone promptly. Ringing telephones are a source of irritation to everyone. Set a goal of picking up the telephone after no more
   than five rings, and make every effort to meet that standard (the telephone usually rings 10 times per minute).

9. Never give a patient a difficult time. If you cannot provide information,
   offer to find someone who can. When you are overloaded, take the
   number and call back, but call back as soon as possible.

10. Be discreet, confidential, and sensitive to the problem. A caller may be
    upset and anxious for reasons that are not obvious. For example, there
    may have been a recent death in the family, or the parent may have
    been up all night with an ill child.

11. If you sense parental concern, ask the caller "Would you feel better if
    Dr _____ saw your child?"

12. Avoid the "May I put you on hold?" habit. Put yourself in the caller's
    place. How would you feel if you were put on hold before you even
    have a chance to respond? If you must put the caller on hold for a
    moment, explain and say, "Will you hold the line please while I check
    that information..." or "while I answer another telephone..." or "while I
    get Dr _____"

Figure 8-4: Staff summary guide to office telephone use.

form can be ordered with a self-sticking adhesive back so a record of the telephone contact can be easily inserted into the patient's chart, or the encounter can be printed on both sides for economy. If a notebook is used, information such as prescriptions called into the pharmacy may need to be transferred into the patient record. Out-of-chart encounter records should be retained for as many years as old medical records.

There are several reasons for written documentation of phone conversations and for retaining records. Salient details of past conversations, as well as the date and name of the office staff member who received the call, can be retrieved quickly. This information is invaluable if the patient subsequently registers a complaint and past history must be separated from intervening events to objectively evaluate the problem. Also, in a group practice, it is helpful to be able to review details of prior telephone instructions when the patient's regular pediatrician is away. If follow-up information needs to be conveyed to a patient or if instructions must be modified, it is helpful to have the patient's telephone number and details of the earlier call readily available. Tabulation of telephone data also provides useful management information about the number and type of calls received.

Telephone personnel

The personnel selected for telephone care represent the vital link between families and the pediatrician. How well this responsibility is performed will have a profound influence on the quality of care, patient and pediatrician satisfaction, and the growth of the practice. Individuals selected for telephone responsibility must be properly oriented from the beginning (Figure 8-4).[2] They are, in effect, the image and voice of the practice. However, care must be taken to avoid telephone burn-out. The extent of training and supervision depends upon the degree of responsibility the pediatrician wishes to delegate; the knowledge, experience, and motivation of the person answering the telephone; and the characteristics of the population served.

If possible, those who answer the telephone in a pediatrician's office should hear themselves speaking with patients using a tape recorder. The staff should be reminded that when they use the telephone, their voices create the image of the practice. The patient who calls cannot see the rest of the staff or the office. The speaker's voice creates the visual picture. A double headset may be installed by the telephone company so that junior staff can listen in to live telephone calls on a telephone with the mouthpiece sealed. Conversely, senior staff can then monitor less experienced personnel as they talk to patients.

References

1. Katz HP. Quality telephone medicine: training and triage. *Policy and Practice: HMO Practice*. 1990;4:137-141
2. Katz HP. *Telephone Triage and Training in Pediatric and Family Practice: A Handbook for Health Care Professionals*. 2nd ed. (Formerly *The Telephone Manual for Pediatric Care*) Philadelphia, PA: FA Davis, Co; 1990
3. Katz HP, Wick W. Malpractice, Meningitis, and the Telephone. *Pediatric Annals*. 1991;20:74-79

Bibliography

Brown JL. *Telephone medicine*. St Louis, MO: C.V. Moseby Co; 1980

Fosarelli P, Katz HP. Residents on the phone. Letters to the editor. *Pediatrics*. 1987;79:311-312

Fosarelli P, Schmitt D. Telephone dissatisfaction in pediatric practice: Denver and Baltimore. *Pediatrics*. 1987; 80:28-31

Group Health Cooperative of Puget Sound. *Nurses' Guide to Telephone Triage and Health Care*. Baltimore, MD: Williams and Wilkins; 1985

Hessel SJ, Haggerty RJ. General pediatrics: A study of practice in the mid-1960s. *J Pediatrics*. 1968; 73:271-279

Katz HP, Mushlin A, Rosen S. Quality assessment of a telephone care system utilizing non-physician personnel. *Amer J Pub Health*. 1978;68:31

Schmitt BD. *Pediatric Telephone Advice*. Boston, MA: Little, Brown & Co; 1980 (2nd Edition scheduled for release in 1992)

Strasser PH, Levy JC, Lamb GA, et al. Controlled clinical trial of pediatric telephone protocols. *Pediatrics*. 1979; 64:533-537

Checklist

✓ Do you review your telephone equipment on a regular basis for function? Newer practice features? Cost saving?

✓ Do you have the telephone company monitor your incoming lines on a regular basis for adequacy?

✓ Do you emphasize telephone courtesy on a regular basis?

✓ Does your staff wait a few seconds prior to putting a patient on "hold," in order to determine if an emergency exists?

✓ Do you regularly review the telephone training techniques in your office for appointment efficiency and availability? Illness advice?

✓ Do you save telephone encounter forms for review at a later time?

✓ Are telephone encounters involving medical problems documented to assure continuity of care and avoid potential professional liability?

✓ Do you monitor your answering service on a regular basis for efficiency? Courtesy? Promptness in phone answering?

Personnel

This chapter describes personnel management principles, including:
- **an understanding of duties and responsibilities via job descriptions**
- **a sufficient number of staff to ensure a smooth flow of patient services**
- **regular performance and salary reviews**
- **staff involvement in office policymaking**
- **creation of a personnel policy manual**
- **laws governing employer-employee relations**

Chapter 9

The pediatric office should be well organized. A competent office staff enables the pediatrician to function optimally. An efficient office can accommodate more patients, and additionally frees the pediatrician to pursue special interests and family life.

Organization is the logical structuring of relationships among staff members to bring the business functions, facilities, and staff into effective relation with each other. It promotes cooperation, teamwork, and direction while limiting the potential for friction.

The need for job delineation and descriptions

Organization involves assigning functions and tasks to employees. It is important to delegate authority appropriately, so tasks can be completed successfully.

Office staff organization requires a thoughtful listing of functions or tasks to be performed. The theme or philosophy of the practice usually determines office needs. For example, a high-volume office setting has different needs than a low-volume setting. Other variables that can affect personnel needs include outside billing services, presence of a laboratory, use of a computer, group or individual practice, and so forth.

When considering the number of employees and expense, some employers like to follow a formula, eg, salaries should only amount to 15% to 20% of the gross income, or there should be three to three and one-half or four employees per pediatrician.[1] However, a personnel formula must take variables in the practice into account in order to determine the staff needed for the "front and back office." A pediatrician with a patient load large enough to keep him or her busy should not be performing tasks someone else can do as well. The pediatrician is better off with overhead at 50% of $200,000 than 30% of $70,000.

If accounts receivable pile up, billing is delayed, insurance claims handling is inefficient, telephones go unanswered or the sign-out area is too busy to accept payment for services, it is likely that the staff is either inadequate or poorly managed. Similarly, when a nurse doubling as a laboratory assistant spends so much time doing laboratory work that nursing assistance is rarely available, priorities and duties should be evaluated and additional "back-office" help secured if necessary.

After office functions or tasks and personnel philosophy are established, an approach incorporating job description, performance evaluation, and salary review should be considered. The job description gives the employee a basic understanding of what is expected. The performance evaluation permits both the employer and the employee to consciously, and sometimes painstakingly, evaluate actual performance. The salary review permits the employer to reward the employee based on performance of added duties, or on extraneous factors such as inflation.

Communication is a key element in any office, regardless of size. Open lines of communication prevent misunderstandings from festering and growing out of proportion.

Pediatric office positions

The major personnel problems in the office fall into two categories: authority and responsibility. Written job descriptions firmly establish lines of authority and define the duties of each position.

The support staff usually is divided into two major groups: the business staff (front office) and the nursing staff (back office).

Job positions within the business section (front office) may include:
1. sign-in reception and switchboard;
2. file clerk;
3. bookkeeper;
4. insurance clerk;
5. typist;
6. exit or sign-out clerk.

One person should be identified as the office manager. This can be someone from the foregoing list or a person hired primarily as a manager if the staff size warrants.

Job positions within the nursing staff (back office) may include:
1. nurse, daytime;
2. off-hours nurse (for extended-hours or after-hours triage);
3. nurse aide;
4. laboratory personnel;
5. specialty nurse, (eg, allergy testing, diabetes education);
6. nurse practitioner.

One of these should be identified as the head nurse.

Generalities for job descriptions

Although the content of each job description will vary, a common format promotes understanding and consistency. Each job description should have five sections. The specific description and content for each section is developed by the pediatrician(s) and the office manager or head nurse. The sections are:

1. Position – job title and individuals supervised;
2. Basic functions – overview of job content and nature of the position;
3. Duties and responsibilities – major activities associated with the job;
4. Principal working relationships – interpersonal aspects of the position, (eg, work alone or deal with others);
5. Standards of performance – quantitative and qualitative standards of performance to be expected.

A written job description (Figures 9-1 through 9-4) makes other aspects of personnel management easier. It:

1. Assists in recruiting: Defining the type of employees needed for the practice narrows the search. For example, is experience necessary or can someone bright and enthusiastic be trained to office philosophy and needs?
2. Assists in selection: Use the job description to review the duties of the job and determine if the applicant can measure up to the necessary tasks.
3. Assists in training: A job description can be used as a training guide.
4. Assists in reducing conflicts: A job description defines areas of responsibility and prevents misunderstandings by defining who has supervisory activity over whom.

It is important to remain flexible about the basic functions. Too much detail inhibits flexibility and creativity for both the employer and employee. There should always be room for the innovative personal contribution to office efforts. However, employees should not be allowed complete freedom, and the job description helps to establish the parameters within which the employee can make appropriate efforts or suggestions.

Job descriptions should not be "frozen in concrete." Although a job description may seem appropriate, changes are inevitable and frequently desirable. Therefore, from time to time the pediatrician should be willing to modify job descriptions as conditions dictate.

Recruiting, interviewing, hiring

Recruiting appropriate employees is essential. The first step is deciding what level of expertise is needed. If you are starting a new office, someone with experience is in order. On the other hand, if you are replacing someone who is leaving, a less experienced person with potential to learn your system might be appropriate.

In a larger office the entire process can be delegated to your office manager and head nurse. How will they find their candidates? The options available to find that special person for your office are newspaper advertisements, educational institutions, local hospitals, employment agencies and word of mouth. Current employees can generate leads. If you are considering using an employment agency, find out who pays the fee, the employee or the employer.

When advertising, construct the ad carefully and don't quote a salary. Many potential candidates can be screened out in a phone interview. Questions should include a job history and references. Some would add a letter indicating why the person is interested in the position.

The prescreening process should identify several likely candidates. A carefully structured face-to-face interview should enable the pediatrician to match the best qualified applicant with the unique requirements of the position and the work environment. The personal interview should be structured to elicit a sense of the candidate's personality. Ask open-ended questions which invite elaboration.

When hiring, be aware of legal considerations which stem from the Civil Rights Act of 1964 (42 USC 2000A). Discrimination in hiring based on race, color, religion, sex or national origin is forbidden. Subsequent legislation has extended this protection to pregnant women and older people. States also have their own anti-discrimination laws which may be even stricter than the federal standards. Lastly, be aware of county and municipal ordinances. There is no law, however, that requires an employer to hire someone incapable of doing the job.

Orientation and training

The job description can be used as a guideline for orientation and training. New employees should carefully read their job descriptions along with the personnel manual. (See Figure 9-6.)

Training for a new employee most often consists of informal instruction, but might also include formal programs (eg, instruction on computer use or laboratory technique). A typical mix of didactic and informal training might include a communication book to be read and initialed for any change in procedure, home study of standing telephone instructions and regular monthly in-service meetings.

Any new employee requires an intense period of on-the-job training. The most discouraging experience a new employee can have is to be expected to perform a job for which they are unprepared. Supervisory personnel should also recognize that everyone learns at different speeds.

New employees should be informed that the initial 2-3 months are a trial period. At the completion of this probationary period there will be a review to inform them of their progress and present job status. It is an unfortunate reality that some employees will never be suited for the position they've accepted. After a reasonable trial, everyone is best served if this is recognized and the employee is terminated or, if possible, retrained in another job.

Often, the completion of a 2-3 month probationary period is interpreted by the employee to be a guarantee of continued employment. Again, it should be clear that an employee needs to perform his or her job in an acceptable manner on a continual basis, and that the completion of a probationary period does not guarantee continued employment.

Performance review

The performance review is a formal, two-way appraisal. It can be performed once or twice a year as desired. In larger groups, if the review is conducted every 6 months, the mid-year meeting can be conducted by the employee's supervisor and the yearly review by the physician manager. The

Job Description

POSITION: Receptionist
REPORTS TO: Office Manager
SUPERVISES: _____

BASIC FUNCTION

Prepares daily log and makes follow-up appointments for patients. Receives and records all payments made in person.

Major Duties and Responsibilities

1. Assembles ledger cards of patients to be seen.
2. Records in daily log services provided and charges for these services.
3. Receives payments or furnishes payment envelope to patients leaving office. Posts payments received in the daily log and on the patient ledger.
4. Makes follow-up appointments as necessary.
5. Provides receipts and insurance information to patients as required.
6. Verifies patient address and phone number.
7. Balances log sheet records with payments on hand at end of work period.
8. Performs other clerical duties assigned by the office manager.

Principal Working Relationships

1. Has contact with patients (responsible party) regarding payment for services. Non-routine questions are referred to the office manager.
2. Coordinates claim form processing with the insurance clerk.
3. Provides balanced daily reports to office manager.
4. Night and weekend receptionists assist nurses with phone and other patient duties as time permits.

Principal Standards of Performance

A. Quantitative

1. Correctly balances daily log sheets.
2. Daily posting and filing of ledger cards.
3. Collection ratio.

B. Qualitative

1. Accuracy in posting daily log and ledger cards.
2. Accuracy in scheduling appointments.
3. Speed and efficiency in processing patient flow.
4. Ability to establish comfortable relationships with patients.
5. Ability to work calmly under pressure.

Reprinted from the Academy's "Personnel Management" Notebook, April 1986.

Figure 9-1: Sample job description for receptionist.

Job Description

POSITION: Insurance Clerk
REPORTS TO: Office Manager
SUPERVISES: _____

BASIC FUNCTION

Completes all insurance and public assistance claim forms and send them to the appropriate party.

Major Duties and Responsibilities

1. Assist patients in completing insurance forms.
2. Answers private line.
3. Furnishes patients with itemized bills when requested.
4. Answers routine questions regarding billing and insurance.

Principal Working Relationships

1. Contacts insurance companies and public assistance department regarding questionable claims.
2. Confers with patients regarding claims and bills.
3. Consults with office manager regarding claims and patient payment arrangements.

Principal Standards of Performance

A. Quantitative

1. Completion of claim forms within 1 week of receipt.
2. Reject ratio of filed forms.
3. Collection ratio on accounts receivable.

B. Qualitative

1. Thoroughness and accuracy in completion of claim forms.
2. Ability to resolve tactfully patient questions regarding insurance and receivables.

Reprinted from the Academy's "Personnel Management" Notebook, April 1986.

Figure 9-2: Sample job description for insurance clerk.

Job Description

POSITION: Office Manager
REPORTS TO: Director of Business
SUPERVISES: Receptionists
Transcriber
Insurance Clerk
File Clerk

BASIC FUNCTION

Has responsibility for the development and implementation of business operating procedures. Controls and monitors all financial activities of the medical practice. Maintains sound management control over the clerical staff and their functions. Ensures courteous and thorough communications with patients by the business staff.

Major Duties and Responsibilities

1. Performs bookkeeping duties, which include:
   - entering checks received in the mail from patients on the daily log and on the patient ledger
   - balancing daily logs
   - preparing daily deposits
   - writing checks for payment of bills
   - preparing payroll for all employees
   - tax deposits.
2. Prepares necessary management information reports and forwards required data to the accountant's office.
3. Maintains inventory control over office supplies and equipment. Orders supplies as required.
4. Recommends the hiring and termination of clerical personnel.
5. Prepares performance appraisals and recommends merit increases for clerical staff.
6. Supervises the daily activities of the clerical staff.
7. Develops and implements annual business goals and budgets.

Principal Working Relationships

1. Informs doctors of business matters on a regular basis. This should include personnel and financial items of importance.

2. Works with the accountant to coordinate accounting activities.
3. Contacts suppliers regarding cost and quality of materials purchased.
4. Coordinates business activities with medical activities through the head nurse.
5. Trains clerical staff in performance of their duties.

Principal Standards of Performance

A. Quantitative

1. Timely preparation of financial reports and data.
2. Cost and level of inventory.
3. Collection ratios.
4. Aging of accounts receivable.
5. Status of insurance claims.

B. Qualitative

1. Ability to maintain accurate and complete financial records.
2. Ability to make sound decisions regarding business and personnel matters.
3. Capacity to supervise effectively and smoothly clerical staff.
4. Ability to motivate subordinates to high levels of performance.
5. Ability to train clerical staff.
6. Capacity to delegate responsibilities effectively.

Reprinted from the Academy's "Personnel Management" Notebook, April 1986.

Figure 9-3: Sample job description for office manager.

Job Description

POSITION: Day Nurse
REPORTS TO: Head Nurse
SUPERVISES: _____

BASIC FUNCTION

Prepares charts and physical facilities for patient visits. Provides routine medical advice to patients by phone. Establishes helpful and friendly relationships with patients.

Major Duties and Responsibilities

1. Check examining rooms daily – clean and stock as required.
2. Prepare patients for the doctors. For example:
   - weigh patients
   - measure patients
   - tests as necessary
3. Clean examining room after patient leaves.
4. Carry out doctors' orders – ie, give injections, make appointments, clean and bandage wounds, do assigned testing.
5. Assist doctors with treatments.
6. Screen incoming calls – decide if doctor needs to see or call patient.
7. Inform parents how to care for and what to expect from well and sick children.
8. Periodically check entire work area including waiting rooms and tidy up as necessary.
9. Record lab test results in patient charts and contact patients as necessary regarding tests.
10. Contact pharmacies to authorize prescribed medication for patients.
11. Pull and process patient charts for next day. This includes such items as:
    - stamping
    - adding sheets
    - updating immunizations
12. Thoroughly clean and stock each examination room weekly.
13. Make patient appointments.
14. Perform filing, phone duty, kitchen clean-up and other duties assigned by the head nurse.

Principal Working Relationships

1. Works very closely with patients in scheduling appointments; escorting and settling in examining rooms; answering routine medical questions by phone and in obtaining basic information for chart preparation.
2. The nurse must have a pleasant phone technique, like children and be very understanding of the patient's fears and needs.
3. Helps doctors stay on schedule by efficiently and quickly preparing examining rooms for patients.
4. Assists doctors with ordered medical tests, procedures and medications.
5. Coordinates and works with other nursing and office staff to ensure smooth processing of patient medical and business data. Performs as part of a total team, providing high quality medical services.

Principal Standards of Performance

A. Quantitative

1. Ability to get patients into examining rooms on time.
2. Accuracy in testing patients and reporting to doctors.
3. Ability to clean and stock rooms properly.
4. Ability to handle most phone calls within an average of 3 minutes.

B. Qualitative

1. Capacity to remain pleasant and helpful to patients under all conditions.
2. Ability to remain calm and professional.
3. Organizational skills to keep track of several patients, tests, etc, at one time.
4. Ability to use office and lab equipment properly.
5. Ability to anticipate physician and patient needs.

Reprinted from the Academy's "Personnel Management" Notebook, April 1986.

Figure 9-4: Sample job description for day nurse.

Performance Review

Employee Name_____

Position _____

Date of review _____ Date of last review _____

Days absent since last review _____

Employee's strengths (comment fully on the employee's
job-related characteristics):

Employee's weaknesses (comment fully on the employee's
job-related characteristics):

Employee's attitude (include such items as initiative, responsibility,
ability to work with other employees, and ability to deal pleasantly
and effectively with patients):

Job skills (include such items as accuracy, record keeping, speed,
thoroughness, and appropriate specific job knowledge):

Rating:

    ☐ outstanding   ☐ marginal

    ☐ superior   ☐ unsatisfactory

    ☐ good

Employee comments:

_____
supervisor/reviewer   date

_____
employee   date

Figure 9-5: Sample performance review form.

process offers four fundamental benefits to both employer and employee:

1. It identifies the employer's strengths and weaknesses.
2. It identifies the employee's strengths and weaknesses. With this review, the employer considers the ability of the employee in a carefully thought-out manner. (This is not a "seat-of-the-pants" evaluation.) Any employee whose behavior is unsatisfactory has an opportunity to find out what the employer considers satisfactory.
3. It can serve as a basis for salary review. A conscientiously complete appraisal clearly identifies the elements of importance in evaluating job performance, and helps clarify any reward system proportionate to merit if this is an office policy.
4. It provides for communication and job feedback. The performance review formally establishes the fact that the employer is willing to communicate with staff members – that someone is willing to listen, even at the highest level of authority. Feedback from employees can be valuable; an employee frequently can suggest constructive improvements in techniques or systems.

The employee should be allowed to review his or her evaluation and there should be space for the employee to add comments. Usually the employee and supervisor/reviewer go over the evaluation together. The employer (or supervisor/reviewer) should ask the employee for ways he or she believes job efficiency can be corrected, new ways to improve the job, and new tasks which can be added to the job. (For an example, see Figure 9-5.)

Salary review

Formal salary reviews, whenever possible, should be conducted at a time different from the performance review. This review forms a basis of promoting understanding about the desirability of the employee receiving fair compensation for the specific job and the work performed. Compensation should be in accord with the limits of the worth of the job and with consideration of such factors as inflation, relative importance of the job to the office, and comparison of salary ranges with other employees. The value of fringe bene-

fits should be discussed during the salary review because benefits are always a part of the total salary structure.

Personnel policy manuals

A personnel policy manual, sometimes referred to as an employee handbook (Figure 9-6), defines the essential, nonmedical office policy information needed by all employees. This information stands apart from the professional information included in job descriptions. All employees should have either a personal copy or an opportunity to read and sign the master office copy. Each should be asked to read it thoroughly and seek clarification on any confusing points. Personnel policy manuals should include a disclaimer stating that the manual is *not* an employment contract, nor a promise of continued employment.

Administrative and policy matters to cover in the personnel manual appear in a "Checklist for the Personnel Policy Manual" found in the box on page 56. This document should be carefully drafted and reviewed; it may be wise to consult legal counsel before distributing the first version or after making any major changes.

Working hours can be defined – hours the employees are expected to be on duty, lunch, break times, and potential odd hours such as Saturdays, Sundays, or early evening. Accurate time records for employees must be kept in accordance with wage and hour laws. Indicate that all employees must check in and check out each work day for payroll purposes; the most accurate way to determine hours worked is a

time clock. Explain that overtime must be authorized and by whom.

Fringe benefits can be defined in the policy manual. List the paid holidays. Most pediatric offices are closed New Year's Day, Memorial Day, Fourth of July, Labor Day, Thanksgiving Day, and Christmas. Additional (religious and other) days may be considered appropriate and should be offered as paid days.

Vacation schedules can be defined in the policy manual. Although vacation schedules vary from practice to practice, an average vacation schedule is 2 weeks after 1 year of employment and 3 weeks after 5 years.

Sick leave policy also should be clearly stated. Most offices give approximately 6 to 10 days a year paid sick leave (not accrued) and grant short leaves for personal emergencies. If additional wages are given to employees for not using the sick days, the staff will be less likely to use the time as extra vacation (some practices also pay for unused vacation days each year). Employees may be sick for longer periods of time than covered; if possible, their job should be protected.

The medical care given to office personnel by the pediatrician and the limits of this care should be described in the policy manual because pediatricians cannot provide all aspects of adult health care.

Other provided employee benefits, such as medical insurance, life insurance, pension contributions, and so forth should be listed in the policy manual. A tax-sheltered Keogh or a corporate pension or profit-sharing plan benefits the pediatrician, and it can be a strong inducement for older, experienced employees. Reinforce this advantage by presenting each participant with an annual statement of his or her plan participation.

Some businesses adopt a cafeteria-style benefits program which enables employees to select appropriate options for themselves. Any differences in benefits between full-time and part-time employees should be carefully outlined in the manual. Reasons for employee termination should also be addressed.

Employment laws

Pediatricians must be attentive to the spirit and letter of local, state and federal employment laws. A succinct sum-

Employee Handbook

Introduction

We want to extend a warm welcome to you as you join the staff of *(insert practice name here)*. We want you to enjoy the experience of working here. Please read this manual carefully. It should answer most of your questions about our personnel policies. We want your working relationship with others in the office to be excellent from the beginning; if you have any questions, just ask.

We have a large number of employees, and we're all human. We will need help and understanding from each other. You are encouraged to speak with each other clearly, honestly, and respectfully. Regular staff meetings are held to work on common problems. Please address any specific concerns about your job, patient care, other employees, or the general running of the office to your immediate supervisor.

Our collective purpose in this practice is to provide quality medical care to the infants, children, adolescents, and young adults we serve. What you say, what you do, and how you say and do it will contribute greatly to the perception families have of us. Many patients and their parents come to us in less than a perfect mood. They may be ill, worried, or even angry. It's part of your job to be cheerful, tactful, and patient even if they don't reciprocate.

As an employee of this office, you are bound by medical ethics. Information entrusted to you by patients, doctors, and fellow employees must be completely confidential. A patient's name as it relates to something that has been heard or has happened in the office should not be mentioned. All of us are responsible for guarding privileged information, and we can be subject to legal action if we violate that contract with our patients.

Structure and Mission

Describe goals and objectives.

Office administration

There are both administrative and professional employees in a medical office. By necessity a high degree of cooperation is required between these two groups. To facilitate smooth running of our office we have formulated a chain of command.

To improve communication and to oversee the running of the office, the physicians have appointed two other essential individuals:

- Office administrator – The administrator is to be responsible for all medical office activities, including accounting and financial procedures. This person is also in charge of all office clerical personnel and answers to the physician director of adminstration. The nursing supervisor will coordinate activities through the office administrator.

- Nursing Supervisor – The nursing supervisor will oversee all nursing functions in the office. This person is to keep an inventory of supplies, order all nursing supplies, and institute a nursing service plan to provide coverage for

patient-contact aspects of the office: telephone, health supervision and sick visits, etc. The nursing supervisor will report to the physician director of nursing.

The office administrator (or designate) and the nursing supervisor have the responsibility and qualifications to resolve the great majority of inner-office problems. In the event that the situation needs further attention, the office administrator will arrange for appropriate mediation with the physician director(s).

In-service meetings

In-service meetings will take place on a regular basis. Every employee will be expected to make every effort to attend, since they will address subjects of general concern and interest. The meetings are expected to be free and open. Any problems concerning patient care, employer-employee relations, or physician-employee relations are fair subjects, but the meetings are not to be a forum to resolve serious personality conflicts. A private setting is in order under these circumstances.

Deportment

A parent or child's first impression of an office comes from their contact with the employees. Employees are expected to present a neat, professional appearance and an open, friendly attitude.

The positive tone of that initial contact must be reflected throughout the visit.

Please avoid discussion of a patient's problem (bill, illness, personal observations) with the patient, his/her parent, or another employee within earshot of others.

Our office has a **no smoking** policy, and we hope that you will not find this to be a major inconvenience. We feel very strongly that we should do as we say; we advise our parents and our patients that smoking is very harmful to their health.

Personal telephone calls

Please keep personal telephone calls to a minimum during working hours. Please have family and friends call during the lunch break only, except for emergencies. When taking a personal call, one of the other private lines must be kept open. If all private lines are in use when you pick up your call, inform the caller you will make contact at another time.

If personal phone calls are thought to be a problem for a particular employee, this will be brought to that employee's attention. Persistence of the situation will be reflected in that person's annual evaluation. Personal calls should be limited to essential matters and be brief.

Lunches and breaks

Lunch is scheduled between *(insert time here)*. One nurse will be required to remain in the office during the lunch hour to assist with emergency phone calls. If an individual physician requires assistance during the lunch hour, the appropriate nurse will be asked to remain until no longer needed.

Figure 9-6: Sample employee handbook.

Working hours

Full-time employees are defined as employees who are regularly scheduled to work *(insert number of hours here)* hours or more in a week. Less than *(insert number of hours here)* hours defines a part-time employee. Working hours may vary for each employee. Employees who are going to be delayed or are sick should call in as early as possible. Chronic tardiness will not be tolerated.

We will make every effort not to keep you overtime. It will, at times, be necessary for hourly employees to work more than 40 hours a week. You will be compensated by being paid time and a half.

Salary

There will be yearly evaluations by one's supervisor. Each employee's compensation will also be addressed on a annual basis around the anniversary date of employment. Cost of living and merit raises will also be considered. Each employee will be informed of their pay change individually. It is expected that this information is to be considered confidential and not to be shared among other workers.

Holidays which fall on weekdays will be paid; those which fall on weekends will not.

Paid holidays for full-time employees are:
(insert list of paid holidays here)

Vacation policy

The following is our vacation policy:
(insert specifics of policy here)

Benefits

(insert specifics of benefits here)

Sick time

(insert specifics of policy here)

Termination

(insert your policy here)

Personnel file

Every employee will have a personnel file. Included in that file will be a copy of the job description. Each employee will be asked to read and sign this job description. The file will also contain copies of annual evaluations and any pertinent information which affects the employer-employee relationship. It will be confidential and kept in a locked cabinet.

IDENTIFYING INFORMATION

Name: _____

Address: _____

Telephone Number: _____

Date of Birth: _____

Social Security Number: _____

Marital Status: _____

Children: _____

If married, spouse's name: _____

Spouse's place of employment, address, and phone number:

_____

_____

_____

Whom and where to call in case of an emergency:

_____

_____

I, _____ , acknowledge that I have received and read the *(insert practice name)* Employee Handbook and that I fully understand its provisions.

I understand that the policies and rules contained in the handbook are subject to change from time to time at the discretion of management and that the handbook is not intended to be, or deemed to constitute, an employment contract.

_____   _____
Signature   Date

NOTES

Figure 9-6: Continued.

Checklist for the Personnel Policy Manual

Administrative dates (taxes and licenses)	Fees	Personal leaves
Appearance and dress code	Filing	Petty cash
Appointment system	Forms and printing	Professional courtesy
Banking procedures	Grievances	Records and record systems
Benefits	Holidays	Referral procedures
Billing procedures	Housekeeping	Salaries and wages
Bonding of employees	Insurance processing	Salary review (statement)
Collection and credit	Mail	Sick leave
Confidentiality	Medications for the practice	Supplies
Disbursements	Office hours	Telephone privileges
Drug samples	Overtime	Termination of employment
Emergency procedures	Pay periods	Time cards
Equal opportunity (statement)	Payroll	Vacations
	Performance review	Working hours

mary of federal legislation can be found in the pamphlet *Personnel Policies in Practice* published by the American Society of Internal Medicine.[1] The following will highlight a few pitfalls that others have identified.

Every office personnel manual should have a section on termination of employment, but one need not explicitly discuss periodic reviews, warnings, probation, reasons for firing (such as violations of confidentiality or embezzlement), bonding of employees or other specifics. Such statements can be used against you by an employee who needs to be terminated. Manuals can be construed as employment contracts. Doctors should give themselves maximum flexibility to fire, subject only to the limitations of anti-discrimination laws. Comprehensive personnel files are a necessity and problems with employees must be documented and kept on file.

The federal Fair Labor Standards Act of 1938 (29 USC 200-219) applies to offices with two or more employees and an annual gross income of $200,000 or more. It requires that the following records be kept:

- Personal information, including name, address, occupation, sex and date of birth (if under 19 years of age);
- Hour and day when workweek begins;
- Total hours worked each workday and each workweek;
- Total daily or weekly straight-time earnings;
- Regular hourly pay rate for any week when overtime is worked;
- Total overtime pay for the week;
- Deductions from, or addition to, wages;
- Date of payment and pay period.

The act requires overtime pay for each hour worked over 40 hours in a week. Overtime must be paid at a rate of no less than 1½ times the employee's regular pay rate. In addition to federal overtime provisions, individual states have overtime statutes. Contacting the US Department of Labor's Wage and Hour Division can give you more complete information. Local telephone directories which do not list a direct number will show a Federal Information Center telephone line, where callers can locate the nearest field for inquiries.

The employer is also required to comply with tax laws. Federal income tax and social security taxes must be withheld from employee wages. States and local governments may levy additional taxes that the employer must collect and deposit. New employees must fill out an IRS form W-4 to determine the number of exemptions to which they are entitled for federal tax withholding purposes. One person in the office should be designated to oversee this process.

An additional payroll-related tax is the Federal Unemployment Tax. Only employers pay it. Forms and additional information can be obtained from the regional IRS office.

It is not possible to detail all the laws which impact employee benefits in this guidebook. The pediatrician must consult an attorney or other professional conversant with these laws. Pension and profit sharing plans may not discriminate against lesser compensated employees.

Conclusion

The pediatrician must devote some time to personnel matters. Even the best systems require hands-on involvement in training, supervision, and communication.

The successful pediatrician shows genuine consideration for employee needs. No pediatrician should be too busy to pay attention to the office staff. A well managed office and competent, effective staff are two key elements of consistent quality patient care.

Reference

1. *Personnel Policies in Practice*. Washington, DC: American Society of Internal Medicine; 1988

Bibliography

American Academy of Pediatrics, Committee on Practice and Ambulatory Medicine. *Personnel Management*. Elk Grove Village, IL: American Academy of Pediatrics; 1986

Klass R. *The Physician's Business Manual*. New York, NY: Appleton Century Crofts; 1981

Laetz CR. The Front Office: A Reflection of Your Practice. *Phys Mgmt*. 1983;23:80-92

How to Hire a Good Office Staff. *Phys Mgmt*. 1984;24:184-198

Scroggins CL. How to Train That New Assistant. *Med Econ*. 1985;62:141-149

Weber R. Delegate Tasks for Maximum Efficiency. *Phys Mgmt*. 1984;24:168-185

Edmonson N. How to Set Staff Salaries. *Phys Mgmt*. 1984;24:182-194

Case J. How to Determine the Right Fringe Benefits for Your Staff. *Phys Mgmt*. 1984;24:120-129

Enright S. How to Fire Someone Without Fallout. *Med Econ*. 1984;61:175-180

Analyzing a Resume. *Med Econ*. 1988;65(1):175

Ballard R. How to Hire Top-Notch Office Assistants. *Med Econ*. 1987;64:136-153

Paxton H. What the Law Demands of You, The Boss. *Med Econ*. 1987;64:225-231

Paxton H. Five Things That Drive Good Employees Away. *Med Econ*. 1988;65:114-121

Harrison D. Starting Your New Staffer Off Right. *Med Econ*. 1989;66:69-75

Checklist

✓ Is your staff adequate?
✓ Do your employees know their job descriptions?
✓ Do you have a policy manual?
✓ Do you schedule performance reviews? Salary reviews?
✓ Do you listen to your employees? Do you hold office meetings regularly?
✓ Do you update employee benefits? Are employees aware of any changes?
✓ Are your employees bonded?
✓ Do your employees feel secure in your office? Do they feel you appreciate them?
✓ Do you have a personnel policy manual for your practice?

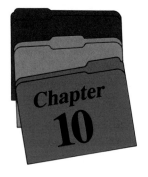

Office Medical Records

The medical record is both a clinical and an administrative document. This chapter discusses workable record systems, including:
- **basic components of administrative and clinical records**
- **chart filing**
- **satellite office record management**
- **organizing medical information and transferring records**
- **handwritten, dictated, or concurrent computer charting**
- **legal and ethical considerations**

The medical record provides both administrative and complete clinical data about the patient and family. (See "Administrative and Clinical Components of the Medical Record" box on next page.) It documents all patient care and provides the basis for charges. It establishes recommended follow-up visits, including immunizations. This chapter will address basic components of the pediatric medical record. Individual practices will quickly identify specialized needs.

Medical record content

Each patient should have an individual record. A family medical record was once quite common, but it is no longer considered the most appropriate format.

The ambulatory medical record consists of administrative information and medical data. An 8½ × 11 inch sheet is the most common vehicle; index cards or odd-sized pieces of paper are to be avoided. Color-coded paper for various purposes (eg, laboratory results, data base information, progress notes) facilitates filing and retrieval. Information should be fastened and filed within the folder in a divided and logical sequence. Loose sheets may become lost or misplaced.

Special concerns

The often hectic nature of pediatric practice requires particular sensitivity in some areas. Medical records regarding allergies, immunizations, medications and telephone consults must be clear and complete. Specific allergies

should be highlighted in the record. Color coded stickers work well, as does prominent notice on the face sheet of the chart. The use of multicolored pens to record or underline laboratory data, injections, immunizations, serious reactions, and parental concerns may be helpful.

Counterpoint

Records inactive for 2 to 5 years are much more likely to be used than those inactive for more than 5 years. Therefore, you may want two inactive locations, one for 2 to 5 years which is close at hand, and one for greater than 5 years at a more distant location.

Immunization reactions must be recorded. The National Childhood Vaccine Injury Act (42 USC 300aa) requires that the lot number of the vaccine and the name of the administrator be documented. Patient information material must be given to the parents of the child before an immunization is given. (See Professional Liability and Risk Management, Chapter 19.) Immunization reactions must be reported. At present, reactions occurring in the private sector are reported to the Food and Drug Administration and those that occur in public clinics are reported to the Centers for Disease Control. A single agency may be named in the future to receive the reports. The report should be documented in the record.

Medication information entries require great care. Drug names and

dosages must be carefully specified. Misspellings or misplaced decimal points can have serious consequences.

Telephone calls must be clearly documented. These notes are often key to a successful defense against alleged negligence. (See Office Telephone, Chapter 8.) Patient complaints and/or physician advice should be noted, along with attempts to return calls, patient response, refusals to comply with therapy, and follow-up plans.

Filing systems

Medical records should be readily accessible. Open-space, shelf-filing systems are generally more efficient than closed files. The files are visible, shelf storage requires less space than cabinets, and shelves are considerably cheaper than cabinets.

Records may be filed alphabetically, numerically, or in a combination of the two (alpha-numerically). Color coding facilitates identification, filing and retrieval. Some offices also make use of different-colored patient folders. System selection is based upon patient volume, billing requirements, computer use, and personal preference. Medical office supply representatives have information on initial or conversion filing systems.

If the medical records system in an established practice does not seem to be serving the practice well, it may be necessary to convert to one of the newer systems. Temporary clerical employees can assist in the conversion. Inactive records can be removed and stored first. Then new and in-use records can be incorporated. Any modification in the forms used to collect and/or record information should be made with a view to potential computer applications. Consultation with a qualified pediatric forms supplier can greatly ease later conversion to a computerized medical record system. (See Computer Systems, Chapter 13.)

Retiring charts to an inactive record area after a predetermined period of 2 to 5 years is greatly assisted by placing color-coded and dated year markers along the exposed folder edge when the patient is seen. Retiring the chart at the time a patient leaves the practice is also helpful.

Inactive medical records of pediatric patients must be kept for long periods of time; they should be placed in a reasonably accessible area. Each pediatrician needs to be aware of the individual state's statute of limitations for professional liability. (See Professional Liability and Risk Management, Chapter 19.) Records should never be misplaced or destroyed. Limited space may require out of office record storage, but all storage should be insured and protected from fire, theft, unlawful access, and environmental damage. Some offices utilize microfilm for storage of old charts. A reasonable charge for time may be made for the retrieval and transfer of information from these records. Prompt access and availability of the information must be assured.

Locating misplaced medical records within the office is often more a problem than it should be. A color-coded tab placed in the open file when a chart is removed can indicate its temporary location, (eg, insurance desk, laboratory, pediatrician's desk, collection and billing, next day visit or nurse call desk). This identification system and the use of color-coded folders can save a great deal of time tracking records.

Satellite office records

Satellite office records can be managed in various ways depending upon the volume of patients and the type of practice. The patient's record should be retained permanently at the primary care site. Transporting records between offices is *not* recommended because the record or its components may become lost. Patients will at times be seen without the chart present. The encounter information should then be recorded on a form that is easily placed

---

Administrative and Clinical Components of the Medical Record

The **administrative data component** in a medical record should include:
1. Name, address, birth date, and telephone number of the patient and parents and/or other responsible party. Include office address and telephone for both mother and father. If the parents are separated, document both home addresses.
2. Name, address, and telephone numbers for local person to reach in an emergency.
3. Each parent's occupation, birthdate (to determine which insurance is primary), place of employment, and social security number. (Include each employer's name, address and telephone number.)
4. Insurance coverage, data to identify each policy by plan name, policyholder, individual identification number, group contract number, and effective date.
5. Family profile, including names and birth dates of siblings.
6. Name of referring physician or agency.
7. Other information useful to the individual practice.

Important: This patient information needs to be updated at each office encounter.

The **clinical data component** of the record should include:
1. A data base form which contains family, social, and medical history. This includes perinatal, developmental, and nutritional notes, comment on illness, injury, hospitalization, surgery, medication reactions, allergies, and past immunizations. A log of illnesses or other health problems is also desirable.
2. An immunization record, maintained in accordance with requirements of the 1986 National Childhood Vaccine Injury Act. An immunization record (separate from the daily flow sheet) should be easily visible somewhere in the chart.
3. Growth charts showing height, weight, and head circumference.
4. Records which document blood pressure, vision, hearing, x-ray, and laboratory data. Some of these can be incorporated in the content of each health supervision visit.
5. Dated note of each office visit and telephone encounter. (See Office Telephone, Chapter 8.)
6. Hospital data, correspondence, consultations, laboratory, x-ray, and miscellaneous reports, each in a defined place in the chart.

Standardized forms for recording administrative and medical components may be obtained from medical stationers or pharmaceutical industry resources.

---

in the medical record. Urgently needed medical information may be transferred by a telephone facsimile (FAX) system. Often a simple telephone call between sites will suffice. Computerized medical records are also a good solution to satellite and parent office record management. (See Computer Systems, Chapter 13.)

Organizing the medical record

The pediatrician must define the family data base information to be used in the practice. This information should be collected at the patient's first visit and updated at appropriate intervals. The data base should include family and personal history, as well as significant medical diagnoses. Developmental, environmental, psychosocial, and behavioral problems that influence the patient's health and welfare also should be included. A standardized, printed format facilitates a uniform, complete report. A summary index form assists reference, transfer, and auditing tasks. (See Figures 10-1 and 10-2.)

History, physical and developmental findings, assessments, plans and treatments should be noted at each health supervision visit. Visit-specific encounter forms are available which also provide information for anticipatory guidance and review of the significant data base. (See Figures 10-3 and 10-4.)

NEW PATIENT QUESTIONNAIRE
TO BE FILLED OUT BY PARENT

Mother's name _____ Age _____

Occupation _____

Father's name _____ Age _____

Occupation _____

If adults in the household work outside the home, what child care arrangements are made for this child?_____

_____

NAME _____

CHART # _____

DATE _____

A. PREGNANCY AND BIRTH:

1. Mother's age at birth _____
2. Did mother have any illness during pregnancy?   No   Yes
3. Did she take any medications other than vitamins and iron?   No   Yes
4. Was the baby on time?   Yes   No
5. What was the birthweight? _____
6. Did the baby have any trouble starting to breathe?   No   Yes
7. Did the baby have any trouble while in the hospital? (jaundice, infections, other?)   No   Yes

   What kind? _____

   _____

B. PAST MEDICAL HISTORY:

1. Where has your child gone for check-ups until now? _____
2. Date of last check-up: _____
3. Date of last dental check-up: _____
4. Has your child had allergic reactions to any medications, foods, insect bites?   No   Yes

   Which ones? _____
5. Has your child had reactions to any immunizations?   No   Yes

   Which ones? _____
6. Any hospitalizations other than for birth?   No   Yes

   For what? _____
7. Any serious injuries?   No   Yes

   What kind? _____
8. Are any medications taken regularly?   No   Yes

   Which ones? _____

C. FAMILY HISTORY:

1. Are the child's parents both in good health?   Yes   No
2. Circle any diseases that this child's parents, grandparents, brothers, sisters, or aunts and uncles have had: anemia, asthma, allergies, diabetes, high blood pressure, heart trouble, tuberculosis, mental illness, drug problems, alcohol problems, inherited illness, venereal disease, cancer, AIDS, others
3. List age, sex, and general health of brothers and sisters _____

   _____
4. Have any of your children died?   No   Yes

D. FEEDING AND NUTRITION:

1. Is your child's appetite usually good?   Yes   No
2. Is it good now?   Yes   No
3. Was there severe colic or any unusual feeding problem during the first 3 months?   No   Yes
4. Do any foods disagree with him/her?   No   Yes
5. For the first 6 months, is he/she (was he/she)

   breast fed or bottle fed? _____
6. If still on formula, which one do you use? _____
7. Does he/she take vitamins?   Yes   No

E. REVIEW OF SYSTEMS:

1. Has your child had frequent ear infections?   No   Yes
2. Any eye problems?   No   Yes
3. Has he/she had any problems with teeth?   No   Yes
4. Does he/she have frequent colds or sore throats?   No   Yes
5. Is there asthma, pneumonia, or recurrent cough?   No   Yes
6. Does he/she have a heart murmur or any heart problems?   No   Yes
7. Any problems with urination?   No   Yes
8. Any problems with diarrhea or constipation?   No   Yes
9. Have there been any convulsions or other problems with the nervous system?   No   Yes
10. Any eczema, hives, or other skin conditions?   No   Yes
11. Has your child ever been anemic?   No   Yes
12. Please list any other medical problems: _____

    _____

F. DEVELOPMENT/BEHAVIOR:

1. At what age did your child sit alone? _____
2. At what age did he/she walk alone? _____
3. Did he/she say any words by the time he/she was 1½ years old?   Yes   No
4. How does this child compare to others

   his or her age? _____
5. Does he/she have any trouble sleeping?   No   Yes
6. What grade is he/she in? _____
7. Has he/she had any trouble in school?   No   Yes
8. Does he/she get along with other children?   Yes   No
9. Circle if your child has had any of the following: nail biting, thumb sucking, bed wetting, problems with toilet training, bad temper, hyperactivity, nightmares, speech problems, problems with discipline, others

G. SAFETY/ENVIRONMENT:

1. Do you live in a private house, apartment, mobile home, other? (CIRCLE)
2. Do you know the hottest temperature of the water in your pipes?   Yes   No
3. Is there a working smoke alarm on each floor in the house?   Yes   No
4. Does your child always use a car seat/seat belt when riding in a car?   Yes   No
5. Are there any smokers in the household?   No   Yes
6. Are there any problems with the condition of your home? (peeling paint, insects, rats, or mice)   No   Yes
7. Does your child always wear a helmet when riding his/her bicycle?   Yes   No

H. DO YOU HAVE A RECORD OF IMMUNIZATIONS?   Yes   No

Figure 10-1: Health questionnaire for a new patient. This form is completed by the parent and retained in the medical record.

Immunization Record/Problem List

IMMUNIZATIONS

	DATE	OPV/IPV (SPECIFY)	DATE	TINE/PPD (SPECIFY)	DATE	RESULT	OTHER	DATE
DPT 1		1					INFLUENZA #1	
DPT 2		2					INFLUENZA #2	
DPT 3							INFLUENZA #3	
DPT 4		3					OTHER	
DT/DPT 5		4						
DT 6		MMR #1		DRUG ALLERGIES:				
HIB 1		MMR #2						
HIB 2								
HIB 3								
HIB 4								

PROBLEM LIST

DATE	PROBLEM	RESOLUTION

Figure 10-2: Immunization record/problem list. This form provides a quick reference and is kept in the front of the medical record.

WELL CHILD CARE CHECK SHEET

AGE	DEVELOPMENTAL TASKS S = Social Fm = Fine Motor L = Language M = Gross Motor	White Bars = Age during which 75% – 100% of children accomplish task per Denver II. (*) Check Age in which task accomplished								ANTICIPATORY GUIDANCE Sa = Safety Fd = Feeding Sx = Symptomatic Rx Fl = Feeling Check if Discussed	PROCEDURES Circle If Done	INIT / DATE
		0	4w	8w	4m	6m	8m	10m	12m			
2–4 wks	S Stares at surroundings* Cuddles* Fm Follows toy to midline Equal movements L Responds to sound, facial activity, activity ceases M Moro* Primitive step* Neck/elbow flexor tone* Palmar grasp*									Sa Car restraints Infant cues Bathing Infant states Bedding Fd Breast-feeding Preparation of formula Propping, burping Volume expectations Sx Thermometer use Bulb syringe Skin care Fl Parents & siblings Parent roles Mom – time for rest	Hgt Wgt HC PKU UA	
6–8 wks	S Smiles, eyes follows person* Fm Palmar grasp fades* Holds object briefly* L Listens to bell, direct regard, coos* M Lifts head (prone) 45° No head droop, susp*									Sa Falls (rolls over) Crib guard Car restraints Fire retardant clothing Small objects out of reach Fd Formula or breast Future solids Sx Colic stools Fl Abdominal sleep, bedtime ritual Return to work, child care	Hgt Wgt HC DPT-1 OPV-1 **Hib**	
3–4 mos	S Smiles spontaneously Talks to self in mirror Fm Hands together Scratches clothes Follows 180° L Squeals, laughs, babbles M Rolls over Head steady, sitting Head up 90°, prone									Sa Crawling: objects out of reach stairway "gate" Risks of walkers, jumpers Fd Review solids Spoon Formula or breast Sx Diarrhea, constipation, vomiting Fl Behavior expectations Toys Schedule Asking for help	Hgt Wgt HC DPT-2 OPV-2 **Hib**	
5–6 mos	S Fm Grasps rattle Regards small object Reaches for object L Turns to voice Imitates speech sound M Prone holds chest up Pull to sit, no head lag									Sa Review crawling: objects, electric outlets, floor heaters Food aspiration (beans) Fd Formula High chair Food selection Feeding techniques – bottle Sx URI, when to call MD Fl Discipline – consistency Play – activity Parenting classes	Hgt Wgt HC DPT-3 **Hib**	
7–8 mos	S Bites Chews Fm Raking grasp Cube hand to hand L Mama-Dada (nonspecific) Combines syllables M Sits – no support Bears some weight									Sa Car seat Stairs Fd Feeding techniques – solids Sx Ear Infection Childhood illness exposure Fl Separation anxiety Baby sitters CPR class	Hgt Wgt HC Optional Visit	
9–10 mos	S Bye-bye Uses cup Peek-a-boo* Holds bottle Fm Thumb-finger grasp Looks for hidden object* L Mama-Dada (specific) One word* M Stands holding on Crawls well									Sa Review poisons (Ipecac) Fd Finger feeding Weaning Feeding techniques – cup, spoon Sx Dental hygiene Fl Experimentation, separation Exploration – play, toys Bedtime ritual	Hgt Wgt HC HCT Sickle PPD Ipecac	
11 mos –1 yr	S Helps with dressing* Toy release* Pat-a-cake* Points* Fm Bangs 2 cubes, puts cube down* L Two words Follows directions* M Walks with help* Stands alone momentarily									Sa Streets Climbing (poisons, falls, windows) Fd Decreased appetite, weaning Eating habits – table foods Sx Vomiting Review Fl Independence testing Consistent limits Self-control Memory versus obstinacy	Hgt Wgt HC Optional Visit	

*denotes items which are not included in Denver II data

Figure 10-3: Well child care check sheet, from 2 weeks to 6 years old. The form is used in conjunction with a physical examination and is printed on heavy weight, tinted paper for easy identification in the medical record.

AGE	DEVELOPMENTAL TASKS										ANTICIPATORY GUIDANCE		PROCEDURES

Header legend:

DEVELOPMENTAL TASKS
S = Social
Fm = Fine Motor
L = Language
M = Gross Motor

White Bars = Age during which 75% – 100% of children accomplish task per Denver II. (*)
Check Age in which task accomplished

| 12m | 18m | 2y | 2½y | 3y | 4y | 5y | 6y |

ANTICIPATORY GUIDANCE
Sa = Safety   Fd = Feeding
Sx = Symptomatic Rx   Fl = Feeling
Check if Discussed

PROCEDURES
Circle If Done

---

1 yr – 18 mos

- S: Drinks from cup; Plays ball; Uses spoon, messy
- Fm: Scribbles spontaneously; Tower 2 cubes
- L: 4 words (other than Mama)*; Jargon*
- M: Walks well, walks backward; Crawls up steps*; Stoops and recovers*

Anticipatory Guidance:
- Sa: Car restraints; Window screens; Running into danger; Scalds
- Fd: Complete weaning; Appetite slump
- Sx: Review mouth-to-mouth resuscitation
- Fl: Imitation of adults; Tantrums; Strong preferences

Procedures: Hgt; Wgt; HC; UA; MMR (≥15 mo); Hib

---

18 mos – 2 yrs

- S: Imitates*; Feeds doll; Removes clothing; Uses fork, spoon
- Fm: Tower 4 cubes; Dumps raisin from bottle spontaneously*
- L: Points to pictures; Combines 2 words; Names picture
- M: Kicks ball; Walks up steps; Throws overhand

Anticipatory Guidance:
- Sa: Water safety; Matches; Sharp or electric objects
- Fd: Proper snacks; Self-feeding
- Sx: Toilet training
- Fl: "No"; Bedtime rituals – naptime; Night terrors; Testing limits

Procedures: Hgt; Wgt; HC; PPD; Hct; DPT-4; OPV-3

2–2½ yrs

- S: Feeds self well*; Puts on clothing; Washes/dries hands, brushes teeth
- Fm: Tower 6 cubes; Bowel/bladder control
- L: Points 4 pictures; Names 6 body parts
- M: Jumps; Throws ball overhand

Anticipatory Guidance:
- Sa: Sibling torment; Car restraints; Play, supervision
- Fd: Good eating habits
- Sx: Constipation
- Fl: Discipline: explanation & consistency; Need for play with peers; Helping out at home

Procedures: Hgt; Wgt; HC; Optional Visit

2½–3 yrs

- S: Names friend; Plays tag; Imaginary friend*
- Fm: Imitates vertical line; Tower 8 cubes
- L: Plurals*; Names 4 pictures*
- M: Balance 1 foot 1 second; Broad jump; Pedals tricycle*

Anticipatory Guidance:
- Sa: Teach child play safety: throwing sharp objects; following ball into street
- Fd: Small portions of food; Fluids
- Sx: URI – Viral infections
- Fl: Decision making within limits; Explaining "rules"; Curiosity; Child care supervision; Choices

Procedures: Hgt; Wgt; BP; PPD; Hct; UA (female); Vision; Hearing

---

3–4 yrs

- S: Separates easily from mother; Dresses with & without help
- Fm: Buttons up*; Picks longer line; Copy ○
- L: Comprehends cold, tired, hungry (2 of 3); Comprehends prepositions*; Recognizes colors (3 of 4)*; Knows full name*
- M: Hops on 1 foot; Balances each foot

Anticipatory Guidance:
- Sa: Supervised use of scissors, pencils; Street crossing; Water safety
- Fd: Table manners; Simple meals
- Sx: Nightmares
- Fl: Genital exploration; Imaginative play and fears; Labeling and categorizing; Sexual identity

Procedures: Hgt; Wgt; BP; PPD; UA (female)

4–5 yrs

- S: Brushes teeth, no help; Dramatic play*; Plays games
- Fm: Draws man, 3-6 parts; Copies square (demonstr)
- L: Opposites (2 of 3): Hot __ Woman __ Big __; Counts 5 blocks
- M: Catches bounced ball; Balances well – 5 seconds; Heel to toe walk*

Anticipatory Guidance:
- Sa: Teaching "outdoors alone" safety: travel to school; neighborhood play
- Fd: Teaching food selection
- Sx: Check regarding: eneuresis; school phobia; tummy aches
- Fl: Teaching respect for feelings and property of others; Home responsibility

Procedures: Hgt; Wgt; BP; PPD; Hct; UA; DPT-5; OPV-4; Vision; Hearing

---

5–6 yrs

- S: Shares with peers*; Knows street address*; Knows parents' names
- Fm: Draws man, 6 parts; Copies square
- L: Defines (7 of 9): Ball __ Beach __ Desk __ House __ Banana __ Window __ Ceiling __ Fence __ Sidewalk __; Composition (3 of 3)*: Spoon __ Shoe __ Door __
- M: Backward heel-toe walk; Skips; Passes all 5 year items*

Anticipatory Guidance:
- Review 5 year items
- Sa: Bicycle helmets; Strangers; Good/bad touch
- Fd: Breakfast habits; Help with food preparation
- Sx: Emergency planning; Colds; Teeth grinding
- Fl: School preparation; Responsibility for "wellness"

Procedures: School form; Hgt; Wgt; BP; PPD; Hct; UA (female); Vision; Hearing; Immunization Update

---

denotes items which are not included in Denver II data

Figure 10-3: Reverse side.

SPORTS PARTICIPATION HEALTH RECORD

This evaluation is only to determine readiness for sports participation. It should not be used as a substitute for regular health maintenance examinations.

NAME _____ AGE _____(YRS) GRADE _____ DATE _____

ADDRESS _____ PHONE _____

SPORTS _____

The Health History (Part A) and Physical Examination (Part C) sections must both be completed, at least every 24 months, before sports participation. The Interim Health History section (Part B) needs to be completed at least annually.

PART A — HEALTH HISTORY:
To be completed by athlete and parent

	YES	NO
1. Have you ever had an illness that:		
a. required you to stay in the hospital?	____	____
b. lasted longer than a week?	____	____
c. caused you to miss 3 days of practice or a competition?	____	____
d. is related to allergies? (ie, hay fever, hives, asthma, insect stings)	____	____
e. required an operation?	____	____
f. is chronic? (ie, asthma, diabetes, etc)	____	____

2. Have you ever had an injury that:
   a. required you to go to an emergency room or see a doctor? ____ ____
   b. required you to stay in the hospital? ____ ____
   c. required x-rays? ____ ____
   d. caused you to miss 3 days of practice or a competition? ____ ____
   e. required an operation? ____ ____

3. Do you take any medication or pills? ____ ____

4. Have any members of your family under age 50 had a heart attack, heart problem, or died unexpectedly? ____ ____

5. Have you ever:
   a. been dizzy or passed out during or after exercise? ____ ____
   b. been unconscious or had a concussion? ____ ____

6. Are you unable to run 1/2 mile (2 times around the track) without stopping? ____ ____

7. Do you:
   a. wear glasses or contacts? ____ ____
   b. wear dental bridges, plates, or braces? ____ ____

8. Have you ever had a heart murmur, high blood pressure, or a heart abnormality? ____ ____

9. Do you have any allergies to any medicine? ____ ____

10. Are you missing a kidney? ____ ____

11. When was your last tetanus booster? _____

12. For Women
   a. At what age did you experience your first menstrual period? _____
   b. In the last year, what is the longest time you have gone between periods? _____

EXPLAIN ANY "YES" ANSWERS _____
_____
_____
_____

I hereby state that, to the best of my knowledge, my answers to the above questions are correct.

Date _____

Signature of athlete _____

Signature of parent _____

PART B — INTERIM HEALTH HISTORY:
This form should be used during the interval between preparticipation evaluations. Positive responses should prompt a medical evaluation.

1. Over the next 12 months, I wish to participate in the following sports:
   a. _____
   b. _____
   c. _____
   d. _____

2. Have you missed more than 3 consecutive days of participation in usual activities because of an injury this past year?
   Yes _____ No _____
   If yes, please indicate:
   a. Site of injury _____
   b. Type of injury _____

3. Have you missed more than 5 consecutive days of participation in usual activities because of an illness, or have you had a medical illness diagnosed that has not been resolved in this past year?
   Yes _____ No _____
   If yes, please indicate:
   a. Type of illness _____

4. Have you had a seizure, concussion or been unconscious for any reason in the last year?
   Yes _____ No _____

5. Have you had surgery or been hospitalized in this past year?
   Yes _____ No _____
   If yes, please indicate:
   a. Reason for hospitalization _____
   b. Type of surgery _____

6. List all medications you are presently taking and what condition the medication is for.
   a. _____
   b. _____
   c. _____

7. Are you worried about any problem or condition at this time?
   Yes _____ No _____
   If yes, please explain: _____
   _____
   _____

I hereby state that, to the best of my knowledge, my answers to the above questions are correct.

Date _____

Signature of athlete _____

Signature of parent _____

Figure 10-4: Sports participation form. A copy of this form is retained in the medical record.

Part C – PHYSICAL EXAMINATION RECORD

NAME _____ DATE _____ AGE _____ BIRTHDATE _____

Height _____ Vision: R _____/_____, corrected _____, uncorrected _____

Weight _____ L _____/_____, corrected _____, uncorrected _____

Pulse _____ Blood Pressure _____ Percent Body Fat (optional) _____

	Normal	Abnormal Findings	Initials
1. Eyes			
2. Ears, Nose, Throat			
3. Mouth & Teeth			
4. Neck			
5. Cardiovascular			
6. Chest and Lungs			
7. Abdomen			
8. Skin			
9. Genitalia - Hernia (male)			
10. Musculoskeletal: ROM, strength, etc.			
a. neck			
b. spine			
c. shoulders			
d. arms/hands			
e. hips			
f. thighs			
g. knees			
h. ankles			
i. feet			
11. Neuromuscular			
12. Physical Maturity (Tanner Stage)	1. 2. 3. 4. 5.		

Comments re: Abnormal Findings: _____

_____

_____

_____

PARTICIPATION RECOMMENDATIONS:

1. No participation in: _____

_____

2. Limited participation in: _____

_____

3. Requires: _____

_____

4. Full participation in: _____

Physician Signature _____

Telephone Number _____ Address _____

American Academy of Pediatrics

Figure 10-4: Reverse side.

Handwritten, dictated, or concurrent computer charting

Many pediatricians continue to handwrite the medical record. This is time consuming and often illegible. Printed data base and office encounter forms, or rubber stamps and different colored pens, can highlight immunizations, phone calls, and allergic reactions. These tools are useful to both the pediatrician and the office staff.

The dictated/transcribed record has infinite advantages in efficiency, continuity of care and medical-legal defense. Dictating records saves time, eliminates legibility problems and expedites reproduction. A portable dictating device, telephone stations, or regular telephone systems can be linked to a compatible transcriber. In smaller offices, the transcription may be performed outside the office by direct telephone transcription or transfer of tapes or disks. Added efficiency frees the pediatrician for direct patient care – an economy that can quickly compensate for the cost of the system and personnel. A brief period of adjustment will be required for those accustomed to handwriting. Don't be tempted to become "wordy" when dictating. Always review transcribed records for errors and initial the entries before they are placed in the chart.

Computers can greatly ease office record and patient care management. Some experts believe that present trends suggest that computers may

someday be the predominant vehicle for all medical and business records. Computerized medical records provide a system for obtaining, storing and printing comprehensive information, transfer and "retirement" of records, and recall of information for process and outcome auditing. (See Computer Systems, Chapter 13.)

Guidelines for Good Record Keeping

- keep medical record entries current
- keep documentation objective
- maintain legible medical records
- maintain comprehensive medical records
- DO NOT ALTER MEDICAL RECORDS

Legal and ethical considerations

Original records are legal documents and should be retained for the time specified by the state statutes in which the practice is located. Medical records should never leave the office or secured storage unless they are summoned by the court. The medical record is a confidential document involving the physician-patient relationship; information in it should not be communicated to a third party without the patient's or parent's written consent, unless it is required by law or necessary to protect the welfare of the patient or community (eg, contagious disease information). Some states have special confidentiality requirements for psychiatric or psychological problems. A valid authorization must be in writing, identify the person clearly, and be properly signed and dated. Information regarding the presence of HIV infection may be protected information in some states.

At no time should information be erased, obliterated, written over, added to or removed from the chart. Errors made at the time of the original recording should be identified by putting a line through the incorrect recording followed by the correct information. Subsequent to that, addendum notes can be added at any time to the chart to clarify previously recorded information. All correction and addendum notes

should be properly identified, timed, dated and author initialed.

The American Medical Association has determined it is unethical to withhold medical records from the new physicians of patients who have left the practice. Records should not be withheld for failure to pay for services, to return, or to follow instructions; nor should parts be withheld without a valid reason. Courts of law have determined that patients have a legal right to their health records. This makes it imperative for pediatricians to be extremely careful about the information included in medical records. Although the medical record, *per se,* is the property of the pediatrician, the patient has a right to review the information it contains. In addition, with appropriate legal steps, the information in a medical record can be obtained for use in litigation or other purposes. Five days is considered a reasonable notice to obtain a medical record. Some physicians request a fee for sending health records to another physician; this is no longer considered to be unethical.

A system should be developed for transmission of health information from one physician to another or for use in hospital admission. A completed summary form can eliminate the need to copy the entire record.

Conclusion

A pediatrician's medical record system requires careful planning and maintenance. Many available systems meet the basic requirements discussed here. Uniform, accurate, legible, detailed, and well organized records are mandatory in today's health care environment. The medical record is the vehicle by which continuity of care is assured, and a legal document which protects the pediatrician and the patient.

Bibliography

A Simple Guide For Pruning Your Records. *Med Economics.* 1989;66:73-78

Bjorn JC, and Cross HD: "Problem-Oriented Practice." Chicago, IL: Modern Hospital Press; 1971

Gordon IB: Office medical records. *Pediatr Clin North Am.* 1981;28:565

"Opinions on Physicians' Records." *Current Opinions of the Judicial Council of the AMA.* Chicago, IL: American Medical Association; 1982:23

Record Retention Schedule. *Medical Executor.* 1982; Winter

Sparer CN: Organizing the physician's office. *Pediatr Clin North Am.* 1981;28:537,543

Counterpoint

Some feel that those who decline opportunities to explore the role of computers for recording medical records, invite frustration. The equipment, information system, training, start-up, and integration costs only increase as such a decision is postponed. The use of qualified, experienced computer expertise will provide safeguards and reduce unnecessary problems. Gradual implementation proceeding from business to medical records will provide the knowledge base and confidence required for success.

Task Force on Medical Liability. *An Introduction to Medical Liability for Pediatricians,* ed 4. Elk Grove Village, IL: American Academy of Pediatrics; 1985

Tufo HM, Bouchard RE, Rubin AS, Twitchell JC, Van Buren HC, and Bedard L: Problem-Oriented Approach to Practice. JAMA, 1977:238:502

Weed LL: Medical Records, Medical Education and Patient Care. Cleveland, OH: Case Western Reserve University Press; 1971.

Checklist

✓ Are you satisfied with your record system?
✓ Can you easily find records?
✓ Are your records efficiently organized for effective day-to-day use by you and your staff?
✓ Do you employ printed fill-in and check-off forms?
✓ Are you using an 8½ × 11 inch, open-space filing system?
✓ Are your parent and satellite record systems compatible?
✓ Do you "retire" your records into an inactive status on a regular basis?
✓ Are you maintaining your records in a proper fashion and in accordance with statutes of limitation of your state?
✓ Is your transfer of medical information timely, useful, and easy to accomplish?
✓ Do you write legibly or dictate your records?
✓ Have you considered using a computerized medical record system?
✓ Are you embarrassed to show your records to colleagues?

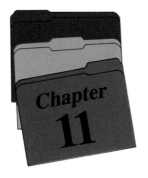

Printing for the Pediatrician

Printed materials are required in all pediatric offices. Consider all of the printed materials utilized by the office: prescriptions, patient information sheets, progress notes, immunization records, stationery, business and appointment cards, patient education materials, birthday notices, telephone encounter forms, "superbills," and newsletters. These printed materials require considerable attention to the following:
- **is the printed material necessary?**
- **how is it best obtained?**
- **can it be updated easily and economically?**
- **does it contain the information you and your patients need?**
- **is it easily readable?**
- **can it be obtained more economically elsewhere?**

Printed materials are a necessary part of any pediatric practice, even if only letterhead and prescription blanks are used. The extent to which print materials are used will vary with the practice, but pediatricians who have not investigated the use of booklets, pamphlets, and information sheets might be wise to do so. Printed materials can enhance a practice in many ways: help educate patients, clarify and reinforce instructions, save time, and serve as a public relations tool.

Preprinted materials are available from organizations – including the Academy – as well as government and private agencies and companies.

Preprinted materials should be carefully read before distribution to assure accuracy, ease of readability and understanding by the parent, and compatibility with the pediatrician's philosophy.

All printed materials should be readable and effectively fulfill a purpose, and they should be well organized. The information should be accurate and written at about a fourth to fifth grade level.[1] The pediatrician should review all printed materials on a regular basis to cull obsolete materials and update or revise current materials.

Any printed materials, and especially those for patients, should look professional. Mimeographed or poorly printed copy may cause the patient to wonder what other areas of the practice also are less professional. All printed materials should include the pedia-

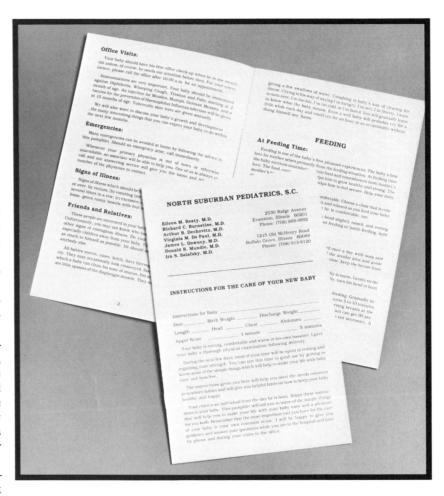

Figure 11-1: Newborn information booklet. The pediatrician gives this to the parents in the hospital. It contains hospital nursery data and important information on caring for the newborn baby at home.

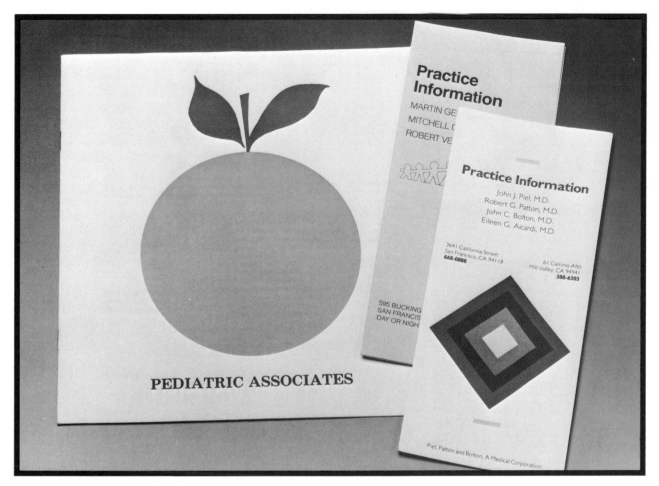

Figure 11-2: Practice information folders and booklets. These are available for patients to take from a display rack in the office, or the pediatrician gives them to parents with an explanation of the practice's services.

trician's name and address, either pre-printed, stamped or labeled.

Printed materials can be a large cost center within any practice. The pediatrician and staff can significantly curtail expenses if these costs are well managed and monitored.

Printed materials handed to parents aid them in the care and treatment of their children. A subtle, additional benefit is enhanced public relations for the parents and the community. Printed materials usually are seen by others in addition to the parents, and they may serve as a silent source of referral for prospective parents or families new in the community who happen to see them. The pediatrician's name becomes familiar to them, and the pediatrician is established as a caring physician who provides quality services.

Printing for use in the business office can include (see also Business Office, Chapter 12):
1. Business letterhead

2. Business cards
3. Appointment cards
4. Encounter forms
5. Forms for response to physician's request for information

Printing for use by patients includes:
1. Parent information booklet.
2. Anticipatory guidance material, eg, health advice, specific illnesses, accident prevention.
3. Newborn infant information, eg, newborn booklet with general information, material on newborn jaundice and advice on newborn feeding (Figure 11-1).
4. Immunization information and consent forms to be read and returned to the office for inclusion in the chart.

Suggestions for basic materials

Introduction to the Practice

A booklet or letter about the practice will provide necessary information and serve as a reference for future health needs. (See Figure 11-2.) Suggested topics include:
1. Name(s) of pediatrician(s), their backgrounds and special interests. (You might also include professional staff if turnover is not an issue).
2. Addresses and telephone number(s).
3. Hospital affiliations.
4. Office hours.
5. Professional services (eg, laboratory, psychologist, social worker, pharmacy).
6. Emergency care information.
7. Payment procedures, billing and insurance or third party information.
8. Health supervision schedule.
9. Ages of patients seen in the practice.
10. Willingness to discuss family problems.

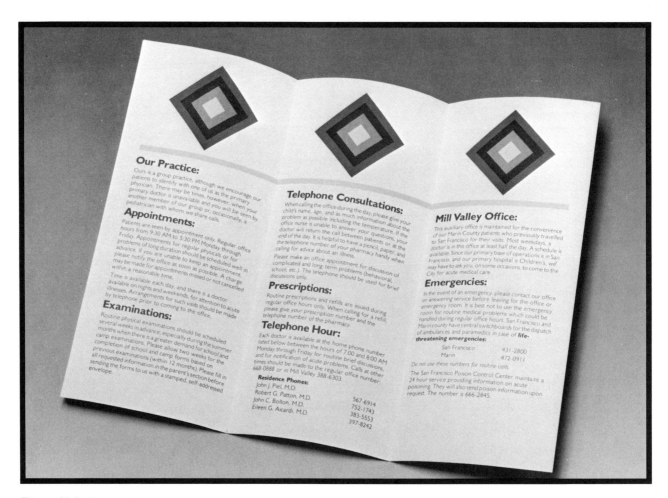

Figure 11-2: Continued.

11. Special information, such as lectures, group meetings, and community resources.

The printing may vary from a simple mimeographed letter to a printed booklet with a logo and special colored paper. **This booklet or letter is best given to the patient by the pediatrician to emphasize the importance of the information and enhance the use of the information by the family.**

Newborn encounter and Information form

Data from the nursery usually is supplied on a form from the hospital and usually also includes delivery information. If the hospital does not supply a separate form, one should be made for all newborn infants entering the practice.

Other forms

Miscellaneous other forms or "prewritten" letters may be useful for the following purposes:
1. Insurance coverage – claim information.
2. Patient responsibility for finances and insurance.
3. Collection statements.
4. Termination of patients from the practice.
5. Professional courtesy "charge" letter.

Examining room forms

These following forms may be used in examining rooms by the pediatrician:
1. Instruction pads with pediatrician's name.
2. Prescription pads.
3. History questionnaires.
4. Excuse forms.
5. Courtesy notes.
6. Immunization information forms.
7. Athletic examination forms. (See Figure 10-4 on pages 64, 65.)

Do-it-yourself printing...or not?

Pediatricians express a variety of opinions on preprinted materials. Some may think that preprinted material works well for them as provided. Others may feel that preparing and designing their own materials is beyond their capabilities and/or too expensive.

Those who wish to become involved with printing their own materials should check with local printers. Printers and typesetters can offer good advice about style of type, design, and layout at a reasonable price.

Plan in advance how the printed materials for patients will be distributed: by mail, to those who ask for information, to those with the problem(s) discussed, by the pediatrician, by the nurse, or on a table in a rack for patients to pick up at will. More than one method of distribution may be appropriate.

Let's say that you have decided to prepare your own material. What steps should be taken to make sure that your efforts turn out just the way you want? Here are some suggestions:

1. Consider using a word processor. If you're not a professional writer, and few pediatricians are, it is likely that you will be altering your copy constantly until you get it right. The ease of working with a word processor – with a spell-check program included – makes the labor of writing much less burdensome. This will allow you to make changes in the future with less effort.

2. If you feel you must, have a professional editor review your material for clarity and grammar. You may find this person within one of your practice's families. Be prepared to compensate such activity.

3. What about printing? Check with a local printing firm to see what best meets your needs. It's likely that photocopying will be cheapest, and if your original copy is of good quality, (the printing sharp, dark, and legible) the results can be acceptable. Booklets can be collated and colors can be selectively used for highlighting. You might want to consider typesetting the title page for an additional touch of style, or even typesetting the entire job if it is within your budget. Make sure your name and office phone number are conspicuously present on the front page. It's good marketing, credit deserved, and the patient will know the origin of the material.

   Whatever the format, print in large quantities for economy. The unit cost is lower, and the materials no doubt will be used faster than anticipated. Even if you have to store the material, the cost savings will likely be worthwhile. A careful inventory control of printed materials is necessary to avoid the extra expense and difficulty in obtaining printing on a rush basis. Pharmaceutical representatives can also be excellent sources of printed materials.

4. Lastly, plan distribution in advance. If you are preparing a newsletter, have your printer prefold it so that envelopes won't be needed. Consider getting a bulk mail permit.

Office pamphlets about the practice should be accessible to everyone. Booklets on special topics should reach your target group. Materials which deal with very specific concerns shouldn't be taken by parents who really don't need them. Try to be selective. Remember your hard work and cost and think carefully about distributing your best self-written material to just the right people.

Conclusion

All pediatric offices require printing and production of office paper goods. These should be readable and look professional. Producing your own educational material facilitates economy, personalization, and specific content. Careful attention to office printing is sound business policy.

Reference

1. Flesch R. *The Art of Readable Writing*. 25th Anniversary ed, revised. New York, NY: Harper-Row;1974

Checklist

✓ Does your printed material fit your budget?
✓ Have you established inventory control for all printed material?
✓ Do you update content on a regular basis?
✓ Is your name, address, and telephone number in a prominent place on all your printed materials?
✓ Are your patient education materials in an attractive rack for patient accessibility?
✓ Do you have a method for appropriate distribution of printed materials?

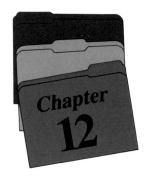

Chapter 12

Business Office

The pediatrician's business office needs to operate with sound, proven, operational, financial, and marketing techniques. This chapter discusses such office practices as:
- **business office layout and location**
- **proper use of printed forms and letters**
- **ensuring accuracy of family data**
- **billing and collections**
- **bookkeeping, including reviewing accounts**

Not all business offices are alike, nor should we expect them to be. However, certain essential functions needed for the smooth transition of the patient emanate from a well-run business office. The attitude and organization of this area make a first and last impression upon the patient. Although you are not usually present in this area as it goes about its business, it will still be perceived as a direct extension of you.

The medical business office usually revolves around the type of billing system used. In the solo pediatrician practice, the function might be handled by a nurse or aide who posts the bills manually. A large multi-practitioner office is likely to utilize more sophisticated, expensive computer equipment. Any system should be quick, accurate and user-friendly to both the office staff and the patient.

Business office location

The physical location of the business office must be carefully selected. It is best located centrally in the office suite adjacent to the waiting room but easily accessible from the health care delivery section. It should be in a place that facilitates patient flow and allows for immediate communication with the medical staff. This area should include the following:
- definite sign in/checkout area
- service/financial counseling area
- accounting or computer space
- adequate present and future record storage
- sufficient work space
- adequate telephone lines

The handling of accounts is one of the most sensitive functions accom-plished by office staff. The exit window should afford sufficient privacy to accommodate patients.

Staffing

Business office staffing will be determined by the size of the practice, the type of insurance filing performed (Medicaid, HMO, PPO, hospitalization only, etc) and whether contract services (such as collection agencies, account-ants, service bureaus) are utilized.

The key to effective staffing is to ensure that someone in authority (the pediatrician, a managing partner or a supervising clerk) actually under-stands the intricate mechanisms neces-sary to accomplish the myriad of tasks performed by the business office. The pediatrician should always be the ulti-mate decision maker, who acts follow-ing appropriate input from all involved personnel.

Cross-training of business office per-sonnel is important for several reasons. First, the office may not generate a suf-ficient amount of work to justify strict division of duties. Second, when per-sonnel are able to perform more than one task, coverage can be provided when the work demand increases in one area or when personnel are absent from work for illness or vacation.

In small office practices, the busi-ness office and receptionist duties may be shared, which can provide a broader base of knowledge among a select group of employees.

Qualifications

Business office personnel should have a desire to serve the practice and its patients with courteous concern. They should be proficient in typing, mathe-matics, and a 10-key adding machine.

With the proliferation of computers into the smallest of offices, it would be important to consider an employee who is familiar with office management sys-tems. Be sure the employee will fit the job description. Do *not* make the job fit the employee.

Training

Training may be done in the office or by outside consultants. It is normally arranged by supervisory personnel. Job descriptions should be clearly defined and personally reviewed with new employees, each of whom should have one copy while a second remains in the personnel file. The performance review mechanism utilized in the busi-ness office should be reviewed with the new employee. Employees in the busi-ness office should be encouraged to avail themselves of the many seminars, tapes, and other educational oppor-tunities offered by insurance com-panies, Medicaid, and others. These services can enable your staff to stay on top of guidelines and regulatory changes made by government agencies and third party payers.

The reception (sign-in) area

In most offices the reception area is adjacent to the business office with a good view of the entrance to the office and waiting area. Smaller offices often consolidate the reception area with the business office. The function of the reception area should be limited to patient registration, minor triage of walk-in patients, telephone answering, patient routing to treatment area, and reminder calls. If the reception area is often chaotic, or patients appear frus-trated when they arrive in the examining room, the receptionist may either be overworked or not tempermentally suited to the job.

The patient sign-in provides an opportunity for the receptionist to assist the business office by obtaining and continuing to update patient demographic data for billing purposes (new address, employment change, change of insurance carrier). The patient encounter form, whether prepared manually or by computer, can be initiated here as a routing slip for the patient. Appointments booked in advance should already have their encounter form and chart available at the receptionist's desk before the patient arrives.

Business office personnel should check the appointment schedule at least 1 day prior to prepare the chart for the visit, review the status of the account and allow for early review of medical records by medical personnel.

Controlling paperwork

Patient flow through the office necessitates paperwork from the time the appointment is made through the rendering of medical care and the full payment of the bill. Intelligent forms design reaps dividends in overall paperwork management; research and effort put into this area is well invested. Working with paperwork rather than against it can lay the foundation for an efficient business office operation.

Forms

Forms and form letters are an integral part of collecting and disseminating information for the efficient operation of a medical practice. Forms should provide information relevant to each area within the clinic and aid in patient flow through the facility. These forms may also enable staff to monitor quality assurance indices (See Improving the Quality of Office Practice, Chapter 27.) Forms used continually and in high volume can be designed in-house with a professional printing company and/or given on bid to several printers. Computer software can sometimes be modified for individual practices to generate forms on an as-needed basis, eventually reducing the cost of printing and encouraging more frequent revision of forms.

Patient registration

Patient registration is of utmost importance to the business office (See Figure 12-1.) This is the primary source of demographic data and should include:
1. Responsible party for account, parents' birthdates (to determine whose insurance is primary), current address, occupation, home and work phone numbers, and social security numbers.
2. Family profile (who lives in the household with the patient and their ages).
3. Patient age, date of birth, and sex.
4. Insurance coverage – including company name, certificate and/or group number, policy number, individual identification number, social security number, and address for claims processing.
5. If a single parent family – type of custody and guardianship.
6. Name of person to reach locally in an emergency, with address and telephone.
7. Name of referring physician or agency.

New patient letter or booklet

The initial encounter in the office is the best time to inform the patient of office policies and billing practices. A new patient booklet or letter given at the initial visit and/or sent after the first visit can introduce patients to the practice. (See Printing for the Pediatrician, Chapter 11.) Some pediatricians include a picture and personal CV as part of this booklet.

Patient charge sheet (encounter form)

The encounter form serves best when it is designed to meet the needs of the individual practice. It can be used as a sequential routing slip from the receptionist to the pediatrician, then to the laboratory or other ancillary services, and end with the patient sign-out desk in the business office.

The encounter form should be designed primarily for efficient use by the pediatrician and other office personnel. A majority of procedures and common diagnoses can be pre-printed on the form using International Classification of Diseases, Ninth Revision, Clinical Modification (ICD-9-CM) codes for diagnosis and Current Procedural Terminology, Fourth Edition (CPT-4) codes for procedures. The

pediatrician then may mark the appropriate codes and sign his or her name. The sign-out staff enters and totals the charges and records any payment presented by the patient.

If the encounter sheet is a carbon or self-carbon form, consider having it produced in triplicate. The first copy is kept by the office for entry onto the day sheet or computer. The second copy may be given to the patient to serve as an insurance claim record, or designated for completion by the business office staff or computer and then mailed for insurance purposes. The third portion could be kept with the chart to reconcile at the end of the day.

Some practices refer to this form as a superbill, because it provides a comprehensive, abbreviated record useful to the practice, the patient and the payer.

An example of content and layout for this triplicate office form defining services rendered, diagnosis, etc, for insurance use appears in Chapter 14, Charging for Services. CPT-4 codes may be changed annually and should be carefully verified each year.

If the practice has a computer service, financial information as well as demographic and insurance information may be pre-printed on the encounter form (eg, the aging of the account and date of the last payment), making it easier for the business office to make collections or obtain payment commitments from patients when they sign out. Sophisticated software also could provide information on the encounter form about drug allergies, immunization records, diagnoses, history, and so forth.

The encounter form in a small office may be a simplified superbill. This is especially true if the patient is not routed for laboratory or other studies outside the physical office area. A different superbill may be used for billing hospital services. (See Figures 14-2 and 14-3 on pages 91 and 92.)

Day sheets

This simple document will help maintain the orderly flow of patients through the office. It should contain each doctor's schedule for the day and may be used by the receptionist to note patient arrival, the nurse and physician in the treatment area, and the cashier as the patient leaves. This may be prepared manually and copied for each user area or generated by computer.

**BEAR DOWN
PLEASE PRINT**

PEDIATRIC ASSOCIATES
PATIENT HISTORY INFORMATION
PLEASE FILL IN ALL THE UNSHADED AREAS ONLY.

**BEAR DOWN
PLEASE PRINT**

MOTHER
OR
GUARDIAN

FATHER
OR
GUARDIAN

PERMANENT
ADDRESS

STREET   APT. NO.

OR
VISITING
ADDRESS   CITY   STATE   ZIP

RESIDENT
PHONE: EMPLOYMENT
PHONE:

FATHER'S
EMPLOYER:

EMPLOYER'S
ADDRESS

SPOUSE
EMPLOYED
BY:

REFERRED
BY:

PRIMARY
INSURED'S
NAME

PRIMARY
INSURANCE
COMPANY

POLICY
NUMBER

COMPANY   PLAN   GROUP   CERTIFICATE

MEDICARE   REL   MEDICAID

OTHER INSURANCE   NUMBER

DATE: /   /

ACCOUNT NUMBER

☐ NEW   ☐ WELFARE

LOCATION

☐ CHANGE   ☐ H   ☐ L   ☐ P   ☐ SPECIAL

☐ DELETE   BILLING ☐   CREDIT ☐
             CODE   CODE

CHILDREN-FROM BIRTH TO 18 YRS. LIST MEMBERS BY BIRTH DATE, OLDEST FIRST:

NAME	SEX	BIRTH DATE	MEMBER NUMBER

DRIVERS LICENSE #

OTHER IDENTIFICATION

THE UNDERSIGNED AGREES THAT ALL SERVICES ARE RENDERED ON A PAID BASIS ONLY. IF COLLECTION BECOMES NECESSARY, THE UNDERSIGNED SHALL PAY ALL COSTS INCLUDING ATTORNEY'S FEES.

MOTHER OR GUARDIAN   S.S. #   FATHER OR GUARDIAN   S.S. #

Figure 12-1: Patient registration form. This form is completed prior to the first appointment and updated as information changes.

Insurance forms

A standardized insurance claim form approved by the American Medical Association's Council on Medical Service and the Health Care Financing Administration, such as HCFA-1500, (Figure 12-2) is recommended. Although most traditional insurance companies accept a superbill, some (including Medicare, Medicaid, and CHAMPUS) require the submission of HCFA 1500 forms. The standardized forms are available in single or multiple copies (pin feeding for computer processing is available) from any medical forms distributor.

Statements

Statement design and function is limited by the billing system. However, the main objective with any statement is to provide the patient with as much information as necessary to pay for the services performed.

A monthly statement that may double as an insurance form reduces requests to the business office for insurance claims filing assistance. Any type of statement must contain:
1. responsible party's name and billing address
2. patient(s) name
3. date(s) of service
4. place of service
5. procedure(s) performed
6. payment(s) received
7. pediatrician's name and provider number
8. balance due

A remittance stub and/or return envelope is helpful. For insurance purposes, a statement should additionally contain:
1. a procedure code (CPT-4 code) for each service performed
2. ICD-9-CM code for each diagnosis
3. patient's insurance group and/or identification number
4. patient's relation to the insured
5. condition due to injury or illness
6. workmen's compensation
7. name and address of insurance company
8. physician or group federal tax identification number, or insurance company identification number
9. signature block for patient to authorize release of medical information

10. optional signature block to authorize insurance payment directly to the physician.

Examples of optional information that may be provided to the patient are:
1. unpaid account aging
2. amount of last payment (by family – not third party)
3. date of last payment
4. family or patient charges and payment year to date
5. payment or credit policies
6. seasonal greetings or messages related to current health topics.

The age of accounts should be maintained and reflected on the statement. Account aging is usually done in 30, 60, 90 day intervals. A means of managing accounts at each of these times should be established policy. The probability of collection on accounts beyond 90 days is small.

Health care information transfer

Health care information transfer forms (Figures 12-3 and 12-4) usually are handled by the business office staff with occasional consultation with the pediatrician. The patient's record also should be checked to:
1. Determine if the patient has an outstanding balance
2. Determine if special collection procedures should be used
3. Attempt to obtain a new billing address if the patient is moving.

It is recommended that no charge should be made for transferring records.

Transfer of patient's records to another physician in the immediate area can occur for a variety of reasons including changes in insurance coverage, but may indicate dissatisfaction with the services delivered by the staff and/or physician. A review of records transferred within a specific geographic area followed by a direct phone contact to inform the family that the records are being transferred and to inquire if there were any problems with your practice may help correct problems that were not previously known.

Patient visits – ensuring accountability

The business office provides a control function to ensure that all patients seen during the day are accounted for and properly charged. However, this control mechanism requires some assistance:

A. **To initiate from the pediatrician in a manual system**
1. The pediatrician records charges and procedures for each patient seen on a day sheet.
2. The business office then balances charge sheets (encounter forms) against the pediatrician's day sheets.
3. If a patient has left the office with the charge sheet, verification of charges may be obtained from the pediatrician's day sheet, with the medical record as a back-up source of information.
4. The charge is then entered onto the patients' accounts.
5. A dummy charge sheet can then be prepared and a copy mailed to the patient.

B. **To initiate from the business office using preprinted charge slips**
1. The receptionist maintains a numbered log of each patient signing in using **preprinted numbered triplicate** charge slips as the office trip ticket.
2. The corresponding number for each patient is written on the patient charge sheet.
3. Before posting charges and again at the end of the day the business office must assemble all charge sheets in numerical order; if a number is missing it is retrieved from the saved third copy sheets or identified by the receptionist's log.
4. The charge is then entered onto the patients' accounts.
5. A dummy charge sheet can then be prepared and a copy mailed to the patient.

C. **To initiate from the pediatrician using preprinted charge slips**
1. Charge sheets with preprinted or computer printed numbers may be used.
2. After the pediatrician records charges on the slip for each patient seen, the third copy of the charge slip is attached to the patient's chart so the nursing staff can save it;
3. Before posting charges and again at the end of the day the business office must assemble all charge sheets in numerical order; if a number is missing it

HEALTH INSURANCE CLAIM FORM

FORM APPROVED
OMB NO. 0938-0008

(CHECK APPLICABLE PROGRAM BLOCK BELOW)

| ☐ MEDICARE (MEDICARE NO.) | ☐ MEDICAID (MEDICAID NO.) | ☐ CHAMPUS (SPONSOR'S SSN) | ☐ CHAMPVA (VA FILE NO.) | ☐ FECA BLACK LUNG (SSN) | ☐ OTHER (CERTIFICATE SSN) |

PATIENT AND INSURED (SUBSCRIBER) INFORMATION

1. PATIENT'S NAME (LAST NAME, FIRST NAME, MIDDLE INITIAL)

2. PATIENT'S DATE OF BIRTH

3. INSURED'S NAME (LAST NAME, FIRST NAME, MIDDLE INITIAL)

4. PATIENT'S ADDRESS (STREET, CITY, STATE, ZIP CODE)

5. PATIENT'S SEX

MALE ☐   FEMALE ☐

6. INSURED'S I.D. NO. (FOR PROGRAM CHECKED ABOVE, INCLUDE ALL LETTERS)

7. PATIENT'S RELATIONSHIP TO INSURED

SELF   SPOUSE   CHILD   OTHER

8. INSURED'S GROUP NO. (OR GROUP NAME OR FECA CLAIM NO.)

☐ INSURED IS EMPLOYED AND COVERED BY EMPLOYER HEALTH PLAN

TELEPHONE NO.

9. OTHER HEALTH INSURANCE COVERAGE (ENTER NAME OF POLICYHOLDER AND PLAN NAME AND ADDRESS AND POLICY OR MEDICAL ASSISTANCE NUMBER)

10. WAS CONDITION RELATED TO:

A. PATIENT'S EMPLOYMENT

YES ☐   NO ☐

B. ACCIDENT

AUTO ☐   OTHER ☐

11. INSURED'S ADDRESS (STREET, CITY, STATE, ZIP CODE)

TELEPHONE NO.

11.a.   CHAMPUS SPONSOR'S :

STATUS   ☐ ACTIVE DUTY   ☐ DECEASED   BRANCH OF SERVICE
☐ RETIRED

12. PATIENT'S OR AUTHORIZED PERSON'S SIGNATURE (READ BACK BEFORE SIGNING) I AUTHORIZE THE RELEASE OF ANY MEDICAL INFORMATION NECESSARY TO PROCESS THIS CLAIM. I ALSO REQUEST PAYMENT OF GOVERNMENT BENEFITS EITHER TO MYSELF OR TO THE PARTY WHO ACCEPTS ASSIGNMENT BELOW.

SIGNED _____   DATE _____

13. I AUTHORIZE PAYMENT OF MEDICAL BENEFITS TO UNDERSIGNED PHYSICIAN OR SUPPLIER FOR SERVICE DESCRIBED BELOW.

SIGNED (INSURED OR AUTHORIZED PERSON)

PHYSICIAN OR SUPPLIER INFORMATION

14. DATE OF:
   ILLNESS (FIRST SYMPTOM) OR INJURY (ACCIDENT) OR PREGNANCY (LMP)

15. DATE FIRST CONSULTED YOU FOR THIS CONDITION

16. IF PATIENT HAS HAD SAME OR SIMILAR ILLNESS OR INJURY, GIVE DATES

16.a. IF EMERGENCY CHECK HERE

17. DATE PATIENT ABLE TO RETURN TO WORK

18. DATES OF TOTAL DISABILITY
   FROM   THROUGH

DATES OF PARTIAL DISABILITY
   FROM   THROUGH

19. NAME OF REFERRING PHYSICIAN OR OTHER SOURCE (e.g. PUBLIC HEALTH AGENCY)

20. FOR SERVICES RELATED TO HOSPITALIZATION GIVE HOSPITALIZATION DATES
   ADMITTED   DISCHARGED

21. NAME AND ADDRESS OF FACILITY WHERE SERVICES RENDERED (IF OTHER THAN HOME OR OFFICE)

22. WAS LABORATORY WORK PERFORMED OUTSIDE YOUR OFFICE?
   YES ☐   NO ☐   CHARGES:

23. A. DIAGNOSIS OR NATURE OF ILLNESS OR INJURY. RELATE DIAGNOSIS TO PROCEDURE IN COLUMN D BY REFERENCE NUMBERS 1, 2, 3, ETC. OR DX CODE
1.
2.
3.
4.

B.

EPSDT   YES ☐   NO ☐

FAMILY PLANNING   YES ☐   NO ☐

PRIOR AUTHORIZATION NO.

24. DATE OF SERVICE		B. * PLACE OF SERVICE	C. FULLY DESCRIBE PROCEDURES, MEDICAL SERVICES OR SUPPLIES FURNISHED FOR EACH DATE GIVEN		D. DIAGNOSIS CODE	E. CHARGES	F. DAYS OR UNITS	G. * T.O.S.	H. LEAVE BLANK
FROM	TO		PROCEDURE CODE (IDENTIFY)	(EXPLAIN UNUSUAL SERVICES OR CIRCUMSTANCES)					

25. SIGNATURE OF PHYSICIAN OR SUPPLIER (INCLUDING DEGREE(S) OR CREDENTIALS) (I CERTIFY THAT THE STATEMENTS ON THE REVERSE APPLY TO THIS BILL AND ARE MADE A PART THEREOF)

26. ACCEPT ASSIGNMENT (GOVERNMENT CLAIMS ONLY) (SEE BACK)
   YES ☐   NO ☐

27. TOTAL CHARGE   28. AMOUNT PAID   29. BALANCE DUE

30. YOUR SOCIAL SECURITY NO.

31. PHYSICIAN'S, SUPPLIER'S, AND/OR GROUP NAME, ADDRESS, ZIP CODE AND TELEPHONE NO.

DATE:

32. YOUR PATIENT'S ACCOUNT NO.

33. YOUR EMPLOYER I.D. NO.

I.D. NO.

* PLACE OF SERVICE AND TYPE OF SERVICE (T.O.S.) CODES ON THE BACK
REMARKS:

APPROVED BY AMA COUNCIL ON MEDICAL SERVICE 6/83

Form HCFA-1500 (C-2) (1-84)   Form OWCP-1500
Form CHAMPUS-501   Form RRB-1500

Figure 12-2: 1990 standardized insurance form (HCFA-1500). This claim form, or its updates, is generally accepted by third party payors.

PEDIATRIC CENTER
1335 South Street
Smithsville, MO 12345

Date _____

Account _____

_____

_____

_____

_____

Please release any pertinent medical records and immunizations for:

Patient name _____

Address _____

_____

Date of Birth _____

(Parent's signature) _____

(Witness' signature) _____

(Doctor's signature) _____

(Patient's signature, if applicable) _____

Figure 12-3: Health care information transfer request form.
This gives the parent's consent for the pediatrician to request
information from prior physician(s).

PEDIATRIC CENTER
1335 South Street
Smithsville, MO 12345

**PEDIATRICS
ADOLESCENT MEDICINE**

Date _____

Re: _____   Account _____

Dear Doctor _____

The above named patient was under my professional care from _____ to _____ .

This patient's growth and development were normal except as noted below:

Significant Past History: _____

_____

_____

Pertinent Laboratory (including TB test)

Date/Result _____

Pertinent X-ray

Date/Result _____

IMMUNIZATIONS GIVEN

DTP 1 _____   Oral Polio 1 _____   MMR _____
                                (Trivalent)

   2 _____   2 _____   HiB _____

   3 _____   3 _____   Hepatitis B _____

Boosters _____   Boosters _____

_____

DT _____

I hope the above information will be of aid to you. If there is further information needed, please do not hesitate to ask.

Cordially,

_____

Figure 12-4: Health care information response form. This contains a summary of clinical information to be sent to a new physician.

is retrieved from the saved third copy sheets or identified by the receptionist's log.

4. The charge is entered onto the patients' accounts.
5. A dummy charge sheet can then be prepared and a copy mailed to the patient.

Preprinted charge sheets can be a great convenience. However, care must be taken to account for numbered sheets that may be voided, destroyed, or prepared in advance for patients who are "no-shows."

The business office should serve as the exit point for the patient. Business office personnel should be prepared to:

1. Present the patient with an itemized bill of that day's procedures;
2. Make an attempt to collect payment for services;
3. Remind the patient of any existing balance;
4. Encourage the patient to make payment arrangements if the balance is delinquent;
5. Discuss any insurance arrangements that are applicable;
6. Give a postage-paid business reply envelope (franked – not stamped) to all patients with a balance.

The bookkeeping function

Effective accounts receivable management requires the establishment of and adherence to sound methods and routines of accounting for business office transactions. Clear documentation and an audit trail of every transaction is mandatory. Methods of accounting for transactions may vary with the type of billing system used, but the key element is that transactions are recorded on a daily basis.

Posting to patient accounts

Charges and adjustments

Within a multiple physician practice, accounting for patient charges depends somewhat on the elected method of accounting for individual physician production and compensation. Most practices choose to record charges segregated by physician. Posting to patient accounts begins after determining that all patient visits for the day have been accounted for. Regardless of the method of maintaining financial records – use of ledger cards, service

bureau, in-house computer, and so forth – it is imperative that:

1. Charges be posted on a daily basis;
2. Records are balanced daily to ensure the validity of the posting;
3. An accounts receivable total is updated daily;
4. The reason for the adjustment to a patient's account is thoroughly documented and initialed by the person making the adjustment;
5. If computer records of accounts are used, there is "backup" and the disk is stored off premises daily.

Payments

It is preferable to balance and post different types of payments separately. Accounts receivable payments may be paid on the day of a visit or may be received in the mail.

Desk receipts are monies collected in the office as either cash or a check:

1. Desk receipt payments should be recorded on the patient charge sheet;
2. A carboned receipt book to record cash payments must be maintained;
3. Posting of desk receipts on the patient account should be distinguished from mail receipts to aid in tracing posting errors and balancing.

Mail receipts are payments that come in the mail from either the patient or an insurance company:

1. Compile a list indicating the account number, account name, payer and amount;
2. Balance the receipts by running a tape of the checks and a separate tape of the listed amounts;
3. Distinguish mail receipts when posting patient accounts to aid in tracing errors and balancing.

Embezzlement

If staffing levels allow, it is prudent to have more than one employee involved in tallying receipts and posting to accounts. It is also important to have a managerial person who does not routinely do clerical work in the business office to prepare the bank deposit. Such division of responsibility narrows the possibility for undetected errors and employee theft or embezzlement.

The chance of hiring a thief or being the victim of fraud is more frequent than most pediatricians would expect. Regardless of the precautions built into the procedures, an experienced thief can "beat" any system. Only a trusted employee can embezzle; someone who is not trusted will be watched more

carefully. The best way to protect the practice is to limit the amount of money that can be stolen and the amount of time a theft can continue.

It is crucial that all personnel who are involved in any way with the receipts should be bonded.

Safeguards against embezzlement

- Do not become so engrossed in the medical aspects of the practice as to lost touch with its financial aspects.
- Insist that the bookkeeper be bonded.
- Before hiring a bookkeeper, investigate his or her background thoroughly.
- Have the accountant perform quarterly audits.
- Run an accounts receivable tally on ledger cards and compare it with the day book. If the two do not agree, there could be a mistake, but it could indicate theft.
- Charge slips, receipts, vouchers, invoices, and checks should be serially numbered. Check to see that none of these are missing.
- Examine cancelled checks. Be sure none are missing and that all payees are known.
- Authorize only two people to handle checks and cash.
- Make a deposit every business day.
- Endorse all checks as soon as they are received.
- Never cash checks for patients.
- Have the accountant drop in unexpectedly on occasion to check books.
- Never authorize anyone to sign checks.
- Never sign blank checks. If necessary, have advance checks made out completely, postdate them, then sign them.
- Use an embossing check protector, and write all checks in indelible ink. Do not use felt-tipped pens.
- If an error is made when making out a check, never correct it. Instead, void the check, leave it in the book, and be sure it is included with the cancelled checks given to the accountant at the end of the month.
- Be sure the face amount of each check agrees exactly with the amount on the corresponding invoice.
- If a check must be made out to an individual, always include the person's title after his name (eg, "John Smith, Tax Collector").
- Check the deposit every day, or at least let the bookkeeper believe this is done.
- Spot check receipts and compare them with entries in the day book

while the bookkeeper is present. If a payment was entered on the patient's ledger card but omitted from the day book, be suspicious.

- Check change and petty cash funds regularly. The change fund should always equal the starting amount. Funds and voucher amounts in petty cash should equal the starting amount. Have an audit performed immediately if a theft is suspected. Do not let the bookkeeper reconcile the monthly bank statement with the checkbook. Let the accountant or someone else do it.
- Have the accountant prepare a balance sheet and income statement at least quarterly. If there is a problem, suspicious drains of $400 or more will probably be evident.
- Have envelopes prestamped (order from the post office) or use a postage meter.
- Consider using a bank service called a lock box depository. Patients mail payments in special envelopes directly to the bank where they are deposited into the practice's checking account. An accounting of each day's receipts is mailed to the practice. Day book entries are made from this data sheet so the bookkeeper handles only the checks received directly from patients in the office.

Billing systems

Patient account billing is kept to a minimum when fee for service is expected at the time of delivery. Increased capitated care and other third party reimbursement systems make it imperative that good billing cycles be established.

Billing systems are usually determined by the size of the practice, staffing levels of the business office, and progressiveness of the pediatrician. Because the optimum billing system depends on a number of subjective as well as objective factors, this book makes no attempt to delineate specifications or comparisons.

Billing

Billing cycles or schedules frequently are determined by the type of billing system established, (ledger card, service bureau, in-house computer, and so forth) the number of statements sent, and the number of business office staff. The most important element is

that billing be done on a routine, consistent basis to:

1. To provide an even cash flow;
2. Send bills on a cycle basis to ensure a cash flow throughout the month;
3. Provide budgeting of payments and continuity of billing to the patients.

Billing cycles are most commonly established at 1 month intervals. For ease of integration into the bookkeeping function, statements are often sent the first of each month. (If using a service bureau, the business office billing cycle may be subject to the dictates of the service bureau's processing schedule.) A 1 month billing cycle can:

1. Include multiple visits on one statement;
2. Allow adequate turn-around time for patient receipt of statement and remittance;
3. Establish a structure for easy aging of account balances.

If multiple cycles within a month are desired, it is customary to split the patient population alphabetically or by divisions within the range of account numbers to ensure that a different portion of accounts are billed on each billing date.

Counterpoint

Some management consultants suggest that the monthly billing cycle call for statements mailed on the 25th of the month, since many people pay their bills in one group on the first of the month. The expectation is that the medical bill mailed just before the end of the month will be available for prompt payment, and the bill arriving later will be put off until the next month.

Insurance billing

Insurance billing for outpatient services for the average pediatric practice is generally a non-productive effort as the majority of these services are not covered by traditional insurance. If possible, the responsibility of submitting claims should be shifted to the patient. In some states, through the effort of the AAP Child Health Insurance Reform Program (CHIRP) legislation, many previously non-covered services are mandated. In this situation

it might be more beneficial to provide insurance billing.

The most efficient mechanism is to provide the patient with a copy of the encounter form (superbill) at the time of the visit for attachment to the patient's insurance and submission to the insurance carrier (See Figures 14-2 and 14-3 on pages 91 and 92.)

The encounter form is generally sufficient for processing by most insurance companies if it identifies:

1) the patient
2) date and place of treatment
3) procedures performed and charges itemized
4) diagnoses
5) physician's name and signature
6) physician or group tax identification number.

All other information noted previously may be provided by the patient.

Patient education may be necessary to eliminate the mailing or dropping off of claim forms. For traditional insurance carriers the pediatrician should emphasize that the patient's insurance is a contract between the patient and the insurance company, not between the pediatrician and the insurance company. The patient should be made aware that the pediatrician expects payments from the patient.

Alternative delivery systems billing (HMO, IPA, PPO)

In the last decade, business offices have had to adjust their policies to accommodate the proliferation of the alternative delivery systems (HMO, IPA, PPO). Individual practitioners or groups now must stay current with the varying requirements of any number of plans. When contracting with a new system be sure to review not only the reimbursement aspects but the means by which the business office must conduct billing. Some plans may require that the office collect a co-payment only. Others may require submission of the entire bill prior to reimbursement. Another group may allow complete collection at the time of services, requiring that patients obtain reimbursement from their insurance plans.

Some plans, although capitated, still require the submission of a claim form for each patient encounter. This provides them with the information they need to establish trends and address cost containment issues. This same information, if appropriately main-

XYZ Clinic Ltd.
1706 Eternity Ave.
Homeland, USA 12345

Dear Mr. & Mrs. Wilbur

Some patients find it difficult to
pay for their medical services in
full at the time they are received.
Therefore, we have established a
payment program that allows medical
fees to be paid in four equal monthly
payments or by a special arrangement.

You have not as yet indicated how you
wish to make your payment. Would you
please write us at the above address
or call us at 312-555-1234 now so a
mutually satisfactory plan can be
arranged.

Sincerely,

Mrs. Rose E. Boyd
Credit Department

Figure 12-5: Sample initial collection letter.

XYZ Clinic Ltd.
1706 Eternity Ave.
Homeland, USA 12345

Dear Mr. & Mrs. Wilbur

All charges with the XYZ Clinic are
due within 30 days of receipt of the
initial billing statement. Our records
indicate that charges on your account
are over 30 days old and are therefore
past due.

If there are unusual circumstances
which have prevented you from paying
these charges and you feel these
circumstances would warrant special
financial arrangements, please contact
the clinic credit department to
discuss agreeable arrangements.

Your immediate attention to this
matter is essential to protect your
relationship with the XYZ Clinic.

Sincerely,

Figure 12-6: Sample second collection letter.

tained by the business office, will provide the data needed to allow each practitioner or group to negotiate a fair capitation or reimbursement. It is imperative that each business office be familiar with the idiosyncracies of each contract so that the patient receives the plan's full benefit and the health care provider is appropriately compensated for services delivered within a reasonable billing interval.

Credit and collections

Credit policy

A written credit policy is necessary to enforce collections and communicate effectively with patients about financial responsibilities. This policy may be displayed at the sign-out area and/or stated in an introductory letter given to all new patients.

Payment by cash, check or credit card at the time of service is the preferred policy. But to accommodate patients who may incur substantial charges or are in financial distress, a payment schedule should be adopted which may be administered by busi-

ness office personnel (eg, a certain percentage of the balance or "X" number of dollars per $100 of the balance to be paid monthly). For patients who request special arrangements, supervisory or administrative staff should be available to counsel patients and structure payment terms. A mechanism for identifying and monitoring patients with special payment arrangements should be established. Color coding accounts or assigning "account type" codes are common identifiers.

The coding system should not be designed to embarrass the patient but to notify the staff. When the "account type" changes, the coding system must change immediately.

The pediatrician should be consulted about collection procedures. A special patient case, family circumstances, or a personal relationship with the pediatrician may dictate the degree to which collection procedures are enforced. Despite the above circumstances it is wise to have a policy of a maximum balance after which the account should revert to a cash only basis. Of course,

this does not apply to patients whose accounts are being paid under a third party payor contract with an HMO, PPO, etc. The business office staff should be aware of building accounts with little or no attempt at payment within any billing cycle. Difficult situations can be averted if alternative payment schedules are proposed to help the patient.

If patients with past due amounts already have been informed of the amount due by mail or at the time of the visit, rebilling may only need to include the date of service, a total charged and paid, and the balance due. Collections can be enhanced by adding small reminder notes to the bills. Many stationery firms sell reminder notices in rolls which can be easily peeled from the roll and attached to the bill.

In general, accounts should be aged in 30-day intervals, with a formula established for the sending of collection letters (See Figures 12-5 through 12-9.) Most accounts less than 60 days old will usually be paid. Serial collection notices should be used after 60

```
XYZ Clinic Ltd.
1706 Eternity Ave.
Homeland, USA 12345


Dear Mr. & Mrs. Wilbur

Your account is long past due and
although we have sent you statements,
we have received no reply.

We did not hesitate in giving you our
service and cannot understand why you
ignore our request for payment. Please
understand that we will do everything
we can to cooperate with you in
clearing the account. We sincerely
hope you will cooperate with us by
letting us hear from you soon.


Sincerely,


Credit Manager

Balance:
```

Figure 12-7: Sample third collection letter.

days. Computer billing is extremely helpful for automatically aging the accounts. A well-structured approach to collection of aged accounts is necessary and should be instituted with the guidance of an accountant.

Telephone collections

Telephone collections must be handled discreetly and must comply with guidelines of the Fair Debt Collections Practices Act (15 USC 1692) to prevent charges of harassment or potential lawsuits. Because of the sophistication of collection techniques now mandated by law, business office personnel not adequately trained and monitored in collection calls probably should leave repeated telephone collection attempts to a professional collection agency.

Collection referrals

Prior to collection referral, medical charts for all delinquent accounts should be given to the pediatrician for review and collection approval.

The charts of patients referred for collection should be filed in a separate area for easy identification. Lists of accounts referred for collection should

be prepared and distributed to appropriate personnel to prevent further nonemergency appointment scheduling without business office approval.

Choosing a collection agency

If a collection agency is used, selection must be based on the same criteria used for employees or other consultants. Because the agency acts as an extension of the pediatrician's office, it is imperative that a business staff member be well informed of the collection methods used and the operations of the agency. An arrangement should be signed prior to placing accounts for collection to:

1. Indemnify the practice from any legal proceedings against the agency;
2. Clearly state commission rates to be paid to the agency;
3. Determine whether commissions will be deducted from collection remittances by the agency, or the entire collection will be remitted to the pediatrician with commissions paid to the agency as an after-the-fact expense;

4. Outline the rights of the pediatrician's office to recall an account from collection;
5. Detail the responsibilities in reporting payments made directly to the business office;
6. State the rights of both parties to cancel the agreement.

Termination of patient care

From time to time it may become necessary to discontinue the care of a patient. This usually is done when the patient's bill goes for collection.

There may be other reasons to stop providing care to a patient; chronic non-compliance with regard to appointments and treatment programs, unwarranted hostility, or threat of a professional liability action.

Some important things to keep in mind are: (1) be certain the need for this action is determined on a case-by-case, family-by-family basis, and (2) be certain that the termination is done legally

Agreement to Remit Payment

Account Number _____ Account Balance _____

_____

Patient Name _____ Address _____

_____

Responsible
Party: Name _____ Address _____

_____

I agree to pay the balance of my account in not more than _____ equal payments at the rate

of $_____ per month, starting on _____ and continuing on the same day of each and every

month thereafter until fully paid, if not paid sooner.

Date _____ Signature _____

If signed by other than the patient, print below: Name, address, and relationship.

Name _____ Relationship _____

Address _____

City/State _____

Figure 12-8: Sample Agreement to Remit Payment form.

and in such a manner as to preclude any possibility of a perception of abandonment. This is usually done through the use of a registered letter with a return receipt requested. The letter should state the plan for termination after a specified time interval with emergency services to be rendered until assumption of care by another physician.

Checklist

✓ Have you evaluated the physical location, layout, and space requirements of your business office?

✓ Is your staff adequate in number and proficiency?

✓ Are staff duties delineated? Is there appropriate training and supervision?

✓ Have your reviewed and evaluated your present business forms?

✓ Do you routinely check the accuracy of and update patient's telephone numbers, addresses, and other data?

✓ Do you have a system of ensuring that all patients seen are accounted for and properly charged?

✓ Do you have a system to identify the origin, routing, and outcome of each business office transaction?

✓ Have you determined the cost effective billing cycle for your practice?

✓ Do you attempt to collect fees at the time of service?

✓ Do you have a written credit policy?

✓ Do you have a payment schedule for patients unable to pay the complete charge at the time of service?

✓ Do you have a system to identify patients with delinquent accounts easily?

✓ Do you communicate with these patients about their accounts before their appointments?

✓ Are patients responsible for filing their insurance claims? If not, does your office process claims in a timely, efficient manner?

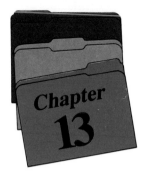

Chapter 13

Computer Systems

This chapter provides an overview of the use of office computers, and discusses:
- **identifying computer needs**
- **selecting hardware and software**
- **professional and business applications**
- **how to introduce computer systems into the office**
- **common mistakes made in purchasing and maintenance**
- **where to go for help**

Computer systems are now so commonplace that they have come to be viewed by most physicians as a necessary ingredient of a successful practice. Computers have their own vocabulary which can challenge the uninitiated. But beneath the foreign terminology, the computer is simply a tool designed to do certain functions, no different in concept from a stethoscope or centrifuge designed to do certain functions. Its uniqueness lies in its ability to do a great many different functions. In making decisions about using computers in practice the pediatrician should first ask what necessary functions are best suited to computerization. The answer to this very fundamental question is different for each physician, and may vary from time to time as the practice grows larger or more complex.

Any physician, whether new or well established, whose practice management challenges fall within the above parameters, should consider a computer solution. A personal practice analysis can determine whether a computer would be a useful tool for your practice. Purchasing a computer to do insurance billing will not solve problems due to inadequate personnel or insufficient training, but it might solve inefficiencies in claims filing due to personnel fatigue or delays in payment due to inaccurate transmission of information.

After making a decision to investigate computer systems, many practitioners will focus on the business functions and delay decisions about computerized patient care functions. This may keep life simple initially, but could be short sighted. Electronic record keeping and other computerized patient care functions are increasingly popular. Some systems come as modules enabling the clinical module to be added when practical. The pediatrician

just starting out may be well advised to introduce a computerized clinical data system from the start in order to avoid the almost inevitable future conversion. The headaches of conversion are generally greater than those encountered starting out fresh.

There are a large number of affordable, well designed office management programs available to the private practitioner.[1] These programs will generally provide, at a minimum, patient billing and insurance claims filing. Added to this basic level of function are options providing the other functions outlined in the chart on the next page. These additional functions may be standard and included in the base price or may be priced separately.

Patient care functions outlined in list II of the chart as A. *Critical information files,* B. *General information files,* and D. *Clinical research using patient databases,* are available to varying degrees in the more sophisticated office management programs or by the addition of relational database programs. These latter programs are essentially generic, and not designed specifically for the medical office. However, they are so flexible and powerful that the practitioner willing to invest the time to customize a record keeping system can do so.

The clinical problem solving functions do require some experience with the use of computers and special equipment. Traditionally most physicians have introduced these functions into their offices only after they have gained some familiarity with computers. However, the rewards to the physician who utilizes such services cannot be overstated. The enhancement in problem solving skills, the ease with which up-to-date information can be obtained, and the resulting improvement in

patient care, more than compensates for the small financial and time investment necessary to perform electronic database searches and utilize CD-ROM.

The mixed clinical and business functions in list III of the chart are no less useful than those in list I or II, but are perhaps less urgent, especially for the new practitioner who is not yet overwhelmed with patients. Nevertheless, one should not lose sight of how easily these functions can be added onto most previously installed systems. The cost is minimal, and for word-processing and electronic spread sheet programs, the possible usefulness spills over into family and community activities.

Definitions

Before talking to a computer salesperson, the pediatrician should be familiar with common terminology.[2]

Hardware refers to mechanical and electronic devices.

Software refers to the programs used to instruct the hardware how to perform.

A **CRT** (cathode ray tube) is the viewing screen with associated keyboard.

A **CPU** (central processing unit) is the essential portion of the computer that executes commands.

ROM means Read Only Memory. Certain program instructions are embedded permanently into ROM and cannot be changed, only reviewed and acted upon.

RAM means Random Access Memory. RAM is the amount of memory (information) a computer can manipulate. This determines the size and complexity of programs the computer can run. The more RAM purchased with a system, the more costly it becomes.

Chip refers to the microelectronic

device in the CPU that is at the heart of the computer and partly determines its speed and power. Terms such as "80286, 80386, 80287 co-processor" are used to denote the power, speed, and function of the individual chip.

16-bit and **32-bit** refer to the number of pieces of information processed at one time. The higher the number the faster the machine and the more costly. The bit number is determined in part by the type of CPU chip purchased. 16-bit machines are sufficient for smaller offices but 32-bit machines are best for larger practices.

12 Mhz, 16 Mhz, 25 Mhz, etc, refers to the speed of flow of information through the machine. The higher the number the faster information is processed. Again, the trade-off is increased speed for increased price.

Modems are hardware devices which convert computer data into a form that can be transmitted via phone to another computer.

BAUD rate refers to how fast a modem transmits data. 2400 BAUD is sufficient for electronic database searches by the physician. 9600 BAUD or higher is best for electronic claims filing and other large data transfers. Not surprisingly, the higher the BAUD number the bigger the price tag.

Networks refer to a combination of hardware and software designed to link several computers together to share information. Larger practices are likely to have a network of one sort or the other. Once installed the operation of the network itself is invisible to the user.

Steps in purchasing a system

The first step is to decide what you want the computer to do for you. Once the practice analysis identifies your needs, the serious shopping should start.

A typical price range to purchase a turnkey system including software, hardware, and installation is generally $7,500 to $10,000 per physician in a practice.

Maintenance contracts (which are essential) usually are about 1% of the purchase price/month for the life of the system.

Within these budget approximations the average physician should be able to purchase a system that will meet his/her needs for 5 to 10 years and perhaps longer.

Always pick the software first, then the hardware. It is the software that determines what the system will do for you. The hardware translates the software's instructions to perform the functions you desire.

Most of the purchase price will be spent on the hardware, so the budget conscious pediatrician will give this component close attention. Keep in mind that higher price may be related to enhanced quality and better performance standards.

The buyer will first have to make some decisions about system size. This includes the number of terminals, the amount of RAM memory, the operating speed (16 Mhz, etc), the number of printers and their speed, the type of equipment needed for back-up of data, and ancillary equipment such as surge protectors and backup power supply, and the number of disk drives and their size.

Present accurate estimates of your practice work load to various computer vendors in order to assess the required system size. Accurate information on the number of patient visits per year, number of insurance claims to be filed per year and rate of new patients entering the practice, enables most medical

---

Typical Functions Performed By Computer In A Pediatric Office

I. Business
   A. Accounts receivable record keeping
   B. Insurance claims filing and follow-up
   C. Billing
   D. Collections activity record keeping
   E. Accounts payable record keeping
   F. Payroll and taxes
   G. General ledger functions
   H. Practice analysis
      1. Individual physician productivity
      2. Profitability of individual services
      3. Practice growth trends
      4. Demographic analysis of referral patterns
      5. "What if?" analysis of proposed financial decisions
II. Patient Care
   A. Critical information files
      1. Immunizations
      2. Key diagnoses from past medical history
      3. Active problem lists
      4. Pharmaceutical profiles
      5. Drug allergy profiles
   B. General information files
      1. Birth data
      2. Demographic profiles
      3. Chart notes
      4. Family history profiles
      5. Genetic and metabolic testing information
      6. Growth data for graphic display
   C. Clinical problem solving
      1. Database and bibliographic searches via modem
      2. Electronic textbooks via CD-ROM
      3. Drug interaction programs
      4. Poison control programs
      5. Recall of specific patients
   D. Clinical research using patient databases
   E. Physician CME via computer (eg, CompuPREP)
III. Mixed clinical and business functions
   A. Word processing
      1. Referral letters
      2. Recall notices
      3. Appointment reminders
      4. Insurance company letters
      5. School forms
      6. Patient newsletters
      7. Patient education
   B. Patient scheduling
   C. Electronic spreadsheet applications
      1. Practice analysis
      2. Clinical research
   D. Relational databases
      1. Clinical research
      2. Demographic research
      3. Patient satisfaction surveys

systems vendors to guide you to an estimate of the system size you need. The answer may be different depending on the software package you wish to buy. System size should anticipate growth.

Attempt to get as many opinions as you can and ask vendors who disagree about your requirements to explain why they disagree. A good additional source of information is the manual, *Computers For The Practicing Pediatrician,* published by the AAP.[2] Also, do not hesitate to get the opinion of a consultant.

Using a consultant

Making the right decision about purchasing a computer can be vital to practice success and personnel satisfaction. Therefore, getting help from a consultant is not a bad idea, particularly for physicians who are not knowledgeable about computers, or who face a number of other practice decisions.

It is best to do the initial needs analysis and then narrow your options before calling in a consultant. Consultants are expensive, and doing the initial analysis yourself will provide a sound understanding of where you are heading. Ask the consultant to answer specific questions – not just to "tell me what to do." You know your practice and your own desires better than anyone.

If possible use a consultant who has worked with pediatricians before, since pediatricians have needs different from other medical specialties. Also, find a consultant who is experienced in medical office software needs. There are large armies of computer consulting firms who have never seen the inside of a physician's office.

Friends or colleagues who may already be using medical office computers can be a valuable source of information. Names of other pediatrician users may be obtained from the computer vendors.

Before signing a contract

Get **written** estimates of costs, installation schedules, training provided, and warranty guarantees in writing from all competing vendors. Never rely on a verbal estimate from a computer salesman. Require that performance characteristics are guaranteed in the sales contract. For example, you could fairly ask the seller to guarantee that the system he proposes selling you is adequate to store all your insurance information for up to 2 years. If the system fails to live up to this specification, the seller will have to give you the extra disk storage capacity to meet this requirement. This allows an accurate comparison of two competing proposals.

Training and installation

Develop a training and installation plan with your computer dealer and key office personnel. Such a plan should clearly delineate the number of hours of free training on the system to be provided by the seller and the conditions under which the training is to be provided. On-site training is best, provided the office is closed so that there are no distractions. It is also useful to have training personnel present on-site in the first day or two of operation to answer questions. They should return periodically to assist with any troubleshooting. Arrangements for ongoing training of new personnel should be made when the system is purchased. Training manuals should be obtained and readily available.

Discuss with office personnel the purposes for which you bought the computer. Assure them that it will not eliminate anyone's job, and clearly delineate who is expected to perform which functions on the computer. You won't decrease the number of people necessary, but you will increase office productivity. This gives employees a sense of personal responsibility, and helps them to concentrate their training appropriately.

Insurance

Computer insurance is a special field in underwriting, and computer equipment may not be covered under your general office policy. Contact your insurance agent to arrange proper coverage before accepting shipment of the hardware.

Data security

The information in a computer exists as electromagnetic particles stored on various media. Therefore it is subject to damage not only from mechanical hazards such as fire and theft but also electrical hazards such as power surges and magnetic interference. In a worst case scenario, it is possible for office personnel to unwittingly erase your data.

It is essential to copy (back up) all the information in the computer and store a copy of the data in a secure place outside the office. Copies should be made daily, usually in the evening after all the patients have left the office.

Although the information contained in a system may seem enormous, it can be copied within minutes onto spare diskettes or tapes. Failure to do this regularly is a serious error.

In addition security codes and levels of authorized access should be clearly worked out in advance so that only designated office personnel have access to sensitive financial or patient management data. Your vendor can easily do this for you at the time of installation.

Finally, the contract should grant you a copy of the "source code" for the program, in the event the vendor goes out of business. This allows you to manipulate the program or to contract others to do this for you even after the original seller is gone.

Maintenance contracts

Maintenance contracts for both the hardware and the software components of your system are necessary. Ideally, hardware and software maintenance should be provided by the same firm, but this is not essential.

Maintenance contracts should specify hours of availability, response times and guarantees to get the system operational by providing substitute hardware in the event of a lengthy repair. Updates to the software program should be provided free, so that all users enjoy the benefits of program improvements as newer versions are released for sale.

Miscellaneous considerations

1. All contracts for purchase, insurance or maintenance should be reviewed by your attorney.

2. If you are introducing a computer into an existing practice, detailed plans for conversion of old data into the new computer system are required. If you are changing from an old to a new computer, a special "data conversion" program may be necessary. This may well be an additional but necessary cost to avoid reentering all old files manually into the new system. Provision of this conversion program should be discussed and arranged with your vendor.

3. If you are installing your first computer system, conversion of hand written ledger cards and other data may take quite some time (months would not be unusual). It is best to run a "dual" bookkeeping system both by hand and by computer for a month or so until the inevitable bugs are ironed out of the new system. Budget for the extra help necessary to perform the conversion and consider the seasonal demands on the office staff common to most pediatric practices when planning the time of installation and conversion. Make sure that you allow sufficient time for conversion, to avoid fatigue developing in your office personnel.

References

1. *Directory of Medical Computer Systems*. Blue Bell, PA: Computertalk Associates, Inc; 1990
2. American Academy of Pediatrics, Committee on Practice and Ambulatory Medicine, Section on Computers and Other Technologies. *Computers For The Practicing Pediatrician*. Elk Grove Village, IL: American Academy of Pediatrics: 1989

Checklist

✓ Have you performed a practice analysis to determine if your practice will benefit from computerization?
✓ Do you have an installation plan which will not disrupt the office?
✓ Will your training program train new office staff to use the system?
✓ Do you know how to use the entire system?
✓ Have you arranged for on-going training so that new staff members will be able to learn to use the system?

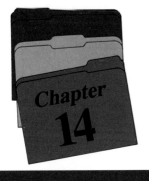

Charging for Services

This chapter focuses on the appropriate steps of the billing procedure. It includes:
- diagnosis and procedure codes
- the superbill
- billing systems
- submitting a bill

Chapter 14

Fees, billing and reimbursements

Reimbursements in medicine have trationally been based on a fee-for-service basis, whether it be barter, cash, or charge card. The introduction of physician salaries by alternative delivery systems removed some of the uncertainty of income for some physicians. Still, proper reimbursement or salary support requires expertise in setting a fee schedule, preparing a bill, and submitting the bill to the patient.

In the past, the patient was responsible directly to the physician for the services provided. The patient saw that the bill was paid, submitted it to the insurance carrier, and obtained reimbursement. The new delivery systems have become the middlemen between patient and physician, often contracting for services at a discount. They require that the bill be sent directly to them, and often advertise that the patient does not have to submit any paperwork for seeing the doctor.

Insurance carriers require two pieces of information regarding medical care of their insureds: why the patient was seen (the diagnosis) and what was done (the procedure). To enable physicians to communicate efficiently with both traditional indemnity and alternative delivery systems, two sets of codes have evolved: diagnosis codes and procedure codes.

Diagnosis codes are currently standardized in the *International Classification of Diseases, 9th Revision, Clinical Modification* (ICD-9-CM).[1] Published and revised by the World Health Organization, it was originally developed as an aid in collecting and comparing illness and disease statistics throughout the world. It nonetheless evolved into the preferred method for submitting diagnosis information to insurance carriers in this country. Medicare has recently mandated submission of diagnosis encoded claim forms for their clients and this trend may be required by other third party payors in the future. The Academy has available an ICD-9-CM diagnosis card listing common pediatric diagnoses which may be obtained from the AAP Publications Department. (See Figure 14-1.)

To assist in the submission of information on medical services, the American Medical Association developed *Current Procedural Terminology,*[2] now in its fourth edition (CPT-4). This compendium contains codes for just about every imaginable medical encounter, grouped into five categories: medicine, surgery, laboratory, anesthesiology, and radiology. Pediatricians generally need only be concerned with the medicine, surgery, and laboratory codes. Payments are based on the procedure codes submitted to the insurance carrier. A working knowledge of CPT-4 is imperative to ensure proper reimbursement for services.

As with any endeavor, certain principles apply. With CPT-4 coding, we suggest the following ten principles.

1. **Design a Superbill.** A superbill is a simple, easy to use method to transmit concise information of patient encounters to insurance carriers. They are at present acceptable to almost all carriers except Medicaid and Medicare, which require the HCFA 1500 claim form. Superbill design and use are described in *Pediatric Procedural Terminology*[3] published by the Academy.

2. **Use Separate Codes for Different Encounters.** With six different codes for established patient office visits, it should be possible to select the appropriate one to describe varying levels of office

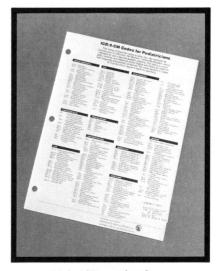

Figure 14-1: ICD quick reference coding sheet available from the American Academy of Pediatrics.

services. In a general pediatric practice, about 20-30 procedure codes will cover 90% of the office or hospital visits.

3. **Set a Separate Fee for Each Code.** It should be obvious that each code should be assigned its own fee. Otherwise the need for multiple codes in a sequence disappears.

4. **Set Fees Independent of Reimbursements.** Your fees should reflect the value *you* place on your services, not what a third party payor remits. Setting your fees to whatever the payor provides may only implement the law of diminishing returns. Many payors only pay a fixed percentage of your billed charges. By only charging the allowed maximum rather than your higher fee, you inadvertently reduce your reimbursement from the payor.

5. **Always Use a Modifier When Altering a Standard Fee.** Modifiers are listed in the introductory sections of CPT-4 and are included

to inform carriers that "this code usage is different." The most common use in pediatrics is that of the reduced fee modifier (presently -52 or 09952) to decrease the charges in certain circumstances. The reduced fee modifier acts to exclude the charge from the physician's profile.

6. **Select Diagnosis and Procedure Codes Yourself.** Since the physician is the *only* person able to accurately relate what was done for a patient, he/she should be the one entering this information on the claim form. It behooves us to choose the most accurate description code(s) possible to the insurance carrier in terms the carrier can understand. Reimbursements depend on it.

7. **Know Local Variations in Reimbursements.** Some carriers may not reimburse you unless you code services in a particular manner. Also some carriers may not reimburse for preventive medicine codes.

8. **Document Patient Services to Justify Codes.** All patient services should be thoroughly documented in the hospital or office record. Attending physicians working with residents who are charging for services need to document their examination of the patient as well as their direction of patient care. In cases where time factors apply (eg, critical care and prolonged detention), documentation of arrival and departure times could prove invaluable.

9. **Inquire About Lowered or Changed Reimbursements.** Carriers occasionally make changes in reimbursements without physician input. Computers sometimes make changes without human input. It becomes important to follow up on sudden changes in reimbursement levels.

10. **Review Your Codes and Fees Regularly.** Since CPT-4 is published at the first of the year and the annual Consumer Price Index is announced shortly thereafter, it is a good idea to review and update superbill codes and charges at this time of year. More frequent review would be required in times of sudden increases in costs, such as the recent escalation in vaccine prices.

Setting your fee schedule

Years ago, establishing a fee schedule was easy. You simply called the physicians in your area and asked them their charges, setting yours in close fashion. Recent Federal Trade Commission (FTC) decisions have held that to do so now is a violation of antitrust laws and physicians are no longer allowed to discuss fees.

Several methods are still available to enable a physician entering practice to develop a reasonable fee schedule:

1. Submit a list of your most commonly used CPT-4 codes to local HMOs, IPAs and PPOs, requesting their current reimbursements. Realize that these reimbursements are often at a discounted rate, so fees should be set to accommodate the discount.

2. *Medical Economics* publishes an annual survey of physician charges.

3. Although physician-maintained Relative Value Scales are now prohibited by federal law, many commercial concerns publish national relative value scales of physician charges. Several of these will isolate pediatric fees by region.

4. In some areas, a fee survey performed by an outside party may be available to physicians entering or practicing in the area.

5. The Harvard Resource Based Relative Value Scale (RBRVS) may become the *de facto* standard once its methodological problems are resolved to the satisfaction of all concerned.

Remember to set your fees using the CPT-4 codes you commonly use in your practice. The considerations listed above should be utilized in your deliberations.

Preparing a bill

In many practices, the physician leaves it to the nurse, receptionist or office manager to prepare the bill for the patient. This practice should be avoided. The physician is the only person who knows what was done in the exam room and should be the person who enters the diagnosis and procedure codes for the patient. He is the one who is also responsible for all billing leaving the office and should be actively involved in the process.

The physician's bill might take several forms, depending on the needs of the practice. A "route slip" may be a simple preprinted code slip on which the physician marks the diagnosis(es), procedures and/or codes and charges which the patient then carries to the receptionist for posting to the account. A superbill itself may serve the same function, with the patient returning it to the front desk for the receptionist to copy appropriate information into the billing system. The patient then completes their copy of the superbill and submits it to the insurance carrier. (See Figures 14-2 and 14-3.)

Billing systems themselves can be simple to complex, done in-house or contracted out. Most single or small pediatric group practices may find the pegboard systems the easiest to manage. Superbills may be designed with carbon strips to work on these systems and decrease the paper flow in the office. However, with the rapid advances in computer technology, serious consideration should be given to computerization of the medical office. Physicians entering practice will find that computers make it much easier to manage patient accounts. Practices using other billing methods will find that computers facilitate analysis of practice financial statistics, diagnostic searches, hospitalization data collection, and implementation of a patient recall system. Some computers can accommodate and store a complete clinical record. Your accountant, colleagues, or medical association may be able to direct you to a system analyst who can help determine your needs in this area. (See Computer Systems, Chapter 13.)

Submitting your bill

Before sending out a bill, the practice must decide on an in-house collection policy. Payment for services at the time they are given minimizes billing costs and is strongly recommended. When the patient returns to the front desk, the receptionist should ask: "Will this be cash, check or charge card?" not "Shall we just bill you for today's visit?" A discrete but obvious sign at the sign-in area will present your philosophy that "Payment is expected at the time of service unless prior arrangements have been made."

A word on charge cards. Although it was once considered unethical for physicians to accept them, this is no

PEDIATRIC CENTER
1335 South Street
Smithsville, MO 12345

Patients Name	First	MI	Last	Insurance	Date	Todays Charges
Subscriber				SS #	Group #	Adjustments
Address		City	State	Zip		Previous Balance
Relationship to Sub.		Date of Birth	Todays Visit	NP	Sib	Payment

ASSIGNMENT: I assign & request payment of major medical benefits to undersigned physician for services described below.

New Balance

SIGNED (Parent if Minor) _____ Date _____

☐ Cash   ☐ Check   ☐ Charge

NEW PATIENT	CODE	FEE	LAB SERVICES	CODE	FEE	IMMUNIZATIONS	CODE	FEE
LIMITED EXAM	90010		URINALYSIS	81000		DPT	90701	
INTERMED. EXAM	90015		HEMOGLOBIN/HCT	85018		DT	90702	
CONSULTATION	90620		THROAT CULTURE	87081		OPV	90712	
			URINE CULTURE	87086		MMR	90707	
WELL CHILD (12-17)	90751		FUNGAL CULTURE	87101		HIB	90737	
WELL CHILD (5-11)	90752		OCCULT BLOOD	82270		PPD	86580	
WELL CHILD (1-4)	90753		PINWORM TEST	87177		TB TINE	86585	
WELL CHILD (0-1)	90754		WET MOUNT	87210		FLU	90782	

ESTABLISHED PATIENT	CODE	FEE	SERVICES/PROCEDURES	CODE	FEE	THERAPEUTIC INJECTIONS	CODE	FEE
BRIEF EXAM	90040		AUDIOGRAM	92551		ALLERGY 01,02	9511	
LIMITED EXAM	90050		IMPEDENCE	92566		EPINEPH 01,02,03	90782	
INTERMED EXAM	90060		EAR LAVAGE	69210		SUSPHRINE	90782	
EXTENDED EXAM	90070		EAR PIERCING	69090		DECADRON	90782	
CONFERENCE	9915		INHALATION RX	94664		GAMMA GLOBULIN	90782	
WELL CHILD (12-17)	90761		LUMBAR PUNCTURE	62270		TIGAN	90782	
WELL CHILD (5-11)	90762		BLADDER CATH	53670		BICILLIN CR, LA	90782	
WELL CHILD (1-4)	90763		CIRCUMCISION	54150				
WELL CHILD (0-1)	90764		LACERATION, FACE	12011				
PREOP EXAM, BRIEF	90200		LACERATION<2.5CM BODY	12001		MISCELLANEOUS		
PREOP EXAM, LIMIT	90215		LACERATION>2.5CM BODY	12002		AFTER HOURS	99050	
PREOP EXAM, COMP	90220					NIGHT CALL AFTER 10 PM	99052	
						SUNDAY/HOLIDAY	99054	
CHDP EXAM			SUPPLIES	99070		SPECIAL REPORTS	99080	

DIAGNOSIS	CODE							
ABSESS/CELLULITIS	682.9	DERMATITIS	692.9	INFLUENZA	487.1	SEPSIS	038.9	
ABDOMINAL PAIN	789.0	DEVELOP. DELAY	783.4	INSECT BITE	919	SINUSITIS, ACUTE	461.9	
ACNE	706.1	DIAPER RASH	691.0	LACERATION	998.2	SPRAIN/STRAIN	848.9	
ADENITIS	289.3	DIARRHEA	558.9	LEARNING DISORDER	315.2	STOMATITIS	528.0	
ALLERGIC RHINITIS	477.9	ENURESIS	788.3	LYMPHADENOPATHY	785.6	STREP THROAT	034.0	
ANEMIA	285.9	EPISTAXIS	784.7	METATARSUS ADDUCTUS	754.6	STYE	373.11	
ASTHMA	493.9	FAILURE TO THRIVE	783.4	MILK INTOLERANCE	579.8	SUNBURN	692.71	
ATTENTION DEFICIT	314.01	FEEDING PROBLEM	779.3	MONONEUCLEOSIS	075.0	SUTURE REMOVAL	V58.3	
BEE STING	989.5	FRACTURE	829.0	MUSCLE PAIN	729.1	TEETHING	520.7	
BEHAVIOR PROBLEM	V71.02	FUO	780.6	NEVUS	224.0	THRUSH	112.0	
BRONCHITIS	490	GASTROENTERITIS	009.0	OBESITY	278	TIBIAL TORSION	736.89	
BURN	949.0	GINGIVITIS	523.1	OTITIS. EXTERNA	380.10	UMBILICAL BLEEDING	789.9	
CELLULITIS	682.9	HEADACHE	784.0	OTITIS, MEDIA	382.0	UMBILICAL HERNIA	553.1	
CHICKEN POX	052.9	HEAD INJURY	854.0	OTITIS, SEROUS	381.4	UMBILICAL, GRANULOMA	686.1	
CONJUCTIVITIS	372.30	HEART MURMUR	785.2	PARONYCHIA	681.9	URI,VIRAL	460	
CONSTIPATION	594.0	HEART MURMUR ORGANIC	745.9	PHARYNGITIS	462	UTI	599.0	
COUGH	786.2	HEMANGIOMA	228.00	PINWORMS	127.4	URTICARIA	708.9	
COX SACKIE VIRUS	079.2	HEMATURIA	599.7	PNEUMONIA	480.9	VAGINITIS	616.10	
CROUP	464.4	HERNIA	553.9	RINGWORM	110.9	VIRAL EXANTHUM	790.8	
CYSTITIS	595.9	HIP DYSPLASIA	755.63	RHINITIS	477.9	VIRAL ILLNESS	079.9	
DACROCYSTIS, NEONATE	771.6	HYDROCELE	603.9	SCABIES	133.0	VOMITING	787.0	
DEHYDRATION	276.5	HYPERBILIRUBIN	782.4	SCARLET FEVER	034.1	WARTS	078.1	
		IMPETIGO	684	SEIZURE DISORDER	780.3	WELL CHILD CARE	V20.2	

Referral

Diagnosis (if not above)

Comments

Doctors Signature

RTO

Figure 14-2: Patient charge sheet, used at each encounter. NCR triplicate contains patient identification, physician identification, and commonly used CPT and ICD codes.

IMPORTANT: Before using any CPT codes listed in this chapter, verify the code in the current edition of the AMA's "Physicians' Current Procedural Terminology" (CPT). Code changes, although minimal, are made yearly.

Pediatric Center
1335 South Street
Smithsville, MO 12345
111/222-3333

Smith,James

1212 Any Street
Anytown,USA

Date_____

43293

FED ID 00-0000000
BC 00000   MEDICAID 0000000

OFFICE VISIT - NEW PATIENT	CPT	FEE
☐ Intermediate	90015	
☐ Comp.	90020	
☐		

OFFICE VISIT - EST. PATIENT		
☐ Intermediate	90060	
☐ Limited	90050	
☐ Comp.	90070	
☐		

OFFICE PROCEDURE
Suture Laceration
☐ 2.5 cm	12031
☐ 2.5-7.5 cm	12032

BURN RX
☐ 1	16000
☐ Small 2	16020
☐ Medium 2	16025

SPLINT
☐ Forearm	29125
☐ Finger	29130

WELL-CHILD VISIT
INITIAL H & P
☐ 12YOA	90751
☐ 5-11YOA	90752
☐ 1-4YOA	90753
☐ 1YOA	90754
☐	

INTERVAL H & P	CPT	FEE
☐ 12YOA	90761	
☐ 5-11YOA	90762	
☐ 1-4YOA	90763	
☐ 1YOA	90764	
☐ DDST	90774	
☐ Nutrition Screen	V65.3	
☐ Titmus Screen	92499	
☐ Audiogram	92552	
☐ Tympanogram	92567	
☐ Tine	86585	

IMMUNIZATIONS
☐ DPT	90701
☐ MMR	90707
☐ OPV	90712
☐ Flu	90724
☐ Pneumococcus	90732
☐ H. Influenza	90733
☐ DT Adult	90718
☐ D & T	90702
☐ Tetanus Toxoid	90703

EENT TREATMENT
☐ Remove Cerumen	69210
☐ Pierce Ears	69090
☐ Fluorscein Eyes	17030

MISCELLANEOUS
☐ Blood Drawing	99000
☐ Supplies Charge	99070

MISCELLANEOUS CONT.	CPT	FEE
☐ Urinary Cath	51010	
☐ Peak Flow	94160	

INJECTIONS
☐ Epinephrine	90782-01
☐ Susphrine	90782-02

LAB
☐ Theophyllin Level	84420
☐ UA	81000
☐ WBC DIFF	85009
☐ HCT	85014
☐ Throat Culture	87060
☐ Urine C&S	87088
☐ Nose Culture	87061
☐ Sweat Test	89360
☐ Stool Guaiac	82270
☐ EKG	93000
☐ PKU.	84030
☐ Pinworm Smear	87177
☐ Strep Screen	86171
☐ Stool Smear	87205
☐ Dilantin Level	84045
☐ Phenobarbital Level	82205
☐ HGB	83020
☐ Cholesterol	82465
☐ Triglyceride	84478
☐ Bilirubin, Total	82250
☐ HDLC	83718
☐ Glucose	82947
☐ Sodium	84295
☐ Potassium	84132
☐ Chloride	82435
☐ CO_2	82374

CARDIOVASCULAR
☐ Functional Murmur	785.2
☐ V.S.D	745.4
☐ A.S.D	745.5
☐ P.D.A	747.0
☐ A.S.	747.3
☐ P.S.	746.02
☐ Tet. of Fallot	745.2
☐ Cong. Hrt. Dis.&Oth.	746.9
☐ Acq. Hrt. Dis.	
☐ Arrhythmia	427.9
☐ Chest Pain	786.52

EENT
☐ Acute Otitis	382.00
☐ Acute Vir. Syn.	079.9
☐ Allergic Rhinitis	477.9
☐ Asthma	493.9
☐ Bronchitis	466.0
☐ Cerumen Impax	380.4
☐ Cervical Aden	683.1
☐ Conjunctivitis	372.0
☐ Cornea Abrasion	370.00
☐ Cough	786.2
☐ Croup	464.4

EENT (cont.)
☐ Enlarged T&A	474.1
☐ Epistaxis	784.7
☐ FB Ear	931.
☐ FB Nose	932.
☐ Gingivostomatitis	054.2
☐ Herpangina	074.0
☐ Infect. Mono.	075
☐ Lac. Duct. Obst.	375.55
☐ Oral Moniliasis	112.0
☐ Otitis Externa	380.1
☐ Pharyngitis	462.0
☐ Pneumonia	482.9
☐ Serous Otitis	381.1
☐ Sinusitis	461.9
☐ Status Asthmaticus	493.1
☐ Strabismus	378.00
☐ Stye (Hordeolum)	373.11
☐ Teething	520.7
☐ Tonsilitis	463.
☐ U.R.I.	460.

G.I.
☐ Colitus Acute	558.9
☐ ABD. Pain	789.0
☐ Anal Fissure	565.0
☐ Colic	787.3
☐ Constipation	564.0
☐ Diarrhea	009.3
☐ Feeding Problem	783.3
☐ Gastritis	535.0
☐ Gastroenteritis	009.0
☐ Hepatitis A	070.1
☐ Hepatitis B	070.3
☐ Impaction	560.39
☐ Ing. Hernia	550.9
☐ Irr. Colon	564.1
☐ Pin Worms	127.4
☐ Swallowed FB	938.
☐ Umb. Hernia	553.1
☐ Vomiting	787.0

G.U.
☐ Cryptorchid	752.5
☐ Dysuria	788.1
☐ Enuresis	788.3
☐ Meatal Sten	598

G.U. (cont.)
☐ Proteinuria	791.0
☐ U.T.I.	599.0
☐ Vaginitis	616.1

METABOLIC
☐ Anemia: FE Def	280.9
☐ Breast Hypertrophy	778.7
☐ Dehydration	276.5
☐ Diabetes	250.01
☐ Fatigue	780.7
☐ Obesity	278.0

MISCELLANEOUS
☐ Abcess	680.9
☐ Down's Syndrome	758.0
☐ Cystic Fibrosis	5188
☐ Apnea	786.09
☐ Unspecified Coag.Dic	286.9
☐ IGG	2793
☐ IGA	27901

ORTHOPEDIC
☐ B.I.T.T.	754.43
☐ Cong. Hip	754.3
☐ Disloc. Elbow	832.0

ORTHOPEDIC (cont.)
☐ FX Clavicle	810.0
☐ FX Finger	816.0
☐ FX Toe	826.0
☐ Metatars Var	754.53
☐ Muscle Spasm	728.85
☐ Osgood Schlaters	732.4
☐ Sever's Kohler	732.4
☐ Sprain	848.9
☐ Tenosynovitis	727.00
☐ Torticollis	723.5

SKIN
☐ Abrasion	919.8
☐ Abrasion, Inf.	919.9
☐ Alopecia areata	704.01
☐ Body Lice	132.1
☐ Burn 10%	948.0
☐ Burn 10%	948.1
☐ Cellulitis	682.9
☐ Contact Rash	692.9
☐ Contusion	924.9
☐ Diaper Rash	691.0

SKIN (contd.)
☐ Dyshidrosis	705.81
☐ Erythema Mult	695.1
☐ Fifth's Dis.	057.0
☐ Folliculitis	704.8
☐ Hand Ft. Mouth	074.3
☐ Head Lice	132.0
☐ Hemangioma	228.0
☐ Impetigo	684.
☐ Ingrown Nail	703.0
☐ Insect Bite	989.5
☐ Lymphangitis	457.2
☐ Monilia Infex	112.
☐ Pityriasis Ros	696.3
☐ Ringworm	110.9
☐ Roseola-	056.9
☐ Scabies	133.0
☐ Scarletina	034.1
☐ Seborrhea	690.
☐ Urticaria	708.9
☐ Varicella	052.0
☐ Warts	078.1

SKIN (contd.)
☐ Weed Rash	692.6
☐ Zoster	053.

NEURO-PSYCH
☐ Anorexia Nervosa	307.10
☐ Concussion	850.9
☐ Dev. Delay	783.4
☐ Headache	784.0
☐ Hyperactivity	314.01
☐ Learn Disord.	315.2
☐ Seizures	345.9
☐ Synostosis	756.0

OTHER SERVICES
☐ Well Child	V20.2
☐ _____	
☐ _____	
☐ _____	

DIAGNOSIS_____
_____
_____

ASSIGNMENT AND RELEASE: I hereby authorize my insurance benefits to be paid directly to the physician and I am financially responsible for non-covered services. I also authorize the physician to release any information required in the processing of this claim.

SIGNED _____

INSURANCE CARRIERS — This form has been adopted to reduce paperwork costs. If any additional forms or itemized bills are required, they will be completed upon receipt of $25.00.

RETURN: _____ Days _____ Weeks _____ Months

NEXT APPT. _____
Day   Month   Date   Time

I DO / DO NOT ACCEPT ASSIGNMENT

Date Symptoms Appeared
Or Accident Occurred _____

DOCTOR'S SIGNATURE _____

ORIGINAL

Figure 14-3: Computer generated patient charge sheet. NCR triplicate contains patient identification, physician identification, and commonly used CPT and ICD codes.

IMPORTANT: Before using any CPT codes listed in this chapter, verify the code in the current edition of the AMA's "Physicians' Current Procedural Terminology" (CPT). Code changes, although minimal, are made yearly.

longer true. Charge cards can significantly decrease billing costs and expedite collection at a cost to the practice of 1%-5% of the amount charged. Inquiries to your local bank, the AAP, or the AMA may provide you with a bank offering a low discount rate. You do not necessarily need to submit your charge card receipts to the bank managing your checking account.

Several considerations must be addressed when submitting a bill. If the patient does not have a practice-accepted insurance contract, the parent or guardian is responsible for the bill, and every effort should be made to collect payment before the patient leaves the office.

If the patient is covered by an alternative delivery system (HMO, PPO, IPA), CHAMPUS or Medicaid, the physician usually must submit the bill directly to the carrier. Many of these patients will have either a co-pay or a deductible for the office visit, which should be collected at the time of service. Nearly all carriers will accept a superbill, but Medicaid and a few others will demand a HCFA-1500 form from physicians caring for Medicaid patients.

If the patient is covered under an indemnity plan (eg, Blue Cross and Blue Shield, Aetna, etc), the parent is usually responsible to the physician for the bill. In this situation, the practice superbill is designed for the patient to submit to the carrier for reimbursement. This is provided to the patient at the time of service.

When both parents are employed, sometimes both may have insurance which covers their children's medical expenses. In most cases, the parent with the earlier birthdate in the year (not the oldest), will supply the primary coverage and insurance should be submitted to that carrier first. Only after benefits have been determined from that carrier can the claim be submitted to the second. This situation presents a considerable headache for most practices, particularly when both carriers are managed health care plans (HMO, PPO, IPA). There are multiple methods of dealing with it; no one system is optimal. Some process the paperwork for both carriers. Most will submit the claim to the first and give the parent a claim form to submit to the second after the first replies, even if both are managed care plans. A few

will refuse to submit either and require the parents to do so.

Divorced or separated families present another complicating situation. Some parents are so hostile to each other that the physician may get caught in the middle. The parent bringing the child in may instruct your office to bill the other for the service. When the bill is sent, the second parent may reply that the first is responsible. To deal with situations such as this, many practices have an office policy that the parent who brings in the child is responsible for the bill at the time of service, thereby allowing the parents to decide how to reimburse each other later. Another approach is to request a copy of the divorce decree which specifies the parent who is actually responsible.

Finally, it should be reemphasized that the same service should be billed at the *same charge* for all classes of patients: private pay, managed care, or traditionally insured. A visit with CPT-4 code 90050 should be billed at the same dollar amount for all. This does not mean a discount cannot be given in certain circumstances, but it should be done through the use of a modifier (-52 or 09952) as discussed in *Pediatric Procedural Terminology*.[3]

Other issues

Most pediatricians feel an obligation to provide services to patients covered by the Medicaid program. Many, however, are unaware of the Early and Periodic Screening, Diagnosis, and Treatment (EPSDT) program, the preventive care portion of the Medicaid program. Generally, because of federal mandates and federal and state funding, reimbursement is available for health supervision services rendered under this program. Pediatricians should contact the state office of Medicaid operations to learn how to participate in the EPSDT program. (Although known as the EPSDT program in most states, it may operate under a different acronym in some.) Billing requirements for EPSDT visits vary from state to state, so be certain that you are in compliance.

With the increasing shift of medical care from inpatient to outpatient settings, pediatricians are rendering more complicated care at home. Outpatient therapy for osteomyelitis, home photo-

therapy for hyperbilirubinemia, and chemotherapy for leukemia and other childhood cancers, are only a few of the conditions which several years ago, would only be treated on an inpatient basis. In order to allow for proper reimbursement of this care, the 1990 edition of CPT-4 established case management services codes at 98900-98922, including three codes for telephone management of cases similar to the above. Because these codes are newly established, it would be proper for pediatric groups to educate their local HMOs, PPOs, Medicaid and other programs in order to gain their acceptance as an alternative to costly inpatient care. The actual use of the codes is an individual physician decision based upon experience with the local carrier.

In every practice there will come a time when patient financial accounts need to be submitted to a collection agency. (See Business Office, Chapter 12.) Most agencies feel that an account submitted after 6 months of nonpayment will be noncollectible; they generally recommend that accounts be considered for collection if no payment has been received within 120 days of billing. Finding a good collection agency is difficult. The recommendations of colleagues, your local medical society and/or the Better Business Bureau should be sought. In some communities, a reputable lawyer may send a letter demanding payment as the last step before a collection agency. The letter, usually at a fixed cost of $5.00 – $10.00, may stimulate a response before surrending 30%-50% of the bill as the fee for a collection agency.

Other considerations in your practice are charges for "no show" appointments and for billing co-payments not made at the time of the visit. After checking with local HMOs, PPOs, and IPAs, you may find that it is permissible to bill a patient a fixed fee for the cost of preparing a bill when the patient "forgets" the checkbook or otherwise fails to pay the co-payment. It may also be possible to apply a "no-show" charge to indemnity, managed care, and private pay situations for patients who fail to cancel an appointment. To maintain office goodwill, it might be advisable to send a warning letter to patients who fail to keep their appointments prior to instituting the charge. In both instances, the practice should display the specific policy at the sign-in area and announce it to the patients when appointments are made.

Much has been written about Professional Courtesy in recent years. The decision to grant this should be made consciously and with care. (See Professional Courtesy, Chapter 28.)

Modifiers

Modifiers instruct insurance company computers that "this one is different" and should result in different claims processing, either through a different subroutine on the computer or by a claims processor. Modifiers can be a 2-digit add-on code or a 5-digit line entry.

Unmodified Bill:

90050	Office Visit	$ X.00

Modified (reduced) Bill:

90050-52	Office Visit	$ Y.00

OR

90050	Office Visit	$ X.00
09952	Reduced Service	− A.00
	Net Charge	$ Y.00

Modifiers exist for a number of services in both the medical and surgical sections and are explained in the introductory remarks for each. Most common for pediatricians are Reduced Services (-52/09952), Unusual Services (-222/09922), Repeat Procedure by Same Physician (-76/09976), and Professional Component (-26/09926).

References

1. *International Classification of Diseases, 9th Revision, Clinical Modification.* Washington, DC: US Dept of Health and Human Services; (PHS) 89-1260 (3 volume set);1978
2. American Academy of Pediatrics, *Physicians' Current Procedural Terminology.* 4th ed. Chicago, IL: American Medical Association; OP:341/8;1990
3. American Academy of Pediatrics, Committee on Practice and Ambulatory Medicine. *Pediatric Procedural Terminology.* Elk Grove Village, IL: American Academy of Pediatrics; 1987

Checklist

✓ Do you use diagnostic and procedure codes as standardized in ICD-9-CM and CPT-4?

✓ Have you designed a superbill?

✓ Have you separate codes for each type of encounter?

✓ Do you carefully document services to justify codes?

✓ Do you review your codes regularly?

✓ Do you prepare your own bill and select the codes for the services given?

✓ Do you charge the same fee for the same service code for all patients?

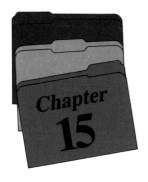

Chapter 15

Practice Payment Systems

Pediatric services are compensated in four general ways: (1) direct payment, (2) traditional health insurance, (3) alternative health care systems, and (4) government programs (CHAMPUS, Medicaid, EPSDT). Payment systems for pediatric care are described in this chapter. Discussion points include:
* **definitions of various systems**
* **comparisons of alternative systems**
* **points to be considered before participating in any alternative plan**

Direct payment

Direct payment continues to provide a significant portion of the pediatrician's income. A survey published by *Medical Economics* in November of 1990 reported that third party reimbursement represented 63% of gross pediatric practice income, leaving 37% to direct pay. Typically, a usual, customary, and reasonable fee for service is charged, and this is paid directly to the pediatrician by the patient or responsible party.

Traditional health insurance

Traditional health insurance directly or indirectly reimburses the pediatrician on a usual, customary, and reasonable fee-for-service basis for procedures covered in the policy agreement. Typically, this coverage is purchased by an employer as a group benefit to employees; some insurance plans are available on an individual basis. Originally, traditional insurance plans were designed to protect the patient or family from large cash outlays for hospital and surgical expenses, but benefits have been broadened to cover more ambulatory diagnostic and treatment services. Reimbursement frequently is incomplete, and additional direct patient payment is necessary.

Coverage frequently is limited by an annual deductible, copayment for services, maximum benefits, or excludable conditions and procedures. Health supervision, preventive care, and new-born infant services are frequently excluded, which can affect services to infants and children.

Additional cost containment conditions in some traditional insurance plans require hospital preadmission authorization, utilization review, and a second surgical opinion.

Traditional health insurance remains a substantial portion of a pediatrician's income. However, because of escalating premiums coupled with diminishing benefits and increasing deductibles, alternatives have been sought by the insurance industry and the payers of health care.

Employer self-insurance

In recent years, an increasing number of employers have rejected traditional group health insurance policies, deciding instead to *self-insure* and fund and/or administer their employees' health care claims themselves. The reasons cited for an employer's decision to assume this substantial financial risk include increasing distress by employers at the continuing and dramatic increases in health care benefits, the negative impact on corporate profitability, and the perception that the "third party payers" are not acting in the company's financial interest.

In 1988, 42% of employees working in companies with over 100 employees which offered health insurance were in self-insured plans.[1] Self-funded plans are not affected by mandated benefits

and other provisions in state insurance regulations. They may not cover pediatric preventive care. Consequently, even in the six states that have enacted some form of the AAP's Child Health Insurance Reform Plan (CHIRP)[2], which mandates the coverage of child health supervision services, the self-insured plans are exempt from the law.

Employer self-insurance, an option available to companies under specified conditions, can be structured for the employee as traditional third party insurance or as an alternative delivery system. Some employers who have adopted a self-insurance approach have developed several such options from which their employees may choose.

Self-funded companies have the option of processing and paying the claims themselves or subcontracting for these services. The majority of employers rely on a third-party administrator (TPA) or a national insurance company to pay claims only, or to pay claims and provide consulting and actuarial services. Fourth party audit organizations have recently appeared on the health insurance scene; these organizations additionally audit the claim for quality of care and efficient use of resources prior to claim approval and payment.

Alternative delivery systems

Alternative delivery systems, in contrast to indemnity insurance programs, insure members/beneficiaries by combining both the delivery and financing of care in one system. Members (patients) are provided the needed medical services directly by contracted providers (doctors, hospitals, etc) rather than receiving reimbursements from insurance. Patients are not charged directly for services. A variety of financial incentives/disincentives, peer review, and utilization management mechanisms are usually put in place to accomplish the dual objectives of assuring the quality of care and containing costs in individual plans. There are many different types of alternative delivery systems; we will illustrate only a few: (HMOs, IPAs and PPOs).

Health Maintenance Organizations (HMO) staff and group models

The HMO is a system of care which organizes physicians, hospital facilities, and other providers by contract to provide comprehensive health care services to a defined population of voluntarily enrolled members. Members pay a periodic (usually monthly), fixed per capita payment which does not fluctuate in relation to either the number or extent of services rendered to the member by health care providers. "Closed" HMOs require that 100% of services required by members be provided by contracted physicians, hospitals, or other providers. "Open" HMOs permit members to utilize non-plan providers. Open HMOs generally pay non-plan providers significantly less than the full cost of the services delivered; the patient is responsible for the remainder.

The federal Health Maintenance Organization Act of 1973 (42 USC 300E) legitimized HMOs and gave them access to the marketplace by requiring that all employers with 25 or more employees offer a federally qualified HMO as an additional option to any health benefit plan currently provided. In return for giving HMOs legitimacy and access to the market, the HMO Act required that HMOs:

1. provide members with a specified set of basic, minimum benefits, including preventive health care for children,
2. permit open enrollment/re-enrollment on an annual basis,
3. have consumer representation on the HMO board of directors; and
4. base premiums for coverage on community expansions (community rating) rather than solely on the

experience of the group purchaser (experience rating).

With the assistance of the federal Health Maintenance Organization Act, HMOs have made a significant penetration into the medical marketplace over the last 15 years. According to Interstudy, a nonprofit health care think tank based in Minnesota, they increased their enrollment by 6.4% in 1989. By mid 1990 there were reported to be 556 HMOs with 33.6 million enrollees.

Primary care physicians participate in HMOs in three ways:

1. as salaried employees of the plan in a staff model;
2. as members of a medical group which contracts with an HMO; or
3. as independent practitioners through an IPA (Independent Practice Association) as discussed in the next section.

Staff model HMOs are usually limited to major site locations and have salaried physicians. Physicians provide care in facilities which are either owned or operated by the HMO, sharing equipment, medical records, and personnel.

Group model HMOs may either contract exclusively with a single multi-specialty medical group organized as a partnership or professional corporation, or with a service corporation, (eg, Kaiser Health Plan and the Permanente Medical Group) or network with many primary care or multispecialty medical groups located within the geographic service area of the plan. While group model HMOs are generally paid on a capitation basis from the HMO plan, individual physicians in the group may be salaried or capitated or paid in accordance with the medical group's income distribution plan.

Some HMOs own their own hospitals; others subcontract with facilities. Some include a full complement of specialists; others refer to outside specialists.

HMO Independent Practice Association (IPA) model

The Independent Practice Association HMO (IPA), an "open panel" HMO, is often considered the "fee-for-service HMO." Like the group or staff HMO, enrollees pay a fixed monthly payment for comprehensive health benefits. The IPA contracts with office-based physicians and reimburses them either on a discounted fee-for-service or capitation basis according to a formula that is agreed upon in advance. IPA physicians are usually in private practice

serving non-HMO patients in their offices as well. (These private practitioners often try to limit their HMO patient population to a certain fixed percentage of the total patients in their practice.) The plan may require a participation fee, and usually seeks to recruit large numbers of private practice, primary care, and specialist physicians in a given geographic area. In some instances an entire physician association or society may contract with the IPA. IPAs may incorporate a variety of mechanisms which act to place the physician at financial risk. For example, IPAs often withhold a percentage of the physician's fees in escrow to ensure the solvency of the IPA corporation. The IPA is responsible for the costs of inpatient hospitalization and use of specialists outside of the system. A variety of physician compensation mechanisms exist, including surplus sharing and return of withhold monies, depending upon the structure of the IPA.

Preferred Provider Organizations (PPO)

Among the new types of health care delivery models, PPOs, or preferred provider organizations, generally provide the maximum freedom of choice for patient and provider. However, the IPA/HMO benefit package is often more comprehensive. PPO characteristics include the following:

- a designated panel of health care professionals and/or institutions that serve as contracted providers;
- an established fee schedule that generally results in a professional discount of as much as 15%-20% from usual, customary, and reasonable reimbursements, generating savings for the employers or insurance carriers who are the purchasers of care;
- medical services provided on a traditional fee-for-service basis;
- a strong emphasis on utilization review and control;
- usually no "lock-in" of the patient to specific health care providers; however, economic disincentives which must be paid by the patient, such as increased copayments or higher deductibles, are often applied if a non-contracted provider or hospital is utilized;
- a lack of formal risk-sharing arrangements between the PPO and the provider, thus differing from the IPA/HMO model.

PPOs are groups of physicians and/or hospitals that contract with employers, insurance carriers, or third party administrators to provide comprehensive medical services on a fee-for-service basis to subscribers. PPOs may be sponsored by a wide variety of individuals and entities; brokers (entrepreneurs marketing to self-insured employers and unions), third party payers (other HMOs or insurance companies), and/or providers (hospitals and/or physicians). PPOs are not insurance plans, per se. They represent a set of contractual relationships between providers, payers, and consumers.

In most states, PPOs may be established and operated under current law without being regulated as an insurer, health service plan or HMO. As of June 1988, the American Medical Care Review Association (AMCRA) could identify 535 operational PPOs operating in 45 states plus Puerto Rico, and Washington, DC.

To participate or not

Pediatricians repeatedly face the need to evaluate opportunities to participate in alternative health care delivery systems. Regardless of whether a pediatrician joins the full-time staff of an HMO or simply adds patients to his or her practice by participating in one or more IPAs or PPOs, he or she can anticipate significant alterations in practice style and perhaps in professional and personal satisfaction and practice income.

It is difficult to generalize about PPOs or HMOs; each plan has its own incentives and disincentives. This discussion will focus on the capitated HMO/IPA model, as it is the format within which most pediatrician/HMO contracting occurs, and the fee-for-service PPO model, as an increasingly popular alternative delivery system. There are three areas of concern to ponder as you read.
1. Specifics of the Contract
2. Pitfalls and problems of individual contracts
3. Legal issues

Preferred Provider Organizations (PPOs)

Physicians who contract with a PPO agree to accept a reduced payment for care or, stated differently, a reduced percentage of the usual and customary charges. Once you understand the dynamics of a PPO, there are certain questions that must be answered.
1. Is there an initial investment to join the PPO? The goal of the PPO developer is to provide proof to the employer or broker that it can provide the largest base of physicians possible for a given geographical area. The appearance of your name in the PPO's book of providers is no guarantee that you will ever receive a patient from the many PPOs with which you contract. Thus, there may be little reason to pay a fee to join a PPO.
2. Do you have hospital privileges at the hospitals used by the PPO? If not, are they available to you?
3. Do the PPO hospitals provide quality care? There may be several hospitals in your area that you have chosen to ignore for quality of care reasons, and these may be the very hospitals used by the PPO. This may place you at legal risk in the event of a medical accident.
4. Some PPO contracts do not let you limit the number of patients sent by the PPO. This may be a problem for your practice if unexpected overexpansion causes you to exceed capacity and inconvenience your patients.
5. Are you limited by contract to a certain group of specialist physicians? Are these the ones you use at present? If not, do they provide quality care? Are they pediatric subspecialists? This clause may potentially increase your professional liability.
6. Are you financially liable for any cost overruns in the PPO? Although highly unlikely, you may be liable for costs incurred by patients if you refer them to physicians not in the PPO registry or to hospitals not in the plan.
7. Are the physicians with whom you share weekend and night coverage members of the PPO? If not, this could inadvertently place you on 24 hour call.
8. Can you be assessed for failure to collect the co-payment due at the time of the visit? This payment is meant to act as a barrier to care and it might be perceived that if the barriers are removed, you should not be entitled to reimbursement for your services. Does the PPO help you to collect the co-payment if the family does not pay? They can contact the patient or refuse to continue the contract if the patients do not pay the co-pay at time of service.
9. Does the PPO contract preclude you from joining other PPOs?
10. What happens if your PPO hospital is full and there are no beds? Where do they go and are you on staff there?
11. What is your liability for continuing care if the PPO fails and declares bankruptcy? Many plans require from 1 to 6 months of ongoing care.
12. Who will market the PPO so that you will receive patients? Are there any costs incurred in this marketing? If so, are they borne solely by the PPO? Will they market your name in an acceptable manner?

Independent Practice Association (IPAs) – capitation programs

IPA contracts differ from PPO contracts in structure, but present some similarities as well as new areas of concern. In an IPA, physicians receive a monthly capitated payment per member. A percentage is often withheld to protect the IPA against cost overruns. While the percentage should be returned if the IPA does well financially, it is possible that it will never be refunded.

It is critical that you understand your role as a gatekeeper in a managed care system and what overutilization by any one member of the team can do to your share in that system. IPAs generally exercise tighter control on referrals than do PPOs, most often through the use of prior authorization and utilization review. This can involve a lot of time and paperwork for your office, and aggravation for your patients, who more than likely will not understand the system.

Physicians who work within capitated managed care systems must follow stipulated policies and procedures. These mechanics are a necessary part of the process and, if understood up front, can ease and expedite the pediatrician's work within a managed care program. Some areas to clarify include:
1. It is often difficult to determine whether given patients are eligible for service in the month they appear. This is especially true in the first week of the month. Many of the plans will send eligibility rosters but some do not. Others will

supply toll free telephone numbers, but invariably they are busy. Often it is more cost effective to see the patient than to attempt an eligibility check. Is there a firm policy?

2. Do you as a physician have any responsibilities to the IPA? Must you participate in utilization review or quality assurance panels? What are the qualifications of the panel members?

3. What is the scope of services to be provided? Do you have any responsibility for house calls? This latter feature is often written into these agreements and you may want it changed.

4. What is the impact of utilization review and quality assurance practice?

5. Are you expected to be more available than you planned to be?

6. It is important to be familiar with grievance procedures for patients and physicians. It is also important to realize that the extra paperwork generated by the management information requirements of the IPA may require that you hire more employees.

7. Probably the most difficult part of functioning in an IPA is the screening required for emergency department visits. There is no question that the emergency room is used as an after hours clinic by many patients and the costs generated by these visits, if left unchecked, could drive any plan to bankruptcy. Thus, it is often necessary to decide whether or not to deny an emergency room visit to a patient at night or on weekends for conditions deemed minor that could be seen the next day in the less expensive office setting. This can create great animosity between physician and patient and could even lead to litigation if incorrect decisions were made medically.

All alternative health care delivery systems share the common goal of cost-containment achieved through cost-effective physician behavior. Cost-containment goals are specified in standards, policies, and rules set forth in the organization's contract with the physician. Whether or not the restrictions and limitations established by the organizations are in the best interest of the physician and his or her patients must be carefully weighed on a contract-by-contract basis. The decision to participate can be facilitated by

a resource kit, *Contracting with Health Care Delivery Systems,* which is available through the Academy.

Legal aspects of managed care or alternative delivery systems

Contracting raises many legal issues. This manual is not meant to speak to the letter of the law, and it would be wise to consult an attorney prior to involving yourself with an alternate delivery system contract. This section is designed to address some of the more common concerns.

Restraint of trade

Specialists who are not on the alternate delivery system rosters will no longer receive referrals from their previous physician base if referring physicians switch to all IPA or PPO modes of practice. This could be construed as restraint of trade.

Liability for specialty referrals

There is potential liability for mistakes made by specialists to whom a pediatrician refers a patient if a court deems that specialist to be incompetent. Pediatricians may be required to vary established referral patterns because of PPO or IPA rules. It is incumbent upon the pediatrician to be sure that the patients are going to physicians with respected medical abilities and that patients are referred to appropriate subspecialists regardless of their participation in the provider panel. The ultimate responsibility for referrals remains with the pediatrician.

Decisions by UR panels

Pediatricians are also potentially liable for utilization review decisions made by IPA review panels or medical directors affecting their patients. Pediatricians can be held liable for untoward events traced to early discharge or failure to authorize a referral for a patient. Physicians have the right to appeal decisions made by the IPA, and must do so if they feel such actions put patients in jeopardy.

Hold harmless clauses

Pediatricians should be sensitive to significant potential liability arising from "hold harmless" clauses.

Hold harmless clauses

Pediatricians are well advised to seek the advice of their professional liability carrier before signing any PPO contract containing a "hold harmless" clause. The following discussion of "hold harmless" clauses is reprinted with permission from an American Society of Internal Medicine brochure, *An ASIM Guide for Physicians and their Staff: The PPO Perspective.*[4]

"In some PPO contracts, individual carriers have asked to have so-called 'hold harmless' clauses inserted (where the PPO itself requires that by contract it be eliminated as a malpractice defendant), to protect themselves from allegations of malpractice by aggrieved patients or their families. These clauses may serve to shift the bulk of the liability risk to physician members of the PPO.

"In addition, the physician's own insurance may not cover 'contractually assumed' liability (where the physician

Avoid Hold Harmless Clauses

Primary Care Physician shall indemnify and hold The Company harmless from any and all claims, lawsuits, settlements, and liabilities incurred as a result of professional services provided or not provided by Primary Care Physician with respect to any Covered Person.

Figure 15-1: Avoid hold harmless clauses.

agrees by written contract to provide medical care). The standard malpractice suit is based on civil tort liability, which is premised not on written contract but rather on the legal duty of the physician to provide such care for his patient as falls within the usual and customary standard. Malpractice policies often won't cover contractually assumed liability, which means that if the PPO insurer is sued, the physician could be held personally liable for the judgment arising from a claim.

"For these reasons it is important that, before signing any PPO contract, you (1) check to see if it contains a hold harmless clause and (2) contact your medical liability carrier to determine if your policy covers contractually assumed liability. It is important to identify who will be liable in the situations described above and to question whether the carrier is attempting to unduly limit its own liability."

Government programs

Medicaid/EPSDT

Medicaid is the largest third party payer for children's health care in the United States, accounting for about 50% of this type of reimbursement. Each state establishes its own Medicaid regulations within the broad limits of the federal guidelines. Pediatricians must become familiar with the regulations in the state in which they practice, obtain a vendor number, and learn to use state billing forms.

Cards which state the dates of eligibility are issued by the local health and human services departments for children who are eligible for the Medicaid program. Medicaid eligibility should be verified if the pediatrician plans to bill the program for services rendered.

The Early and Periodic Screening, Diagnosis, and Treatment program (EPSDT)[5] is an integral part of Medicaid and emphasizes the delivery of routine preventive services and subsequent follow-up care. In some states physicians must obtain certification to serve as EPSDT providers and assure that all screening tests are done. Compensation may be higher for physicians who provide comprehensive care rather than only screening.

Discussion with the state Medicaid staff may help the pediatrician understand local procedures and the extra resources available to those attempting to provide comprehensive pediatric care to Medicaid patients.

CHAMPUS

As stated in Chapter 33, Uniformed Services Pediatrics, all active duty and retired military dependents are eligible for care at any military facility if there is available space and personnel. Since the military cannot provide care for all the dependents, it contracts this care out to civilian physicians and hospitals through a program known as CHAMPUS (Civilian Health and Medical Program of the Uniformed Services). Military families are cared for by private practice physicians who sign up as CHAMPUS providers. Reimbursement is based on the fee-for-service system; military families are responsible for a yearly deductible and a 20% copayment for sickness visits, with the remaining charges paid by the government. Health supervision visits and immunizations are covered only for the first 2 years of life. In general, pediatricians providing care through the CHAMPUS program have found it to be a satisfactory arrangement. Any pediatrician who would like to become a CHAMPUS provider can contact the regional CHAMPUS office.

In August 1989, the Champus Reform Initiative established an experimental program in California and Hawaii to deliver CHAMPUS care in the private medical care sector through a variety of managed care products, including a PPO (Champus Extra) and an HMO (Champus Prime). The program offers financial incentives to military families to switch from standard CHAMPUS and requires physicians to accept reduced reimbursement in order to become providers. If this program is successful, the Department of Defense plans to expand it to other states.

Considering an HMO, IPA, or PPO?

Listed below are 13 points to be considered when assessing any alternative health care delivery system. Also, an attorney and an accountant should review all pertinent documents before an agreement is finalized.

- Does the plan cover outpatient children's services for health supervision, illness, and emergency care? If not, it does not serve children or pediatricians well.
- What is the deductible? Is it by visit, illness, or year? Is it by individual or by family? High deductibles make for inadequate coverage for children's outpatient services.
- Is a discount asked of you? An equal percentage discount for all physicians has a disproportionate impact on the specialties with high overhead. Are you asked to compete with other providers for discount rates periodically?
- Is the reduced fee significant enough to require an increase in volume that might compromise the quality of care you can deliver?
- How much of an increase in patient load will result from joining the plan? Will this increase make you a "captive" of the plan?
- Will pediatricians have a significant voice in policy discussions or in operations? Who has the greatest medical input? What is the role of administrators in control of the plan?
- How is utilization review accomplished? Is it by peers, a commercial utilization review company, or some other means? Can there be retrospective denial? Does this leave you liable?
- What appeal mechanism exists if you disagree with financial, diagnostic, or coverage decisions? Will appeals require that you obtain legal services?
- What hospitals will you be permitted to utilize? Who are the referral specialists in the program? Do they include pediatric subspecialties? Which laboratory and x-ray facilities are contracted?
- How much additional work and stress will this create for the office staff? Are special billing forms required? How do you obtain approval for referrals?
- Is there a "stop-loss" ceiling to limit your liability for excessive patient care costs?
- Does capitation reimbursement realistically relate to the intensity of age-related services? Is the capitation provided for different age-groups? Is it reduced by a withhold? If so, how is the withhold reconciled?
- Does the plan have an exclusivity clause? Is there a hold harmless requirement?

References

1. *Employee Benefits in Medium and Large Firms.* Washington, DC: US Department of Labor, Bureau of Labor Statistics Bulletin #2363; June 1990

2. American Academy of Pediatrics, Committee on Child Health Financing. *Strategy for the Child Health Insurance Reform Plan: Legislation to Mandate Coverage of Child Health Supervision Services.* Elk Grove Village, IL: American Academy of Pediatrics; 1989

3. Flexible HMOs show enrollment gains: Interstudy. *AHA News.* 1991;27:3

4. American Society of Internal Medicine. *An ASIM Guide for Physicians and their Staff: The PPO Perspective.* Washington, DC: 1986

5. Early and Periodic Screening, Diagnosis and Treatment (EPSDT) Program (42 CFR 400,441). 49 *Federal Register* 43653

Checklist

✓ Is it time for you to consider systems other than direct payment and traditional health insurance for your practice compensation?

✓ Are you thoroughly acquainted with existing and prospective programs in your locale?

✓ If you are considering an alternative payment system, does it offer you a style of practice compatible with your professional and personal aspirations?

✓ Have you examined contracts offered by these systems? Have you discussed these contracts with an attorney? With an accountant?

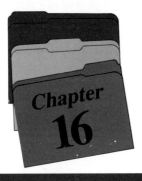

Marketing

Marketing is an important element in the success of any medical practice, and the utilization of marketing practices is vital to any pediatric practice. This chapter:
- **defines marketing**
- **describes marketing techniques**
- **discusses why and how to market a pediatric practice**

Chapter 16

Pediatrics in the 1990's is a part of the "new world" of competition. The practice of quality medicine alone, although essential, no longer guarantees success. As professionals, we would like to believe that patients intuitively recognize quality, that they are and remain loyal to their physicians, and that word of mouth will build and maintain a practice. This is not always true.

The number of physicians has almost tripled in the past decade. In 1960 we graduated 7000 physicians from US medical schools; today almost 17,000 graduate each year.[1] These additional physicians plus foreign medical graduates plus allied health professionals performing medical tasks appear to have created an engorged provider force. (The 3.7% annual growth of medical providers far outstrips the population growth of 0.85%.)[2]

A pediatrician trend is not clear at present. Pediatric residents in 1989 numbered 6353, compared to 6190 in 1987. This is an increase, although a selective look at graduate choices shows that primary care specialties are growing less rapidly than subspecialties.[3] The small increase in resident trainees is believed due to increasing numbers of foreign medical graduates entering into the accredited pediatric training programs.

Competition is ever present. Solo, small group, and large group practices alike will need to understand how a steady stream of newly well-trained pediatricians, family practitioners, and allied health providers, as well as large organized systems of health care, will impact their practices.

As the ultimate consumer of health care, the patient can pick and choose. The perception that all doctors are well-trained, have appropriate empathy, and have similar fees, leads the consumer to select or continue the association with a specific practice on the basis of per-

sonal experience. The events which shape this personal assessment may or may not be significant from the physician's perspective. Physician choice may be medically related, but just as often is office related, personnel related, or availability related. Convenience has taken on a new and more important meaning for patients. Third party payors, like Health Maintenance Organizations, try to increase their profitability by limiting patient demand and dealing with cost-conscious providers. They are likely to pick and choose on the basis of their perception of the cost effectiveness of the practice's operational patterns.

For all these reasons, marketing, the process of making the public, your peers, and purchasers of health care aware of your services, is now a necessity. Finding out what the public wants and needs, or anticipating desired services and creating a need while matching your services to that need, is another definition of marketing.[4]

For physicians, the most frequent misunderstanding in this area is to see only a "part of the whole." Marketing is not just an advertising or promotional scheme, although these are its most visible components. It is more accurate to view this approach as an overall "marketing game plan" or "marketing umbrella" with several crucial components.[5]

Assessment of the practice demography, patient perceptions of the practice, and an unbiased appraisal of the strengths and weaknesses of your own practice as well as those of your competitors, is the start of the "game plan."

The plan should be goal oriented – with the end points realistic and measurable.

Professional goals to examine include the types of patients that the practice would prefer (eg, private, Medicaid, HMO, or a mixture in agreed

proportions); possible changes in the age distribution of patients; modifications of existing services or the creation of new types of care; and variations in the hours and days offered for care.

The staff must be aware of the plan from the outset. Budget time and money for ample discussion, commitment to the effort, assignment of duties, and later accountability for the information obtained. Staff cooperation and enthusiasm is key to the successful marketing effort.

First, define the market. Who is out there? What are their ages and where do they live? Is the community stable or are people leaving? Where are the prime hospital newborn locations? Where are they building new communities, new schools, and new hospitals?

Next, what is the actual market? Is it primarily private patients, or is it heavily Medicaid, HMO, or PPO? Does it fit your desired patient mix? What are the family work and occupation habits? Are there predominantly two income families? How will that affect their willingness to accommodate the present office location and office hours?

Assessing patient perceptions with a patient survey (Figure 16-1) will quickly determine patient opinions, attitudes, and perceptions about you and your practice. Patients appreciate sensitivity to their opinions, and the use of a questionnaire in the reception area or exam room – filled out before leaving and deposited in a "neutral" receptacle – is very effective. This survey approach should be done on a regular basis with all patients to continually sample the degree of satisfaction with the practice.

If a patient leaves the practice, don't neglect a courteous telephone call to inquire about the reason for their decision. Valuable insights are obtained through such "exit interviews."

We'd Like to Know

We want to know your opinions about our practice and the services we offer. To make sure we are meeting your needs, please provide the following information.

1. There are a number of reasons for selecting a certain physician to care for your child. Please check the *major reason(s)* you selected our practice.

    ☐ Convenient office location

    ☐ Hospital affiliation

    ☐ Health care plan

    ☐ Recommended by friends or relatives

    ☐ Referred by another physician

    ☐ Referred by hospital or clinic

    ☐ Advertising (please specify) _____

    ☐ Yellow Pages listing

    ☐ Other (please specify) _____

2. Please indicate how frequently you have experienced each of the following with our office.

	Frequently	Sometimes	Rarely	Never
Difficulty scheduling an appointment when desired	☐	☐	☐	☐
Difficulty reaching the office because the office phone is busy	☐	☐	☐	☐
Being placed on "hold" for an extended period when calling the office	☐	☐	☐	☐
Slow return of after-hours calls	☐	☐	☐	☐
Slow return of calls during office hours	☐	☐	☐	☐
Unfriendly/ discourteous staff member	☐	☐	☐	☐
Difficulty parking at the office	☐	☐	☐	☐
Long waits at the office in the reception area	☐	☐	☐	☐
Long waits in the examining rooms	☐	☐	☐	☐
Billing errors	☐	☐	☐	☐

3. Which of the following time periods are the most convenient for scheduled appointments in our office? Check all that apply.

	Morning	Afternoon	Evening
Monday	☐	☐	☐
Tuesday	☐	☐	☐
Wednesday	☐	☐	☐
Thursday	☐	☐	☐
Friday	☐	☐	☐
Saturday	☐	☐	☐

4. Some pediatric offices have two waiting rooms, one for "well" children and one for "sick" children. Please indicate the importance to you of separate waiting rooms for "sick" and "well" children. (Please circle one number.)

Not Important				Very Important
1	2	3	4	5

5. Some pediatric offices have separate waiting rooms for adolescents and children. Please indicate the importance of having a separate waiting room for adolescents. (Please circle one number.)

Not Important				Very Important
1	2	3	4	5

6. Additional comments _____
    _____
    _____
    _____
    _____

Thank you for taking the time to fill out this survey. Our aim is to continue to provide you with quality health care services.

Figure 16-1: Sample patient satisfaction survey.

PEDIATRIC CENTER
Educational Videocassette Library Club

Pediatric Center is pleased to announce an exciting new service we are introducing to our practice.

In just a few weeks, we will be offering a wide range of approved parent/child educational videocassettes, at no charge to you, our valued patients. Now you will have available answers to commonly asked questions on breastfeeding, care of the newborn, infant development, safety issues, and CPR techniques just to name a few.

How does it work? It's easy! Simply ask our receptionist for a list of the videocassettes, choose one most suited to your needs (only one videocassette per week please), and as you check out after your visit, ask the cashier for your cassette. You will be required to leave an imprint of a major credit card (MasterCard, Visa, American Express) which will be voided upon return of the tape. There will be a late charge of $1.00 per day up to a maximum of $25.00 (the cost of the tape). You will be asked to sign a consent form for the above. Please return the tapes to the cashier (check-out receptionist).

We strongly encourage you to take advantage of this exceptional video library. If you have any questions after reviewing the films, please feel free to ask your pediatrician for further explanation.

As always, we would appreciate any comments or suggestions you may have regarding this new service.

The following is a preliminary list of tapes we'll have available to you:

Baby's First Months – What Do We Do Now? — Practical, informative videos for new parents featuring your very own Pediatric Center doctors.

Diapers & Delirium — Support and advice to new parents on how to remain sane with the arrival of a new baby.

Helping Your Baby Sleep Through The Night

Infant Health Care — First year guide for new parents – hosted by Dr T. Berry Brazelton.

Infant Development — First year guide to growth and learning hosted by Dr T. Berry Brazelton.

Breastfeeding – The Art Of Mothering — Approved by the American Academy of Pediatrics.

Baby Alive — Vital information to keep your infant and young child safe and secure. Hosted by Phylicia Rashad.

Kid Safe — Entertaining video *for children* – teaches them safety issues in the house.

How To Save Your Child Or Baby — Practical demonstration of CPR and the Heimlech manuever.

Sincerely,

PEDIATRIC CENTER

Figure 16-2: Explanation of educational videocassette library.

The Four *P*'s of Marketing

Price
- Evaluate local fee schedules.
- Understand the use of CPT-4 and ICD-9-CM codes.
- Have a specific financial policy clearly understood by staff and patients which is helpful to patients whenever appropriate.
- Establish sound procedures for filing insurance claims and assisting patients in filing claims.
- Review claims and payment procedures with all payors on a regular basis. This can help in two ways. It can assist adequate cash flow for the practice by avoiding conflicts with payors and it can avert the need for resignation from the plan's provider panel with resultant disruption in continuity of care for some of your patients.

Place
- Regional demographic data is usually available at your local hospital.
- Review current patient demographics on a regular basis to be aware of subtle changes to your practice catchment area.
- Evaluate the office regularly for staff appearance, staff manners, office decor, office cleanliness, parking accessibility, appearance of equipment, and ancillary facilities (eg, laboratory and x-ray).
- Continue to emphasize with both patients and staff the attitude that the "patient needs and wants comes first, ahead of technology, ahead of cost." No marketing effort will ever succeed without satisfied patients and the sense that the office is vitally interested in their welfare. Obviously, the office staff is key in this effort.

Promotion
Printing (See Patient Education Materials, Chapter 26.)
- Consider producing a patient information booklet to describe not only office and services, but also practice policies. Consider highlighting physicians and staff with appropriate biography and pictures.
- Think about producing a regular newsletter. It can be a simple one page form discussing common diseases and/or common problems ranging from measles to thumb sucking and sleep disorders.
- Develop a logo and use it.
- Utilize brochures from the AAP and pharmaceutical companies, or produce your own.
- Use practice-identifying labels on ALL brochures and printed materials that leave your office.

Personal Notes
- "Notograms" (triplicate forms) for quick, personalized replies.
- Remember to send thank-you's for referrals to physicians, patients, pharmacists, and pharmaceutical representatives. Thank-you and progress notes to obstetricians after first office visit are important courtesies.
- Birthday cards can be sent out as reminders for health supervision visits.

Telephone
- Check on office availability and adequacy of the number of phone lines for incoming calls.
- Assure that staff employs proper telephone answering techniques, eg, "hold" only after caller approval.
- Provide telephone access in reception areas for local calls.
- Incorporate practice information and promotion with appropriate music – professionally done – while caller is on "hold."

- Initiate telephone call backs – same day or next day initiated by doctor or staff – for follow-up on patient welfare.

VCR
- Place a monitor in the reception areas.
- Utilize for education and/or entertainment value during delay until entering exam room.

Audiotape
- Self-made tapes can be used in exam room prior to pediatrician entrance. These might describe development, newer advances in child care, special messages, health advice, or anticipatory guidance.

Group Discussion
- Sponsor group sessions regarding infant care, child development, or adolescent issues. Consider teen-only and parent-only sessions regarding teen issues. Some groups could feature a nutritionist or psychologist.

Public Speaking
- Make appearances before the public through various forums, including schools, PTAs, civic organizations, and charity events.
- Give educational lectures to other physicians, nurses, medical students and health professionals. It is especially useful to speak to residents, who are tomorrow's referral sources, as well as community family physicians and OBs to improve present referral base.

Yellow Pages
- It is estimated that 7% of new patients results from direct advertising in the "yellow pages."

Product
- Extended hours – Weekend and special hours when necessary for teens and young adults, and availability for working parents.
- Satellite offices.
- Transportation (coordinate and make available when necessary).
- Car seat loaners.
- Videotape and book library for loan to patients. (See Figure 16-2.)
- Flowers to new mothers on arrival home.
- Social services in office.
- Free care when civic need arises.
- Community service
- Athletic event availability school health activities.
- Office pharmacy.
- Office lactation consultant.
- Office developmental testing.
- Office nutrition program with available nutritionist for free group discussions, and private referral when special need arises.
- Computer usage – A computer can facilitate the creation of several ideas listed earlier including newsletters, thank you programs & birthday programs. Other uses might include a recall system, health maintenances notices for patients with specific disorders, special immunization notices, and appointment reminders.

The above are only a few generally utilized suggestions. The list can be easily expanded by your office staff with ideas that are specifically tailored to your particular practice, if you provide the staff with appropriate time and motivation to contribute to your marketing game plan.

Once demography, patient perceptions, and comparable market strengths and weaknesses have been assessed, it is time to develop the actual marketing plan, both short term (tactical plan) and long term (strategic plan). This might include entrenchment (to concentrate on satisfying your present patients), market development (eg, becoming more expert in behavioral problems), or diversification (eg, emphasizing adolescent sports medicine). In reality most good marketing plans combine elements of each. A successful marketing strategy also works on the "market-mix" which consists of "The Four *P*'s of Marketing," shown in the box on the preceding page. Price, place, promotion, and product each play a role. Reorganization and prioritization of market-mix can benefit almost every practice, if it is evaluated with an appreciation that even the "best situation" can be improved.

For those who wish to expend additional financial resources to promote their practice, there are numerous marketing professionals in the community who will be pleased to assist you in this endeavor. Seek out a professional who is properly referred and who is familiar with physician office practices and the medical marketplace. Find someone with whom you feel compatible. Be prepared to met a professional's price. Just as you budget for office supplies, staff salaries and rent, this expense should be seen as part of your office financial plan.

Conclusion

Marketing is not just another word for advertising. Marketing is putting the needs of patients first, and developing services that truly satisfy those needs. This includes appropriate pricing and development of good payor relationships as well as creating communication programs that help patients and their families understand the services of your pediatric practice.

In an era when increasing numbers of health care providers create an intensely competitive environment, accompanied by a demand structure that includes better educated and more sophisticated and selective consumers (with fewer children per family), an effective marketing program is essential to a healthy pediatric practice.

References

1. Etzel SI, Egan RL, Shevrin MP, Rowley, BD. Graduate Medical Education in US. *JAMA*. 1989;262:1029
2. Jolly P, Hudley D. *AAMC Data Book*. Washington, DC: Association of American Medical Colleges; 1990
3. Rowley BD, Baldwin DC Jr, McGuire MB, et al, eds. "Graduate Medical Education in the United States." *JAMA*. 1990;264:7;822-832
4. Blackwell R, Johnson W. Marketing Your Pediatric Practice. *Pediatric Basics*. Fremont, MI: Gerber Products Co; 1986
5. Brown S, Morley A. *Marketing Strategies for Physicians*. Medical Economic Books; Oradell, NJ: 1986

Bibliography

Performance Marketing in Medicine. Columbus, OH: Ross Laboratories; 1986.

Peters T, Waterman RH Jr. *In Search of Excellence*. New York, NY: Harper and Row; 1982.

Checklist

✓ Do you know your practice market, including demography and its changing trends?

✓ Do you discuss courtesy at all office staff meetings?

✓ Do you talk to and with patients rather than at them?

✓ Do you use letters or brochures, patient education materials which are imprinted with your name, address, and phone number?

✓ Do you make your printed materials a complement to your professional care as well as helpful to your patients?

✓ Does the public see you at meetings or on television, hear you on the radio, or read about you in the newspaper or in patient newsletters?

✓ Do you publicize practice changes, hours of availability, community interests, and so forth?

✓ Do you do justice to your marketing program with your time and money? With staff time?

✓ Would your practice benefit from extended hours? A satellite office?

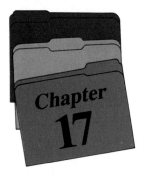

Professional Advisors

Chapter 17

As the owner of the business, the pediatrician is responsible and liable for the nonprofessional as well as the professional aspects of the practice, and must seek consultation or advice from other professionals. This chapter will consider:
- **the selection of an accountant**
- **the selection of an attorney**
- **the use of management services**

Many pediatric groups find ways to share responsibility for different aspects of the business side of practice. While this strategy is effective in creating areas of doctor supervision and accountability, it by no means eliminates the need for professional advice and consultation from professional advisors.

The pediatrician sometimes forgets that his or her practice is a business. Unfortunately, medical practices have been among some of the poorest run businesses, due at least in part to the absence of training in business matters in medical school curricula. As a business owner, the pediatrician is responsible for overseeing nonmedical activities and business procedures. The pediatrician must see that the business aspects of the practice function at the same high level as the medical care. A schedule should be established for regular reviews of the business practices.[1]

Pediatricians cannot be expert in all nuances of front office systems, CPT-4 coding changes, government code changes, paperwork requirements, "marketplace" demands and public relations. Even those pediatricians who specialize in various business aspects will often find that professional advice is still needed. Sound financial, legal and management decisions are all part of a successful pediatric practice. If the pediatrician believes that the mixture of medical services and business techniques in the practice does not seem to be productive, satisfying, and efficient, the services of other professionals may be necessary.

Some advice is needed on an ongoing basis (accounting), some advice is needed under special circumstances (legal), and some advice is needed infrequently (management consultant). The pediatrician should establish a good relationship with reliable consultants when beginning practice. Although the

services of these consultants may appear to be costly, the amount of money they eventually will save the practice more than offsets their cost.

Consultants should be contacted in the planning stages of any endeavor. Unfortunately, many pediatricians mistakenly attempt to save a fee and put off contacting a consultant until the need is urgent. Those who procrastinate in seeking qualified advice may lose, or spend, an enormous amount of money.

This chapter will provide an overview of accounting principles to help the pediatrician understand the day-to-day operations of the business and provide information about bookkeeping and accounting practices. This includes how to protect income and choose an accountant. The types of legal services needed and the benefits of a management consultant also will be discussed.

Finding a consultant

Some general principles can be applied to the search and selection of any new advisor for the practice. Seek referrals from a variety of sources including other physicians in the community, friends and advisors whose judgment you respect, and financial professionals you trust. Some experts suggest that you should look for advisors who have at least 5 years experience in order to be able to evaluate their performance record.[2]

Once you have compiled a list of prospective consultants, perform the initial screening by telephone until the list is narrowed to two or three candidates. Then arrange a personal interview with each candidate. A 30-60 minute "get acquainted" consultation is usually offered free of charge. Seek an advisor who listens closely and asks insightful questions; he or she is more

likely to understand and respond to *your* objectives. Look for a responsive, individualized approach, rather than a well-rehearsed "canned" sales presentation. Also evaluate the individual's ability to work with other advisors for your practice.

Once you have hired the advisor, review the individual's performance regularly. Remember, *you* are the employer. If the advisor fails to perform to your satisfaction, or if the two of you do not work well together because of personality differences, consider terminating the relationship and beginning your search anew.

Accounting and financial considerations

The practice is a means of financial support; therefore, the pediatrician should be concerned with matters that provide income. Most pediatricians have had little or no training in business and finance. Still as business owners, pediatricians will have to realize that the supervision of a business office cannot be delegated entirely. In fact, the wise accountant, who sets the basic bookkeeping procedures in motion, includes provisions for supervision by the pediatrician. The uninvolved business owner is as readily troubled as the uninformed business owner.

The accountant

The accountant is the primary economic advisor to most practices. No professional works more closely with a doctor than the accountant. Pediatricians rely on them for status reports, advice on practice finances, retirement plans, personal and business taxes, and

Accounting System Components

- Establishment of a basic, productive accounting system.
  - Set up a system of collection, charges, and patient account balances, and develop reports from this data.
  - Set up a system of supplies, levels of inventory and responsibility for ordering and payment of bills.
  - Set up controls so books balance daily.
  - Establish records of accounts receivable by age (30-60-90-120 days or account balances).
  - Establish a ledger for petty cash.
  - Establish records for payroll and employee benefits.
  - Establish methods for assistance with and filing of insurance claims, and provide for recording of insurance claims and receipts for these claims.
  - Establish a system for compliance with government requirements (eg, IRS, unemployment, Social Security)
- Establishment of controls to eliminate mistakes and "control" theft. Though no system is foolproof, certain basic techniques are instituted by the accountant to deter error and temptations.
- Establishment of proper collection systems at the office sign-out desk, because fees collected at the time of service is the preferred arrangement. Systems are established that result in the multiple recording of monies owed and monies received so proper credit is issued and monies are arranged in a proper, bankable manner.
- Establishment of a sound and efficient billing system, whether with a "peg-board" multiple-carbon system or by computer. The accountant, with the pediatrician's helpful observations and attentiveness, is in a position to evaluate the efficiency of billing procedures, (prompt statement mailings and so forth) and can review present office procedures to suggest improvements, or changes in an inefficient or outgrown system.
- Establishment of practice statistics – generating reports of expenses (comparable to preceding years and months), of net income (again comparative), and of numbers of procedures and services and their downward or upward trend. It is extremely helpful for future planning or present thinking or rethinking of practice habits to be accurately informed about any pattern in office visits, laboratory procedures, emergency room demands, numbers of newborn infants, and productivity of individual physicians or nonphysician health care providers.
- Review of personal tax planning – guidance in legal tax avoidance, establishment of withholding guidelines, determination of taxable income, preparation of income tax returns, filing for extension of due dates, and representation before the Internal Revenue Service.
- Review and advice for financial planning for retirement in either a corporate or noncorporate setting, with advice on pensions, Keogh accounts, Individual Retirement Accounts, office real estate, property and equipment (rent, buy, lease, or purchase), and so forth.
- Review and advice of your insurance program (with qualified insurance consultation) assure that the tax implications of life, disability, and hospitalization insurance (personal or office-related) are what they are purported to be.
- Advice in establishment of an investment program and investment philosophy.
- Advice to the family, with specific guidelines for family financial planning and budgeting of income. This function is invaluable in placing the family income in proper perspective, including projected expenses and financial responsibilities. This constructive support, which ensures that each marriage partner understands financial reality, can eliminate the turmoil and discord that results from either a lack of sophistication in financial matters or disregard of basic and sensible rules for spendable income.

---

individual investments. The relationship should be comfortable, direct, and truly confidential. The pediatricians should always set aside adequate time for the meetings with the accountant in order to discuss in detail all aspects of the practice.

The selection of an accountant can be as important as the selection of a new physician associate, but frequently there is little to go on. The types of available accounting services range from large accounting firms to accountants in solo practice. The accountant's experience with other medical practices probably is the most important consideration.

It is important to maintain a realistic perspective: the amount of money earned may be less important than the amount of money kept after taxes and expenses. The accountant's primary function should be to ensure that the pediatrician keeps as much money as he or she is legally entitled to keep. A competent accountant can begin to offer financial advice even before a practice is launched. Should the pediatrician go into solo practice or join a group practice? Should the practice be incorporated? Should the pediatrician construct a building (with or without space for other offices) or rent or buy space in an existing building? Should the pediatrician join an existing group practice on a salary basis with a buy-in option? Should the pediatrician lease, finance, or buy equipment and furnishings?

Systems for the payment of office staff, (eg, tax withholding and benefit package) payment of bills, and billing patients are preferably established by an accountant. Ongoing management can be assigned to an in-house bookkeeper (or office manager), who then can report to the accountant.

The accountant will establish and monitor a system to collect payments, monitor accounts receivable, maintain supplies and accounts payable, and balance the books each day. The system will provide for payroll, insurance claims filing and governmentally required records and reports. (See Accounting Systems Components for details to be included in accounting systems.)

The services of an accountant also are vital for tax planning purposes. Discussions must be held between the pediatrician and the accountant about tax planning before the tax year begins to ensure that each year's financial goals are met. The accountant also can assist in estate planning and personal financial planning as well as development of the best approach toward retirement planning.

All the services an accountant performs may be negated unless regular communication is established. Meetings on a regular basis (at least two to four times a year, and more often when the need arises) provide for a review of the office functions, financial records, practice trends, and practice or personal problem areas. Areas of concern can be voiced at these meetings, or new ideas can be discussed. Communication with the accountant is essential in helping him or her gain insights into the practice and the pediatrician's personal needs.

Attorneys and legal considerations

A business attorney is an indispensable consultant. This individual or firm must be highly skilled in legal practice regarding small businesses or professional corporations and their related financial and tax matters. Seek an attorney who has special expertise in medical practices and has a number of physician clients.

The pediatrician must take an active role in developing a relationship with the attorney: good communication and a clear understanding of your problems and objectives are prerequisite. The pediatrician must make requests in a timely manner, because the attorney needs adequate time to research the law, and prepare a case or course of action. Too often the pediatrician signs a contract, then asks an attorney for a review and opinion, frequently with disastrous consequences. Proper legal opinion and the successful practice of preventive law depends on giving the attorney adequate time for preparation. In addition, the pediatrician must give the attorney all the facts; information should never be withheld because of embarrassment or fear. The information on which the attorney's opinion is based must be accurate and complete.

The attorney is a counsel, a draftsman of legal documents, and advocate if the need arises, a negotiator in the pediatrician's behalf, and a resource for specific information. The attorney can act most effectively in all these capacities only when there is a significant input by the pediatrician into this relationship.

Examples of legal services performed by an attorney include providing working agreements and contracts, handling real estate or property matters, and making buy-and-sell arrangements. The attorney, in consultation with the accountant, can provide advice on tax problems, partnership, associations, corporations, employment contracts, estate plans, life plans, pension and profit-sharing plans, retirement plans, and so forth.

Law, like medicine, is becoming so specialized, that the need for consultation on specific legal matters beyond the expertise on the business attorney may arise. Some specialized areas of law which might benefit from review by an expert attorney in the field could include malpractice, estate planning, collection services, partnership/group practice contracts, real estate purchase and lease agreements, and complex business ventures such as mergers.

Experienced lawyers (and CPAs) often delegate work to younger associates in the firm. The pediatrician needs to determine who will be ultimately responsible for performing the legal work. If it will be a legal associate, the

---

Counterpoint

Traditionally, pediatricians have drawn on the advice of an attorney, accountant, insurance broker and investment advisor in managing their finances. But like medicine, the financial services industry has become increasingly specialized. A business and personal financial planner can coordinate the services of these professionals and help the pediatrician devise an effective overall strategy.

Financial planners examine all aspects of your business and personal financial picture. Their fees can range from several hundred to several thousands of dollars, depending upon estate and investment planning requirements.[3] A complete analysis should dissect your financial position in detail, and make recommendations for income tax planning, insurance coverage, investment strategy, retirement funding, and estate planning.

A financial plan is a strategy to reach long-term financial goals, and the planner meets regularly with clients to monitor and update it. More than 250,000 people now call themselves financial planners,[3] and choosing a competent, ethical planner requires the same care as finding an attorney or accountant.

Four out of five financial planners receive commissions on the investment and insurance vehicles they recommend.[3] Some feel that commissions can influence advice, and recommend working with a planner who charges a flat fee, generally $50-$150 per hour or 1%-2% of assets.[3] Others maintain that a commission basis motivates the ethical planner to follow your progress more closely. Either way, it is best to consult your attorney, accountant and other trusted financial advisors, as well as check references and credentials before signing on with a financial planner.

The National Association of Personal Financial Advisors, 1130 Lake Cook Road, Suite 105, Buffalo Grove, IL 60089 (800/366-2732) offers a free guide to selecting a financial planner as well as a list of planners who work on a flat fee basis.

The Registry of Financial Planning Practitioners, maintained by the International Association for Financial Planning in Atlanta (404/395-1605) lists planners who have passed certain examinations and cleared reference checks. Planners designated as Certified Financial Planners (CFP) or Chartered Financial Consultant (ChFC) have met certain requirements established by the industry.

pediatrician should meet with that person. Attorney fees vary with community standards, experience, and the degree of expertise the problem commands. The hourly rate for attorney and associates, and amount of retainer required, should be addressed during the initial interview.

Practice management consultants

Management consultants are professional problem solvers. A management consultant can assist the pediatrician in improving cash flow, increasing income, and reducing taxes. An effective consultant can recommend solutions that improve employee motivation and training, physical facilities and planning, medical records, and paperwork procedures and can share financial systems and controls with the accountant. A management consultant also can keep the pediatrician abreast of the implications of inflation and help relate fees to changing costs.

Clearly, not every pediatric practice needs a management consultant – at least not on a regular basis. If the pediatrician has an aptitude for business, he/she may well get by with no more outside help than that provided by the advice of the accountant and lawyer. In a group practice, the old adage "too many cooks spoil the broth" is truly appropriate. It is imperative that the group designate one pediatrician as the managing partner for all the business affairs of the practice.

The number of practice management firms is estimated at more than 500, with at least one in every state. As discussed earlier, the best sources of referral are physician and dentists locally who have utilized a consultant's services. If you are unable to obtain a suitable referral, the AAP Division of Pediatric Practice can provide more in-depth background information on the selection of a practice management consultant. Listings of those experienced in medical-dental management are available from The Society of Medical-Dental Management Consultants (800/826-2264) and the Society of Professional Business Consultants (312/922-6222).

References

1. Klass R. *The Physician's Business Manual*. New York, NY: Appleton-Century-Crofts; 1981:91
2. Boroson W. *Physician's Guide to Professional and Personal Advisors*. Oradell, NJ: Medical Economics Books; 1982:74-82
3. Schurzer AI. Your Crucial First Step Toward Financial Security. *Med Econ*. 1990;67:20

Checklist

✓ Do you understand the functions of an accountant and what an accountant can do for you?
✓ Are you willing to commit undivided attention during meetings with your accountant?
✓ Do you seek your accountant's advice in a prospective fashion in financial, tax, and investment matters?
✓ Are you willing to commit time to the supervision of your business office?
✓ Are you familiar with the assistance a business attorney can provide?
✓ Do you work closely with your attorney(s) in a prospective fashion in legal matters pertaining to both your practice and personal or family matters?
✓ Are you familiar with the functions of a management consultant?

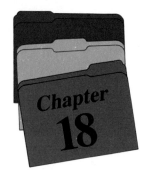

Insurance – Personal and Practice

All businesses need insurance protection for all types of risks. A total insurance program for both practice and personal needs will be discussed in this chapter. Areas emphasized are:
- categories of protection needed
- varieties of insurance available
- the advantages and disadvantages of different insurance forms
- organization and maintenance of a useful program

Insurance is a method of handling the risk of economic loss resulting from unpredictable events.[1] Insurance pools the risks of many to cover the financial losses of a few.

The prudent pediatrician will seek advice from knowledgeable advisors, such as bank officers, accountants, attorneys, and professional insurance agents before purchasing insurance. Good advice sought in a timely fashion from an economic advisor is never a mistake.

Pediatricians should think of insurance in three broad categories – **Personal, Professional,** and **Business.**

Personal insurance

The pediatrician's personal insurance portfolio should incorporate life, disability, medical care, and hospitalization coverage.

Life insurance

Life insurance should be purchased for its protective value rather than as a vehicle for investment. The major risk that life insurance protects against is economic loss from the early death of the family provider. The highest level of protection is necessary in the younger years of practice before savings and prudent investments are accumulated. If sound investment programs are combined with sensible life insurance policies, money should be available at all stages of life in the various amounts needed.

Life insurance proceeds are designed for quick release by the insurer, and are not held by court proceedings. These funds can:[2]
1. Provide emergency funds for living and funeral expenses.
2. Provide a readjustment period for the spouse and/or family.
3. Pay off a home mortgage.
4. Fund a child's education.
5. Provide funds to buy out a partner's spouse. (A special policy can be purchased to offset such a buy-out.)
6. Pay estate taxes.

The amount of life insurance protection needed will vary with age, family status or anticipated family obligations, and other sources of wealth. This changing need for protection mandates that coverage levels and types of protection be reviewed every few years and adjusted as necessary. The decision to increase or decrease amounts and types of coverage should be weighed carefully.

There are three basic types of life insurance policies; term, whole life, and annuity.

Term life insurance[1]

Term insurance provides the maximum death benefit for the lowest initial premium outlay. Protection is issued for a limited period of 1, 5, 10, or more years. Premiums increase with the age of the insured at the end of the time period (term) if the policy is renewed, and some require new evidence of insurability for renewal. The policy expires if the insured survives the term and does not renew. The premiums for term life insurance are initially the least expensive, but term life policies do not have a cash surrender or loan value.

In later years the term life insurance premiums may be prohibitively expensive – and the pediatrician is well advised to balance the less expensive insurance purchased in the early practice years with a sound prudent savings program. This philosophy may provide alternative emergency funds for the estate as family obligations lessen.

Whole life insurance[1]

This type of insurance product is a combination of a term life policy and a savings account. The premium is based on the age of the insured and usually remains the same over the years. These policies accumulate cash value and also loan value, and are usually paid up in 10 to 15 years.

Traditionally, interest rates on the monies present in a whole life policy are conservatively low because they are not market driven; specific cash values are guaranteed. However, newer versions of whole life policies are interest-sensitive. Usually the cash value of the policy equals the total premium in 7-10 years. Whole life insurance is more expensive than term in earlier years, but accumulated savings coupled with stable premiums translate to a better value as years unfold.

A newer variation of the "whole life" product is called universal life or flexible life insurance. These policies provide protection and generate interest, but the interest rate is market sensitive so that the policyholder could realize a higher cash value. Higher savings accumulations result from slightly lower premiums in times of high interest in the market place, and conversely lower savings accumulations result in times of lower interest rates. In times of lower interest rates, you will probably be asked to contribute a larger premium outlay. These policyholders are sometimes allowed to increase coverage without evidence of insurability in exchange for certain premium consideration at the time of application.

Again the pediatrician is well advised to seek competent advice before purchase of these products.

Endowment or annuity[1]

Endowment policies are primarily savings accounts, with little emphasis on death benefits. An annuity's death benefit is only the return of your funds at interest. The face amount of the policy usually is payable at the end of a specified contract period or when the policyholder dies, whichever occurs first. High premiums in the early years of these policies may not be appropriate for the young pediatrician, but endowments and annuities are integral elements of overall estate planning.

Annuities are frequently used for tax sheltered savings or asset-protection to accumulate retirement funds. In any event, competent advice from an impartial third party consultant is imperative.

Disability insurance[1]

Disability insurance provides cash benefits to replace earnings lost during periods of incapacity because of injury or illness. Benefits can be paid for a short or long term or for life. Benefits are not taxable if premiums are paid by the insured. If the premiums are paid by a practice or corporation, the benefits will be taxable to the individual as ordinary income. The goal should be to obtain the highest amount of coverage affordable at a time when premiums are the lowest and health is the best.

The definition of disability is important and differs among companies. In considering disability:

1. Obtain the company's definition of both total and partial disability. Your agent or company will provide this in a letter or brochure.
2. Ask how long the benefits will be paid in the event of a total disability.
3. Ask if partial disability is covered.
4. Find out if the ability to practice pediatrics or a pediatric subspecialty is specifically covered.
5. Ask whether disability is specialty specific. If a pediatrician loses the use of his/her arms, but can still practice in administrative medicine, will disability payments be denied?
6. Determine the length of waiting period required before benefits begin.
7. Determine the policy benefit limits.

Individual policies are issued in relation to your earnings. Therefore, individual policies which take into account other disability coverages will limit benefits if you have other individual or group insurance. Individual disability income insurance should be purchased first, and group policies should be purchased subsequently.

Actuarial statistics show that each of us is much more likely to suffer an illness or accident-related disability than we are to die at an early age. The practicing physician who does not carry adequate disability insurance is taking an unnecessary risk.

Disability insurance benefits vary with the policy. A simple traditional policy guarantees payment of a fixed amount over a specified time with no provision for inflation or changed earning status. Many newer policies contain highly desirable clauses which automatically increase the benefits payable according to an inflationary index.

It is critical to purchase a policy which guarantees income regardless of the nature of the disability. Traditional policies paid benefits only if the policyholder was entirely incapable of doing any useful work whatsoever. It is now possible to purchase policies which define disability as the inability to perform one's own occupation. This allows a disabled pediatrician to continue to work in some other endeavor and still receive benefits. Even better, however, are "income replacement" policies which grant benefits solely on the basis of a provable decrease in income secondary to an illness or accident. These permit the disabled pediatrician to continue practicing on a reduced scale and still collect benefits regardless of future health. The policyholder is not forced to sacrifice all the time and training necessary to practice pediatrics simply to collect on a disability policy. Income replacement disability policies are highly recommended.

Business interruption insurance

Business office overhead coverage provides cash benefits for regular expenses incurred in the conduct of the insured's business while he or she is disabled, but the insured's salary, and usually other family member salaries, are excluded. The benefit amount is the actual overhead expense incurred up to a limit specified in the contract. Premiums are tax deductible. The limit should be set high enough to cover employees salaries, and rental of temporary space and equipment.

Other issues in disability insurance

Waiting period

How long does the disability have to last before the insurance company starts to pay benefits? The longer the waiting period, the lower the premium. Typical waiting periods are from 30 to 90 days, but might be as long as 180 days or even 365. The decision hinges on the individual's ability to essentially self-insure for short term. It is often suggested that insureds consider purchasing policies with different waiting periods.

Residual benefits

Residual benefits, an option that can be purchased for an additional premium, pays benefits when the insured returns to work full-time but incurs a loss of earnings because of diminished capacity. This assures income commensurate with previous earning capabilities.

Noncancellability

With a noncancellable policy, the insurance company cannot cancel the policy nor raise the premiums as long as the premiums are paid. Policies with this feature are more expensive than group policies, which can be cancelled if the underwriter cancels the coverage of the group. It may be wise to purchase a separate, individual, noncancellable policy for a portion of coverage and a group policy for the balance of coverage.

Guaranteed renewability

If the policy is guaranteed renewable, the insurance company guarantees the premium rate, usually for one year, and will renew the policy without further evidence of insurability. Premium can be increased for an entire "class" of insureds but not for an individual. A noncancellable, guaranteed renewable policy is suggested.

Preexisting conditions

All policies underwrite preexisting conditions carefully. Therefore, preexisting conditions should be stated on the application. If a health problem is disclosed on the application and the company issues the policy without waivers for that condition, the policy will cover any disabilities arising from that condition. The company may charge an additional premium and also cover the condition. There is also a possibility that preexisting conditions will not be covered. Check with the agent about how the company underwrites disclosed preexisting conditions.

Contestable period

A contestable period is the period of time during which the company can cancel coverage or refuse to pay a claim if the claim is caused by a condition intentionally omitted from the application which would have caused the company to issue the policy differently.

Exclusions

Some conditions (exclusions) may not be payable. Check with the agent about exclusions.

Medical care – hospitalization

This insurance is available in two forms, the traditional indemnity insurance, or coverage within a managed care system.

The traditional indemnity insurance (hospital, physician fees, excess medical expenses, catastrophic, major medical) is subject to a deductible amount, possibly with specific limitations on each element of expense. Choice of physician and medical facilities is at the discretion of the policyholder. This type of insurance offers a wide range of options, (dental insurance, pharmacy, etc) which affect premium costs.

Managed care insurance, as part of an alternative delivery system, is sold primarily to employers for groups of employees. It offers much the same type of protection and available options. It is usually less expensive than traditional indemnity insurance, and incorporates certain characteristic cost containment features. These include limited choice of providers and locales for service and required prior authorization for specialty referrals, elective admissions, special testing, or some types of therapy. Other cost containment measures usually include requirements for outpatient testing, outpatient surgery when practical, and hospital utilization management to insure hospital necessity. There may also be physician practice and referral pattern monitoring, and use of co-payments.

As with all types of insurance the purchaser should obtain competent advice to understand coverage limitations, and know any special conditions which affect payment. Exclusions, pre-existing illness limitations, health supervision coverage and maternity coverage are among specific aspects to explore.

Professional liability insurance (malpractice)

Professional liability coverage is available on either a claims-made or an occurrence basis.

Claims-made basis

Claims-made insurance covers claims made while the policy is in effect. Claims are covered if the claim is made and reported during the policy period.

These policies provide protection only during the dates specified in the policy. However, claims-made policies offer tail coverage (often very costly) to protect against claims made after the policy expires.

If a pediatrician allows a claims-made policy to expire and does not buy "tail" coverage, he or she is uninsured for claims made after the termination of the policy. The policy should contain guarantees about the availability and the price of the tail coverage. For example, the tail coverage should be available regardless of whether the insurance company or the pediatrician terminates the policy.

Occurrence basis

Although the claims-made policy is usually less expensive, many physicians prefer the occurrence policy. This policy covers any errors or omissions which take place while the policy is in effect, even if the claim is made long after the policy expires. This is especially important to pediatricians, because a young patient may file a claim after reaching majority, which could be years after the occurrence.

A disadvantage of the occurrence policy is that limits purchased today may be inadequate in the future when a claim is actually made. In choosing limits, the pediatrician should be aware that future liability is affected by inflation, by the number of lawsuits and by the dollar value of judgments. It is important to retain proof of insurance through the period covered by the statute of limitations for each state of practice.

Occurrence-based malpractice insurance generally has a higher yearly premium than claims-made basis insurance, since the insurance company must agree to insure you for the rest of your life against any action occurring during the term of the policy.

Insurance companies offer free risk management seminars to teach physicians and small business owners proven techniques which lessen the probability of a costly malpractice action. Completion of such a course often earns the participating physician a reduction in his or her malpractice insurance premium. An active quality assurance/risk management program should exist in the pediatrician's office. (See Professional Liability and Risk Management, Chapter 19.)

Business insurance

Business insurance is often complex. Proper coordination prevents excessive or inadequate coverage and can result in significant cost savings. The pediatrician should seek the help of a single, established, and knowledgeable agent who is experienced in small business and professional insurance to coordinate and plan the coverage purchased.

Property insurance

Office contents (and the building, if owned) should be insured on a replacement cost rather than an actual cash value basis. If there is a loss, old property can be replaced with new property, and the insurance company will not deduct depreciation expense from the settlement. In calculating the limit of the office contents, include the value of improvements, such as remodeling. Coverage should be on an "all-risk" basis.

Make sure that items owned by an individual and not by the corporation or partnership, are also insured. Such property may be covered by writing a separate policy for the individual, leasing the property to the firm, or naming the individual as an insured on the firm's policy.

Valuable papers

Valuable papers insurance covers the cost to reconstruct important papers, records, files, and documents; it also may apply to computer data. Keep documents which cannot be replaced in a safe or safety deposit box and other important records in fireproof containers.

Floater

Equipment the pediatrician carries (eg, otoscopes, house call bags) may be insured on an all-risk basis and at all locations under a physician's equipment floater. This equipment probably would not be covered by personal homeowner or automobile insurance because it is business, not personal, property.

Fine arts
A fine arts floater will cover valuable art and antiques in the office. The insurance is prospectively written for negotiated value and frequently is based on a sales receipt or appraisal. Valuables should be itemized.

Money and securities
The office policy can include coverage, subject to a deductible, for money and securities used in the business, both in the office and in transit to the bank.

Off-premises property
Consider off-premises coverage for business property, such as dictating equipment, which could be damaged while in transit.

Accounts receivable
Accounts receivable coverage is available to make up for bills which cannot be collected because the records are destroyed by fire or another covered loss. Even with this insurance, try to keep a current copy of accounts receivable in a safe location, eg, fireproof storage or duplicate computer information.

Office liability
Office liability insurance in its simplest form covers bodily injury and property damage to others arising from the business. Malpractice is excluded. The best liability coverage is comprehensive, general liability with a broad form endorsement. This insurance includes such extras as off-premises activities and coverage for libel, slander, and false arrest. Employees can be included as additional insureds.

Automobiles
Automobile insurance includes liability, medical payments, uninsured motorist protection, and physical damage insurance. Careful review with an insurance agent will assure proper and sufficient coverage.

Automobiles owned or leased by the corporation or partnership and automobiles which are not owned or leased by the business but are used for business purposes should be covered. This can be done with so-called "nonowned and hired car" insurance. Because physicians in partnership may be responsible for damage arising from one another's professional and business activities, all partners must carry adequate liability insurance on their personal automobiles. Partnership automobile liability insurance is available for this purpose.

Loss of earnings
Temporary loss of income because of a loss, such as fire, should be covered.

Employee dishonesty
All employees should be bonded, particularly those who handle money.

(ERISA) plan coverage
Bond the trustee of a profit sharing or pension plan as required by Employee Retirement Income Security Act (ERISA) and other applicable laws. Also consider fiduciary errors and omissions insurance to cover trustee negligence.

Workers' compensation
Insurance to cover injury to employees is required by law. The premium, based on annual compensation, is ordinarily subject to audit at the end of the policy.

Computer insurance
The increasing use of computers in private practices to handle business accounting, insurance claims filing, and patient record-keeping functions, makes their role an increasingly vital one in the economic health of a practice. Since the computer deals with a medium (electromagnetic impulses) which is vulnerable to destruction, an entirely new type of insurance called "Data-Processing" or "Business Computer" insurance has been developed.

If your practice operates a computer, it should be insured by a separate policy issued by a company and an agent knowledgeable in the technical field of computer insurance. The standard office contents All Risk policy will often specifically exclude computer equipment from coverage. It must and should be covered by a separate policy.

In purchasing such a policy, consider the cost of replacing the hardware and the software, the cost of lost collections and/or business if the computer is destroyed, and the cost to reconstruct lost data files if they, too, are lost.

In dealing with computers, it is critical to "self-insure" with frequent (preferably daily) backup copies of all the data in the computer. The backup copies should be stored on diskette. This "archive" diskette, containing all the practice financial information, should be stored at another site to protect it from any disaster which might occur at the primary business site.

Excess liability (or umbrella coverage)

Excess or umbrella coverage should be an essential part of all insurance packages. An umbrella policy increases dollar limits of liability over and above the basic policy limits. A typical policy provides a $1 million extra coverage, but others can be obtained for $2, $5, or even $10 million of excess. Since the cost is relatively low because the insurance does not cover the base policy amounts, there is no reason not to have an umbrella policy.

The applicant for umbrella insurance will have to provide specific details of all underlying coverage, ie, name of insurance company, policy numbers, dollar amount of coverage, and expiration dates. The limits of minimal coverage necessary are stated in the declarations of the excess liability policy.

Umbrella coverage is strongly advised for automobile, office, liability, personal, and malpractice insurance.

Other considerations

The Academy has studied the insurance needs of pediatricians and makes available group policies to provide insurance coverage of loss of life, loss of earning power, loss of property, and loss from liability.

The total insurance program should be reviewed on a regular basis with an insurance broker, accountant, and attorney. This assures proper coordination of individual and group policies to provide maximum sensible insurance coverage.

The pediatrician will need many insurance policies. Each should be stored safely, and monitored carefully. This assures ready updates, avoids unnecessary and expensive duplication, and keeps important policy information in one reference area.

Sample forms for recording insurance information are given in Figures 18-1 through 18-3. Completion of these or similar forms is vital to an effective insurance program. These records should be updated on a regular basis.

LIFE INSURANCE

It is suggested that policies and most recent policy anniversary premium notices should be examined personally, if possible. The following information should be recorded on this page.

POLICY NUMBERS				
NAME OF INSURANCE COMPANY				
ISSUE AGE				
INSURED				
OWNER OF POLICY				
TYPE OF POLICY				
PREMIUM COST AND MODE				
CASH VALUE				
EXTRA BENEFITS (e.g. waiver of premium, accidental death, etc.)				
AMOUNT OF BASE POLICY				
DIVIDENDS (VALUE & OPTION)				
TERM RIDER(S)				
LOAN OUTSTANDING				
NET AMT. PAYABLE AT DEATH				
BENEFICIARIES AND SETTLE-MENT OPTION ELECTED				
1st to				
2nd to				
POLICY NUMBERS				
NAME OF INSURANCE COMPANY				
ISSUE AGE				
INSURED				
OWNER OF POLICY				
TYPE OF POLICY				
PREMIUM COST AND MODE				
CASH VALUE				
EXTRA BENEFITS (e.g. waiver of premium, accidental death, etc.)				
AMOUNT OF BASE POLICY				
DIVIDENDS (VALUE & OPTION)				
TERM RIDER(S)				
LOAN OUTSTANDING				
NET AMT. PAYABLE AT DEATH				
BENEFICIARIES AND SETTLE-MENT OPTION ELECTED				
1st to				
2nd to				

Figure 18-1: Sample form for recording life insurance information.

HEALTH INSURANCE

It is suggested that policies should be examined personally. The following information should be recorded on this page.

DISABILITY INCOME				
DISABILITY INCOME POLICY NUMBERS				
NAME OF INSURANCE COMPANY				
INSURED				
OWNER OF POLICY/ PREMIUM PAYOR				
PREMIUM COST AND MODE				
TYPE OF CONTINUANCE OR RENEWAL PROVISION				
DEFINITION OF DISABILITY				
MONTHLY DISABILITY INCOME				
ACCIDENT				
SICKNESS				
PARTIAL DISABILITY				
ACCIDENT				
SICKNESS				
WAITING PERIOD				
ACCIDENT				
SICKNESS				
BENEFIT PERIOD				
ACCIDENT				
SICKNESS				
SUPPLEMENTARY BENEFITS				

(continued)

Figure 18-2: Sample form for recording health insurance information.

It is suggested that policies should be examined personally. The following information should be recorded on this page.

MEDICAL EXPENSE				
MEDICAL EXPENSE POLICY NUMBERS				
NAME OF INSURANCE COMPANY OR SERVICE TYPE PLAN				
INSURED				
OWNER OF POLICY				
PREMIUM COST AND MODE				
TYPE OF CONTINUANCE OR RENEWAL PROVISION				
TERMINATION DATE FOR CHILD COVERAGE				
BASIC HOSPITAL				
ROOM RATE				
NO. OF DAYS				
HOSPITAL EXTRAS				
OTHER BENEFITS				
SURGICAL				
MAXIMUM				
TYPE OF SCHEDULE				
MAJOR MEDICAL				
DEDUCTIBLE				
PERCENTAGE PARTICIPATION (COINSURANCE)				
INSIDE LIMITS				
OVERALL MAXIMUM				

Figure 18-2: Reverse side.

References

1. Hubner S, Black K Jr. *Life Insurance*. New York, NY: Appleton, Century and Crofts, Meredith Corp.; 1969
2. Gregg D. *Life and Health Insurance Handbook*. Homewood, IL: Richard D. Irwin, Inc.; 1964

Bibliography

Committee on Medical Liability. *An Introduction to Medical Liability for Pediatricians*. 4th ed. Elk Grove Village, IL: American Academy of Pediatrics; 1989

Checklist

✓ Have you enlisted the help of a competent insurance broker as well as an attorney and/or accountant to advise you of your insurance needs?

✓ Did you fill in current information for all the insurance forms displayed in this chapter?

✓ Will you review and update these forms on a yearly basis?

✓ Are your policies in a safe location?

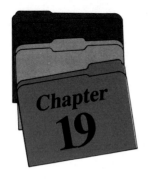

Professional Liability and Risk Management

Chapter 19

An effective risk management program enlists the help and raises the awareness every member of the health care team. Good risk management:
- **identifies and responds promptly to incidents that may result in potential liability and initiates efforts to protect against future risk**
- **systematically monitors practice patterns**
- **includes adequate insurance protection**

CASE #1. Dr H.D. saw a "drop-in" 3-year-old at 1600 hours with a history of mild URI for 2 days, reduced fluid intake and a fever of 39.6°C. Her mother had planned an overnight trip, and simply wanted her "checked out." The remainder of the history and physical were within normal limits; symptomatic therapy was prescribed, but no antibiotics.

At 0715 the next day, Dr H.D. got a phone call from the state capitol some 80 miles away; the 3-year-old had had a terrible night and had been vomiting since 0400. She was febrile, ("I forgot the thermometer!") and seemed to be "really different." He advised immediate dispatch to the nearest ER, which he called and alerted. On arrival, the LP was positive. Successful treatment was instituted promptly, but the child emerged with significant hearing loss. Her parents initiated negligence action.

CASE #2. Dr L.L., a member of a three person pediatric group, had been alerted about an impending "repeat C-section" and was in attendance; the 2250gm infant appeared to be well, and was transferred to the observation nursery. There he continued to do well, according to a nurse responding to a call-back at 1750 hours, just as the office was closing. Dr L.L. advised the nursing staff that she was on call that evening and could be reached via beeper. At 1900 hours, the infant's clinical condition began to change, with rapid onset respiratory distress, a fall in body temperature and sudden fluctuating pallor. Repeated attempts to contact Dr L.L. brought no response. When the night staff came on duty at

2240, a call was placed to one of Dr L.L.'s associates, who came in immediately and made a tentative diagnosis of Group B strep sepsis. Therapy was unsuccessful and the infant expired. A suit was filed against both the physician (whose beeper battery had "gone dead") and the hospital.

CASE #3. Dr H.M. received a telephone call from the mother of a long-standing patient at about 2200 hours. Her 9-year-old son had come home from school complaining of malaise. He had lounged about for several hours and declined dinner. His mother had not been alarmed, since "flu" was running rampant at school. He had retired at the usual time, but awakened suddenly with abdominal discomfort and nausea, and had vomited once.

"No! There is no area of tenderness like there was with Larry when he had his appendix out," his mother declared. Despite her certainty, Dr H.M. asked to see the boy but the mother declined, and seemed reassured that the course was indeed compatible with the flu. She promised to call back if things got worse.

Allegedly, things didn't get worse until the next afternoon, when instead of calling, the mother took the child to the nearby ER because of sudden onset "pain like Larry had!" He was admitted and successfully treated surgically without complications – excepting a physician's gratuitous comment that Dr H.M. was "guilty of malpractice for not having seen the patient at the time of the original phone call." No suit followed, but the subsequent medical staff credentials committee inquiry was stressful and time consuming.

These three actual cases are presented to illustrate the physician's dilemma.

It is an unfortunate fact of today's pediatric practice that a professional liability claim or suit may be brought against you. No longer is pediatrics among the "safe" specialties, and the incidence of claims against pediatricians is rising. While hospitals and emergency rooms continue to predominate as the most likely sites of potential liability, office practices are seeing increasing pediatric claims. It is a myth that only "bad" doctors get sued. In fact, the highest frequency occurs in the mid-career practice years to respected, board certified, and competent pediatricians.

In 1987 and 1990, the American Academy of Pediatrics conducted two surveys which analyzed pediatricians' experiences with medical liability.[1] Survey results showed an 8.9% increase in the percentage of pediatricians who said they had a claim or suit brought against them for malpractice. In 1987, 26.9% of respondents reported that a claim or suit had been filed against them for malpractice; in 1990, 29.3%. The average number of years in practice among pediatricians who had been sued remained stable; 18.0 years in 1987 compared to 18.6 years in 1990. The average time lapse between the occurrence of an incident and when a claim was filed increased by almost 25%; from 30.2 months in 1987 to 37.9 months in 1990.

The proportion of pediatricians reporting cases that were either settled out of court or dropped later by the plaintiff decreased in 1990; 31.2% of pediatricians reported their cases were settled out of court in 1990 (compared to 36.7% in 1987) and 29.8% of pediatricians reported their cases were dropped later by the plaintiff (compared to 35.9% in 1987). Conversely, survey results showed increases in two related areas during this time period. In 1990, nearly 10% of pediatricians reported their cases were defended successfully in court as compared to 0.5% in 1987. The 1990 survey also found that more than 29% of pediatricians reported cases still in progress, as compared to 24.9% in 1987.

As in 1987, the majority of 1990 respondents (53.1%) reported that a claim or suit was initiated by a patient who was not seen regularly by the pediatrician. Nearly a third of those were coverage situations.

Survey data by specialty were also collected, and in 1990 nearly 56% of those pediatricians reporting a claim or suit for malpractice were in general pediatrics. Also in 1990, slightly more than 34% of those pediatricians reporting a claim or suit for malpractice indicated other subspecialties, with clusters in neonatology (8.0%), surgery (5.5%), and allergy (5.0%). No other subspecialty represented more than 3% of pediatricians reporting a claim or suit for malpractice.

Common sources of claims and suits

Certain pediatric activities appear to generate more claims than do others. Perinatal catastrophes, "failure to diagnose," (especially meningitis), pharmaceutical misadventures, improper procedures or immunizations, and missed anomalies head the list. In hospital cases, often the attending physician, consultants, and residents are named when a suit is filed. Unfortunately, involvement in suits is often triggered by careless remarks or criticisms by one physician of another. Attorneys engage in a process called "discovery" in which, by naming everyone whose name appears in the record, they attempt to determine who is responsible for the alleged negligence. As this process unfolds, many of the uninvolved named defendants may be dropped. Even if you are named but not involved, beware of what you say or do, since you may inadvertently harm the defense of your colleagues, or may even succeed in involving yourself. Always seek legal advice in such matters.

Risk management – loss avoidance

A good risk management program is good medicine and effective risk management helps in preventing lawsuits.

At least one member of every pediatric group should participate in local loss prevention education. Health care associations and insurance carriers sponsor programs and produce materials to help the practicing physician identify vulnerable practices and act appropriately. These groups are able to analyze claims on a physician and group basis and develop approaches to minimize recurrence.

Risk management education centers on several basic themes. A recent review of lawsuits filed in Washington state[2] identified key areas which all pediatricians need to address.

1. Physician-patient communication

It is thought that caring physicians are less likely to be sued, even when a negligent act has occurred. An apology, which admits no responsibility for the imprecise science of medicine, along with your considerate and supportive efforts, strengthens your relationships with the patient and family at a crucial time. They will understand and remember that while you are not perfect, you are caring and compassionate in their time of need.

Faulty interactions with patients and family members set the stage for allegations of negligence. When a problem arises, think about and analyze what happened. Then devise a plan to prevent recurrence. Reflect on your spoken, written and body language; raised eyebrows can trigger a negligence action. Then devise a plan to prevent recurrence. A startling number of pediatric malpractice suits relate to telephone management. Keeping the anxious parent on "hold" is fraught with problems. A delay in response to a call on the "beeper" can exasperate the distraught ER nurse. When dealing with patients in the office, remember that a piece of paper with a written instruction can serve as a valuable adjunct to verbal advice.

The pediatrician should conduct a periodic critical analysis of what might be done to improve patient communication, and seek to raise staff awareness through example and formal instruction. Be certain that your staff members conduct themselves professionally at all times. They should demonstrate consistent professional support, not only toward one another but toward all health care professionals.

2. Informed consent

Today's patients, including children and their parents, expect to participate in health care decisions. This is known as informed consent, which should always be obtained prior to treatment and documented in the medical record. To accomplish this, the patient/parent cannot give informed consent unless he or she understands (1) the procedure; (2) the attendant risks; and (3) the alternatives. The pediatrician should share risks and benefits of all treatment alternatives, including, if reasonable, the "wait-and-see" route. Patients should be encouraged to ask questions. This ensures that the patient has enough information to make an informed choice. In addition, pediatricians should check state laws concerning informed consent.

In pediatrics, immunizations are a sensitive area. Not too long ago, physicians relied on "implied consent," eg, many assumed that the patient consented by virtue of coming to the office. Today, especially for immunizations, implied consent is no protection against an allegation of professional negligence. The 1986 National Childhood Vaccine Injury Act (42 USC 300aa) made no specific reference to informed consent requirements, but provided for development of vaccine information materials by the CDC. Once these are finalized, pediatricians will be required to distribute them when administering a vaccine. Until these are finalized, the "Important Information" statements on immunizations developed by the federal Centers for Disease Control (CDC) and used by public health facilities can be employed in the private setting. Information material does not take the place of informed consent.

3. Clinical and laboratory error

Under this rubric falls "failure to diagnose," which is aimed not so much at the outcome as at the process. The pediatrician who visits the patient with abdominal pain, conducts a careful

Suggestions for Pediatricians That May Help Prevent Medical Liability Lawsuits[6]

1. Maintain complete, accurate and unaltered records which can be defended in court.
2. Document all conversations with parents regarding significant complications of treatment.
3. Establish rapport with patients and both parents if possible.
4. Make follow-up telephone calls to patients or parents when you are more than usually concerned about the patient's condition.
5. Provide written instructions to all allied health personnel in your office regarding the extent of their responsibilities, and provide frequent, periodic, in-service training for personnel.
6. Provide adequate supervision for any staff members who perform medical office procedures, especially injections.
7. Provide legible written and/or printed instructions to patients when treating illnesses.
8. Insist on consultation when necessary for good patient care, and document this recommendation. Welcome consultation when requested by a parent or patient.
9. Answer all patients' or parents' questions to their full understanding and satisfaction.
10. Respect the patient's right of privacy regarding release of medical records. Obtain written consent prior to releasing any medical records to anyone, including third party payers. Remember that patients have the right to receive copies of their records, whether or not their bill is paid.
11. Never guarantee the outcome of treatment; either orally or in writing. "Don't worry," or "He'll be all right" may be perceived as verbal contracts.
12. Avoid criticizing treatment by other health care personnel in the presence of patients or parents.
13. Be willing to discuss fees when necessary and avoid overzealous fee collection methods. Frank, compassionate discussions about the fees and reasonable solutions for their payment may prevent a lawsuit.
14. Keep all records until the expiration of the statute of limitations, plus the time under the discovery rule applicable to children. (This period may be as long as forever.)
15. Be sure to display prominently in the chart all the patient's known drug sensitivities. Routinely ask patients or parents about drug sensitivities prior to all injections and prescriptions. Mention the name of the drug when writing a prescription. And watch out for decimal place dosage errors.
16. Inquire about current medicines the patient may be receiving before prescribing another medication.
17. Maintain a properly stocked emergency cart in your office. It must be properly organized, labeled, and readily accessible so there is no delay in administering emergency treatment.
18. Pelvic examinations without a female attendant present is inviting risk in all circumstances. Generally, complete physical examinations may require the presence of a third party.
19. Treatment by telephone involves risks and should be performed only with extreme caution. Treatments prescribed by telephone should be carefully recorded in the patient's chart.
20. Patients with chronic illnesses should be seen regularly to ensure proper supervision.
21. When multiple providers are involved in the care of any child, one physician should be designated as "primary" to coordinate the care of the child.
22. Maintain professional skills through continued medical education.
23. If you send a seriously ill child to the hospital emergency department, strongly consider accompanying the patient until he/she is in the hands of staff at the receiving facility.

examination and reexaminations as indicated, and performs appropriate laboratory and radiologic tests, can "miss" the diagnosis and still not be considered culpable of malpractice if the process was thorough and complete. Therefore the pediatrician should establish a protocol to ensure consistent standards for quality laboratory work. All laboratory and x-ray reports should be reviewed and initialed by the responsible pediatrician. Equally important, all staff members should follow a prescribed method to conduct, communicate and record laboratory and x-ray tests.

Good practice management respects the process component and its documentation. We all function as components of a health care system, and in any system, components can fail. Poor communication among pediatricians who cross-cover, unreported laboratory results, answering service errors and misplaced medical records are among elements of "systems failure" that can set the stage for a malpractice action.

4. Perinatology

Perinatal care has an intense emotional aspect. A century ago, the public and the profession "expected" many mothers and more babies to have major problems as a natural consequence of the birthing process. Today, those expectations have changed, and parents are deeply shocked by any untoward perinatal event. Pediatricians must be particularly sensitive to parents' anxieties and expectations.

5. Medications

Many medications have a very small window between pharmacologic effectiveness and toxicity. Many of their names sound the same. Many are available in multiple dosage forms and many interact in the human body with unexpected results. Pediatricians cope with enormous variations in body size and therefore dosage amounts: the chance of error is both real and ever-present. Studies show that the likelihood of error is a function of the square of the *number* of drugs that are being used, so care in prescribing is imperative.[3]

6. Documentation

Information in the medical record must be accurate, thorough and complete. Height and weight should be recorded methodically. The pediatrician should take the time to note instinctive observations regarding health status. Is the infant alert and playful? Does the child maintain good eye contact? Did you discuss and share allergy warning stickers and other patient education materials? The most automatic observations and informal discussions can enlighten third parties in retrospect.

It is equally important to note what did *not* happen. Did a parent decline to come in for recommended consultation or fail to comply with a specific regimen? Did you discuss your reservations regarding third party denial of a recommended procedure? Are you monitoring a potential problem which will not be evident for some time to come? Write it down!

The modern medical record is a therapeutic history as well as a document that frequently finds its way into legal proceedings. Third party payors, utilization reviewers, quality assurance coordinators, disciplinary board examiners, judges and juries have an interest in the contents. Numerous people are making entries, to document events, conversations and telephone instruction. Legibility is imperative and abbreviations must be clearly defined. A dictated and accurately transcribed entry is far superior to a terse scribble. Documentation of telephone calls, including after-hour and on-call communications, laboratory and x-ray results, and hospital admission and discharge summaries, merit special attention. (See Chapter 10, Office Medical Records.)

7. The role of the expert witness

The courts rely upon expert witnesses to help juries understand the standards of practice as applied to a given case. The expert witness must take care to ensure that such testimony is accurate, thorough and impartial.

The Academy has developed guidelines for members who assume the role of expert witness.[4] These should be reviewed in detail by those who anticipate involvement in litigation.

Briefly, the guidelines specify that experts should have current experience and ongoing knowledge in the clinical areas under examination. They should be familiar with practices at the time and place of the episode, and the details of the occurrence. Testimony should evaluate performance in light of generally accepted standards, and should not exclude any relevant information to create a view favoring either party.

The Academy points out that an expert evaluation will distinguish between medical malpractice, for which a physician may be held culpable, and medical malooccurrence, a reflection of medicine as an inexact science. It will seek to determine whether an alleged substandard practice was causally related to an undesirable outcome.

Expert witnesses should comply willingly with requests to submit transcripts of testimony for peer review.

8. Peer review

Peer review is fundamental to quality assurance and effective continuing medical education. Both government and private peer review came under scrutiny in the late 1980s, when censured colleagues accused members of peer review bodies of conspiracy to limit competition.[5] The Federal Trade Commission, as well as "injured physicians," sought legal remedies. Some suggested that physicians participating in peer review could be liable.

To address this, the federal Health Care Quality Improvement Act of 1986 (42 USC 11101) holds harmless peer review participants who show good faith and meet due process requirements. That Act also established the National Practitioner Data Bank, a central masterfile of disciplinary actions and malpractice awards or settlements. Medical licensing and disciplinary boards, hospitals, malpractice insurance entities, and professional associations must report to this data bank any final disciplinary actions or payments resulting from alleged malpractice. Hospitals must consult the bank at least every 2 years for reports on staff members.

9. Ambiguous situations

Professional liability insurance carriers often have conflicting policies about coverage for activities beyond the scope of your usual practice. It is important to clarify your carrier's policy provisions concerning that, as well as voluntary, nonemergency work as a medical advisor to community groups, day care centers, summer camps or athletic teams. Coverage for ancillary services, such as an office pharmacy, should also be discussed. Many states hold physicians harmless for "good samaritan" emergency care except in the case of gross negligence.

10. State statutes and professional standards of care

Each state regulates physicians under a body of law commonly known as its medical practice act. Courts judge medical malpractice cases in accordance with a professional benchmark termed the "standard of practice" or "standard of care."

At one time, the courts followed a "community standard," which held that physicians would be liable for treatment, or lack of treatment, which violated standards of practice of reasonably competent physicians in the same or similar circumstances with comparable training and experience. More recently, with the wide dissemination of advanced technologies and information about medical treatments, the courts have generally held all pediatricians to a national standard of care.

The pediatrician has a duty to understand and meet state statutory requirements related to medical practice, as well as national and community standards of care. A breach of that duty, if it is the cause of measurable damage to the patient, may constitute malpractice. State statutes can be obtained from your state medical society, and material on guidelines for care through the chapter, district, and national offices of the Academy. It is also wise to review the Academy's Medical Liability Manual.

Professional liability insurance options

Professional liability insurance should not be considered discretionary. Without it, personal assets are at real risk. Liability insurance is designed to pay for the cost of defending you as well as indemnification in the event you have a judgment or settlement entered against you. The various liability insurance options are described below. The Academy can assist you in determining how to identify carriers and what limits of coverage are advisable.

Liability insurance generally takes two policy forms: the traditional (and increasingly rare) "occurrence" policy and the more contemporary "claims-made" vehicle.

An occurrence policy is purchased to cover all events or claims occurring while the policy is in force, regardless of when they're filed. If a physician who retires in 1995 is sued in 1998 for an event in 1992 when he had an occurrence policy, he's covered. This traditional policy form has become less readily available in the wake of exploding malpractice awards and dwindling reinsurance.

A claims-made policy is issued yearly and covers claims which occur and are filed during a covered year. Initial premiums may appear to be significantly lower than quoted averages, because the claims-made premium structure matures over the first 5 years of coverage. Claims-made premiums do increase dramatically in each year of this maturation process.

The claims-made form requires purchase of a "tail" policy upon retirement, which will protect the pediatrician from liability for past events. (In each state, a "statute of limitations" stipulates the number of years allowed to file suit after alleged injury occurs.)

Claims-made insurance also provides "nose" policies covering prior events for those changing claims-made carriers. Also, some build tail coverage into the annual premium, so that long-term policyholders are automatically awarded a tail policy upon retirement, without paying a premium.

Coverage and carriers

Coverage levels

Pediatricians planning to join a group practice should discuss the issue of professional liability insurance, including (if the policy is claims-made) who pays the tail. Ordinarily, every member of a group is insured by the same carrier for the same amount of coverage, and the group is also insured collectively.

Most practices, hospitals, medical staffs and alternative delivery systems (HMOs, PPOs) require that each member obtain a specified level of coverage, so that none are exposed to needless financial risk.

Coverage options

Malpractice insurance coverage options fall into three categories: self-insurance programs (either physician or hospital/group sponsored), commercial insurance programs, and risk retention groups.

Physician-owned companies, which represent 65% of the market, are a form of self-insurance. Most are

organized within a given state, often by the state medical society. Most of these companies have fared well and have adequate reserves for anticipated liabilities. Most are nonprofit, so any excess reserves which accumulate accrue to benefit the insured physicians. Physician-owned companies are generally managed conservatively. Their underwriters avoid risk, and shy away from aggressive marketing or severe premium discounting. Some hospitals and large groups have established "self-insurance" programs, reserving money to pay out claims up to a certain dollar amount.

Another alternative is coverage from one of the remaining "commercial" insurance carriers. Some companies have developed arrangements with state medical associations to provide many of the options provided by physician-owned carriers, such as dividends and premium discounts for participating in "risk management programs." Others tie the malpractice coverage to the physician's total insurance package.

Both the self-insurance carriers (including hospitals) and the commercial carriers depend on "reinsurance," ordinarily from London-based conglomerates, to provide your total malpractice coverage. That market plays a surprisingly large role in setting premiums and reserves.

In the past few years, another option has appeared – the "risk retention group." Set up under the federal Risk Retention Amendments of 1986 (15 USC 3901A) a risk retention group permits groups of professionals to pool their risks. These companies can obtain licensure in one state and then do business in any state without falling under the jurisdiction of local insurance commissioners. This option should be carefully researched and examined. Areas to investigate include adequacy of capitalization, ability to obtain reinsurance and protection under state "guarantee funds" should bankruptcy occur. Contact your state insurance commissioner for more information.

Working with your insurance carrier

Careful research into carriers and coverage levels will pay off quickly in the event of a claim or suit. The right coverage and appropriate carrier are all-

important when a professional liability action is threatened. And full cooperation can greatly expedite your case.

What to report

Early reporting of suspected claims permits the carrier to build a defense when events are fresh; as in most things, there are no penalties for being early!

Notify your insurance company immediately of unanticipated complications, requests for medical records of possible problem cases, or contacts from attorneys. (However "informal" they may be, let your insurer handle them). If you feel that a patient is dissatisfied, or a patient fails to follow-up for further treatment of complications, document that in the chart and notify your carrier. Let your carrier know of any request for a deposition, however innocuous it may seem, as well as any instances when a possibly dissatisfied patient fails to pay the bill for services. (Do not agree to write off your bill or offer compensation.) And finally, report receipt of any legal notice or document, whether or not you are a named defendant.

Assisting your claims examiner

The insurance company will assign your case to a claims examiner, who will attempt to gather all pertinent data. Often, physicians are asked to prepare a narrative summary or what has happened; do this while events are fresh in your mind.

When contacted by an attorney, you will likely be asked to forward a copy of the medical record, x-rays, slides or specimens. (Never release records without written authorization from the patient.) A review of your record will undoubtedly reveal defects; avoid the temptation, however, innocent, to add or delete information. *Never* alter a medical record. Your records will be examined by forensic document specialists, and if any tampering is revealed, your case is hopelessly compromised. Retrospective notes or memos in the patient's chart are equally inappropriate. Establish a separate litigation file for notes pertaining to the case, and lock it in your desk or take it home to avoid inadvertent release of its contents.

Before meeting with your claims examiner, thoroughly review your record. Be a devil's advocate; look for potential weaknesses and construct counter-arguments. Reflect honestly on your clinical judgment, and identify the best authorities in the field who might provide expert support for your actions.

Working with your defense counsel

The insurance company will assign an attorney to represent you. Be candid with your attorney; surprises at trial can be catastrophic. Expect time consuming written questions, depositions and other legal procedures.

Your defense attorney will advise you about proper conduct in discovery and at trial. Trust your counsel and take any advice to heart. The legal system is highly complex and you have much to learn from your attorney. Cooperate fully and make it clear that you are eager to assist him or her in building a successful defense.

At the risk of being redundant

The first rule of insurance relations applies to all carriers and policy forms: the pediatrician who suspects a problem or learns of "intent to sue," should immediately contact his/her malpractice carrier. Never contact the patient or plaintiff attorney, and never alter the medical record. Your carrier is best qualified to advise you on the appropriate approach to minimize exposure or avoid worsening the problem.

The following points are recommended in the event of a threat of a malpractice claim or suit.

1. Report immediately to your insurance carrier. After reporting, discuss it only with your claims person or attorney assigned to your case.
2. Be an active participant in your defense. Meet with your attorney early on and cooperate with his or her requests. Review the alleged incident in detail, and assist with research on the problem. Offer to interpret medical terminology and procedure, and to identify qualified experts for the defense.
3. NEVER ALTER A RECORD!
4. Never independently offer settlement to the patient.
5. Never talk with the plaintiff's counsel unless your attorney is present to represent you.
6. Establish a separate litigation file under lock and key. Do not place documents pertaining to litigation in the patient's file. (Preserve attorney/client privilege).
7. Sign no documents except on advice of counsel.

8. Immediately forward "notice of intent to sue," "summons and complaint," and subpoenas to your insurer upon receipt. They require timely responses.
9. If the patient remains under your care, continue to provide your very best care. Do not discuss the pending lawsuit with the patient or family.
10. DO NOT PANIC. The process is long and arduous (4-5 year period from claim to adjudication is not unusual). Prepare yourself and your family to deal with this hardship and attempt to minimize its impact on the quality of your lives.

A word about stress

Professional liability comes with the territory; the finest practitioner on earth is vulnerable to a medical malpractice suit. A solid risk management program can enable the pediatrician to anticipate potential maloccurrence and guard against it, but no course, book or lecture can prepare the pediatrician for the emotional impact of a professional liability action.

Recognize that this is a time of great stress, which can continue for years before it is resolved. Seek support from your spouse and interested professional associates. Anticipate a time consuming process which can be both mentally and physically draining. Do not dismiss the value of physician support groups; the opportunity to share experiences can yield valuable insights. Assign to yourself the task of maintaining a healthy equilibrium in your personal, family and professional lives, and make that goal a daily priority.

Consult the American Academy of Pediatrics

There are support services available for pediatricians and their families undergoing this trauma. For further detailed information on what to do in case of a lawsuit and how to coordinate with your insurance company, review the Academy's *Introduction to Medical Liability for Pediatricians*. This 12-page booklet which provides a comprehensive, clear overview of professional liability issues and concerns. While no booklet can take the place of continuing education courses and professional risk management advice, this publication introduces concepts and vocabulary in

an accessible, straightforward format.

Copies are available to members at a cost of $5.00; the booklet is item MA0022 in the Academy's publications catalogue. Orders may be placed through the AAP publications department, PO 927, Elk Grove Village, IL 60009-0927.

Summary

Every pediatrician's routine should incorporate a loss avoidance mentality. Establish and periodically refine a system which promotes awareness of professional liability and effective risk management for colleagues and staff. Carry appropriate insurance and take the time to understand what it covers. Learn to recognize and avoid situations which can lead to the perception of medical negligence.

It is unlikely that pediatricians' exposure to medicolegal interventions will disappear in the foreseeable future. Educating yourself about your legal responsibilities, engaging in quality practice and loss prevention activities, caring about your patients and their families, and keeping excellent records will stand you in good stead in this environment.

References

1. American Academy of Pediatrics, Department of Research. Periodic Survey of Fellows, #10; 1990 and #2; 1987
2. Robertson W. *Medical Malpractice: A Preventive Approach*. Seattle, WA: University of Washington Press; 1985, 79 & 85.
3. Vere DW. Errors of Complex Prescribing. *Lancet*. 1965:1:370-373
4. American Academy of Pediatrics, Committee on Medical Liability. Guidelines for Expert Witness Testimony. In: *Policy Reference Guide: A Complete Guide to AAP Policy Statements Published Through December 1989*. 3rd ed. Elk Grove Village, IL: American Academy of Pediatrics; 1990:209-210
5. Patrick v. Burget, 56 USLW 4430 (US May 16, 1988)
6. Robertson WO, Parker W. The Medical Practice Survey. *Med Malpractice Prev*. 1986;1:39

Bibliography

American Academy of Pediatrics, Committee on Medical Liability. *An Introduction to Medical Liability for Pediatricians*. 4th ed. Elk Grove Village, IL: American Academy of Pediatrics; 1989:9,28

Checklist

Certain basic practice habits, such as those listed below, help to reduce the likelihood of a lawsuit:

✓ Cleanliness, neatness, and professionalism.

✓ Considerate, efficient, and well-trained staff.

✓ Availability for patient access at all times.

✓ Prudent and considerate billing practices.

✓ Careful telephone, prescription, and record management with prompt lab and x-ray follow-up.

✓ Effective communication with the patient and family members.

✓ Consents/refusals for all but the simplest treatments and procedures, explaining in simple risk/benefit terms.

✓ Objective documentation of everything significant. (Document actions taken and actions not taken, and why.)

✓ A good faith effort to follow up missed visits.

✓ Entirely honest and genuinely sympathetic discussion of any patient dissatisfaction, including an unfavorable outcome.

✓ Consultation whenever in doubt.

✓ Appropriate conduct when terminating a patient care relationship. Discuss your decision in person, and document the conversation in the medical record. Follow up with a certified letter, return receipt requested. Allow the patient reasonable time to find a new physician, and talk to the new doctor if you wish. Transfer records promptly.

✓ A professional office environment. Delegate inter-office communications, continuing education programming, routine inservice training (such as CPR review), and emergency cart maintenance to qualified, physician-supervised staff.

✓ Respect for patient privacy. It is crucial that the pediatrician establish procedures to guard against inadvertent release of information without proper consent.

Section III

Clinical Essentials

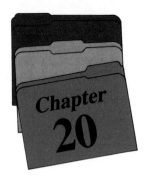

Chapter 20

The Health Supervision Visit

This chapter focuses on the Academy's health supervision guidelines which recommend that:
- a prenatal visit to the pediatrician is desirable
- all of the components of a health supervision visit need to be included in the visit
- relevant anticipatory guidance is especially appropriate for adolescents
- anticipatory guidance and accident prevention should be emphasized

Goals and content of the health supervision visit

A major foundation of pediatrics is its preventive orientation. Pediatricians work toward disease prevention rather than focusing solely on the treatment of an illness through the traditional disease oriented visit. This has been accomplished through health supervision visits, which specifically address preventive issues and teach health promotion activities.

Pediatricians spend almost 25% of their time engaged in health supervision visits. The Academy has developed its own recommendations for preventive care, (Figure 20-1) which represent a consensus of standards which should be met in providing care for a child.[1] Obviously the needs of individual children and their families vary considerably, and physicians and pediatricians may have to vary the content and frequency of these visits to better address their needs.

It is important to have overall goals for a health supervision program. Such goals should include:

1. Health supervision should enable the child to reach his or her full potential. This will maximize the child's level of function, enhance the child's ability to contribute to society, and minimize any burden on society due to a dysfunctional state.

2. Health education should be enhanced with short-term and long-term goals. Short-term goals

include accident prevention, infant and childhood safety, and poisoning prevention. Long-term goals include education regarding development of atherosclerosis, obesity, smoking avoidance, and encouragement of physical fitness.

The foundation for effective health supervision visits can be established by an introductory visit to the practice. Most often this takes the form of a prenatal visit. Such a visit is used to introduce a family to the practice, to establish a line of communication so that parents understand how and when to reach the pediatrician and to enable parents and children to have questions answered in a prompt, efficient manner. This visit also allows the pediatrician to establish the importance of health supervision visits throughout childhood. In addition to prenatal visits, pediatricians should consider offering an orientation interview to families who are new to the practice.

The health supervision visit includes a comprehensive assessment of pediatric development. In addition to the traditional interim and dietary history, physical examination, immunizations and screening tests, it is essential to assess a child's psychosocial development. Further, anticipatory guidance is crucial to enable parents to deal with problems which will occur as the child progresses through development. The physical exam in the health supervision visit is a procedure designed to elicit evidence of disease. In contrast, the physical exam in an acute care visit supports the history and/or demon-

strates the severity of disease.

A health supervision visit should include:

1. A history designed to assess not only physical but interactive problems;

2. A complete physical examination;

3. A developmental and dietary assessment;

4. The enhancement of parenting skills and promotion of productive child-parent interactions;

5. Positive support for parents, especially single parents and parents working long hours;

6. Anticipatory guidance;

7. Specific appropriate screening tests; and

8. A comprehensive plan to ameliorate identified problems, enabling the child to develop to his or her fullest potential.

Providing effective health supervision within the framework of a busy pediatric practice requires organization, effective teaching aids, and innovation. Teaching materials should be given to patients and their families at each visit to orient the discussion during the visit around issues germane to children at that stage of development, and emphasize important issues raised at the visit. The AAP has developed an excellent series on injury prevention targeted by age-group from infancy through adolescence. The Injury Prevention Program (TIPP) sheets are available from the Academy upon request. Appropriate use of these materials, placed in the chart by staff when the visit is sched-

RECOMMENDATIONS FOR PREVENTIVE PEDIATRIC HEALTH CARE
Committee on Practice and Ambulatory Medicine

Each child and family is unique; therefore, these **Recommendations for Preventive Pediatric Health Care** are designed for the care of children who are receiving competent parenting, have no manifestations of any important health problems, and are growing and developing in satisfactory fashion. **Additional visits may become necessary** if circumstances suggest variations from normal. These guidelines represent a consensus by the Committee on Practice and Ambulatory Medicine in consultation with the membership of the American Academy of Pediatrics through the Chapter Presidents. The Committee emphasizes the great importance of **continuity of care** in comprehensive health supervision and the need to avoid **fragmentation of care.**

A **prenatal visit** by first-time parents and/or those who are at high risk is recommended and should include anticipatory guidance and pertinent medical history.

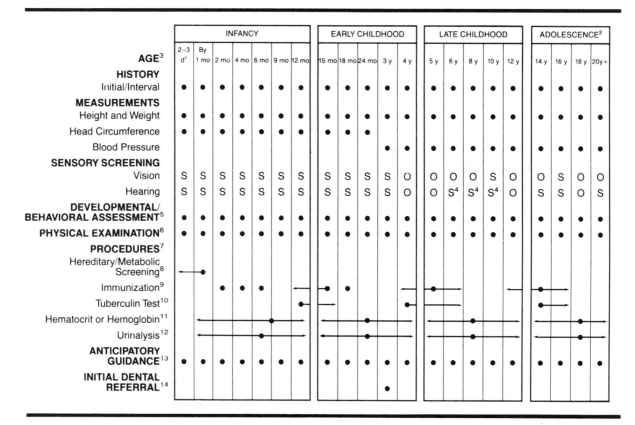

1. For newborns discharged in 24 hours or less after delivery.
2. Adolescent-related issues (eg, psychosocial, emotional, substance usage, and reproductive health) may necessitate more frequent health supervision.
3. If a child comes under care for the first time at any point on the schedule, or if any items are not accomplished at the suggested age, the schedule should be brought up to date at the earliest possible time.
4. At these points, history may suffice: if problem suggested, a standard testing method should be employed.
5. By history and appropriate physical examination: if suspicious, by specific objective developmental testing.
6. At each visit, a complete physical examination is essential, with infant totally unclothed, older child undressed and suitably draped.
7. These may be modified, depending upon entry point into schedule and individual need.
8. Metabolic screening (eg, thyroid, PKU, galactosemia) should be done according to state law.
9. Schedule(s) per *Report of the Committee on Infectious Diseases*, 1991 Red Book, and current AAP Committee statements.

10. For high-risk groups, the Committee on Infectious Diseases recommends annual TB skin testing.
11. Present medical evidence suggests the need for reevaluation of the frequency and timing of hemoglobin or hematocrit tests. One determination is therefore suggested during each time period. Performance of additional tests is left to the individual practice experience.
12. Present medical evidence suggests the need for reevaluation of the frequency and timing of urinalyses. One determination is therefore suggested during each time period. Performance of additional tests is left to the individual practice experience.
13. Appropriate discussion and counseling should be an integral part of each visit for care.
14. Subsequent examinations as prescribed by dentist.

NB: **Special chemical, immunologic, and endocrine testing** is usually carried out upon specific indications. Testing other than newborn (eg, inborn errors of metabolism, sickle disease, lead) is discretionary with the physician.

Key: ● = to be performed   S = subjective, by history   O = objective, by a standard testing method

The recommendations in this publication do not indicate an exclusive course of treatment or serve as a standard of medical care. Variations, taking into account individual circumstances, may be appropriate.

AAP News, July 1991   RE9224

American Academy
of Pediatrics

Figure 20-1: American Academy of Pediatrics recommendations for preventive pediatric health care. This schedule outlines preventive care recommendations for pediatric patients.

uled, provides a context to discuss the patient's specific issues. Separate materials for children and parents may be desirable and complementary.

In group practices, it may be possible to have one member of the group concentrate on health supervision visits on any one day while other members deal with acute care problems. Nursing personnel and other physician extenders may be particularly adept with anticipatory guidance issues and can enhance the efficiency of the process. Some practices address anticipatory guidance problems during group sessions in which families with children of the same age are invited to participate with the pediatrician. A combination of these methods should enable a busy pediatrician to meet the needs of children and families in his practice.

Screening procedures should be anticipated and used for appropriate populations of children.[2] Meticulous documentation of newborn screening should be readily available. Cholesterol screening should be employed in all high risk groups at the present time and its applicability to the general pediatric population in the future depends on additional research information. Free Erythrocyte Protoporphyrin (FEP) and lead screening, as well as sickle cell screening should be considered and used when appropriately indicated.

Documentation

Many objectives are attained during a health supervision visit. Appropriate documentation is critical to record progress and plan for future objectives. The needs of the child can only be met through appropriate record keeping. In addition, third party payors and regulatory agencies have called the benefits of the health supervision visit into question. Documentation detailing the impact of a visit can potentially support the pediatrician's work as child advocate.

All of these aspects of the health supervision visit are addressed in the Academy's manual, *Guidelines for Health Supervision II*. (Figure 20-2.) These guidelines consist of two books: a comprehensive guideline for health supervision providing general background information and a more concise health supervision booklet to guide the pediatrician through specific age related visits. A complimentary copy of this set is available to all AAP Fellows upon request.

Promoting the strengths of children and parents

One of the important outcomes of health supervision is the establishment of a productive physician-patient/family relationship. When health supervision is an important part of the practice, the pediatrician is seen as an authority to seek out during times of stress in the family. This is appropriate, as the pediatrician can best interact with the myriad of other care providers in a community who may work with a child.

To establish this relationship, the health supervision visit must also address the needs of the child's parents. Appropriate recommendations must be made for families in which both parents work. The pediatrician should help single parents find support systems which enable them to meet their needs as well as those of their children. Changes in parental behavior which are constructive must be praised and families who are doing well should receive recognition on a regular basis.

The interaction between children and their parents is readily assessed during the visit. Observing behaviors in the examining room can often serve as a mechanism to reflect upon the adequacy or inadequacy of interaction with parents.

In families with two parents it is important to involve both in the health

Figure 20-2: American Academy of Pediatrics Guidelines for Health Supervision II. *This publication outlines the health supervision components of each preventive care visit.*

supervision visit and to assess the participation of both parents in active parenting. Families who have one dominant parent should be helped to become balanced. To enable a family to succeed, the visit to the pediatrician should be designed to assist parents in growing, developing and learning, so they can reach their full potential in caring for their children.

Anticipatory guidance materials

Total implementation of the health supervision guidelines including anticipatory guidance materials may result in a significant alteration of the pediatrician's practice. Many issues cited in the guidelines are not routinely recognized in some offices during health supervision visits. To integrate all of the material into a practice may take a considerable amount of time. In addition, a complete health supervision visit is time consuming. There may be significant pressures on the pediatrician to shorten the visit to focus on acute problems in other patients. Successful health supervision visits require innovative scheduling and use of all of the personnel in the practice, as well as educational aids to help deal with the large amount of material incorporated into each health supervision visit. (Also see Patient Education Materials, Chapter 26.)

References

1. American Academy of Pediatrics, Committee on Practice and Ambulatory Medicine. Recommendations for Preventive Pediatric Health Care. *Pediatrics.* 1991
2. American Academy of Pediatrics, Committee on Psychosocial Aspects of Child and Family Health. *Guidelines for Health Supervision II.* Elk Grove Village, IL: American Academy of Pediatrics; 1988

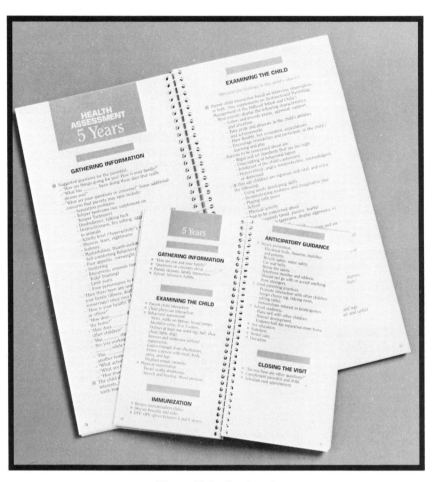

Figure 20-2: Continued.

Checklist

✓ Are the Academy's health supervision guidelines implemented within the practice?
✓ Do you provide anticipatory guidance at each visit?
✓ Do you emphasize the need for continued health supervision as children become older?
✓ Do you provide education aids at each health supervision visit?
✓ Is there time to address new issues raised at each visit?
✓ Are the components of the visit appropriately documented?
✓ Do you encourage prenatal visits?
✓ Are you using the Academy's TIPP Program?

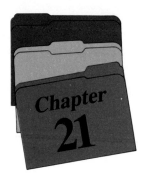

Chapter 21

Office Laboratories and Other Services

The office laboratory is an important part of a pediatric practice. The chapter discusses such aspects of the lab as:
- its location in the office
- guidelines for purchasing equipment
- the importance of trained personnel
- quality control
- examples of types of tests done in many pediatric offices
- safety guidelines
- waste disposal
- the need for a physician lab director

This chapter also discusses the use of an office laboratory in detail, and briefly addresses x-ray and diagnostic services and office-based medication dispensing.

The past 10 years have seen a tremendous increase in the number of laboratory tests that can be done in the private pediatric office. Prepackaged reagents, easier quality control, new testing procedures, and simpler machines which increase the speed and efficiency of testing have contributed to this trend.[1]

Therapeutic decisions in pediatrics have always been based on the history and physical exam of the child. However, those decisions, now more than ever before, are aided by access to laboratory tests that can be done in the office. Both patient convenience and more effective medical care may result when laboratory tests are performed in the physician's office. Office testing provides rapid access to results for the pediatrician and convenience for patients. Coordinated, simplified billing for clinical and laboratory procedures is possible. A potential for increased compliance exists when laboratory tests are performed simultaneously with the office visit. In some communities, laboratory testing in the pediatrician's office will fill an important unmet community need.

It is important, therefore, that pediatricians plan their laboratories carefully. Planning should take into consideration the lab's location, the specific tests that will be performed in the office, quality control measures,

and which personnel should be involved in performing the actual laboratory tests. While the size of the lab, as well as the number and complexity of tests it performs, will vary from office to office, certain factors should characterize all pediatric labs.

Location

The laboratory should be convenient for patients, doctors, and office personnel. Whenever possible, it should be centrally located. A separate blood drawing area contiguous to the lab is desirable. Otherwise, blood drawing should occur in the examining room. The laboratory does not need to be a large room, but should be of sufficient size to accommodate equipment and procedures. Many labs utilize two parallel counters to house the various pieces of equipment. Once calibrated, laboratory equipment should not be moved. A sink is absolutely essential in a lab, as is proper ventilation.

Basic guidelines for choosing equipment

Office laboratory equipment should yield quick, reliable, cost effective, and reproducible results, with a "hard-

copy" print-out. Personnel should be able to perform the tests with a minimum of difficulty.

Laboratory equipment purchases are justified by improvement of patient care, increased office efficiency, and increased patient satisfaction. Obtaining results quickly allows the doctor to make timely decisions about optimal patient treatment; busy parents also appreciate the convenience.

Cost analysis must be done prior to purchasing any equipment, as costs are often greater than the initial purchase price indicates.[2,3] Costs include: (a) supplies (such as syringes, needles, and the necessary equipment for quality control); (b) interest payments when the machine is not purchased outright; (c) maintenance costs (about 10% of purchase price per year); and (d) labor costs, including the personnel needed and time required to perform the laboratory tests, especially if complex testing equipment requiring a certified medical technologist is being considered. Cost analysis should include an assessment of what portion of the practice population will be eligible for office lab tests, since some third party payors require that all lab tests be performed in a contracted reference laboratory.

The decision to purchase an automated machine should be financially justified by projected daily usage. The question which should be considered is: Are these tests medically justified this frequently? Medical indications, not financial ones, should always be the reason for ordering tests.

Once a decision to purchase equipment has been reached, it should be tested carefully in the office prior to final acquisition.

Personnel

There is no question that the accuracy of the laboratory procedure is most affected by, and dependent upon, those

---

Basic Equipment and Tests Required for a Pediatric Office Laboratory Service

Basic Equipment
Microscope
Urine centrifuge
Incubator
Refrigerator
Hematocrit centrifuge or
    hemoglobin analyzer
Culture media
Test kits for individual tests
Single test or multitest machine
    for chemistries and CBCs

Basic Tests*
Urine
Urinalysis (Dipstick
    & Microscopic)
Urine Pregnancy Test
Blood
Blood Glucose Stick
Hemoglobin or Hematocrit
WBC & Differential
Platelet Count,
    Reticulocyte Count
Sedimentation Rate
Sickle Screen
Stool
Occult Blood
Microbiology
Cultures (Throat, Urine, Fungal)
Microscopic Evaluations
    (Pinworm Prep, Vaginal Wet
    Drop Preparations, KOH Prep,
    Gram Stain)
Immunologic
Kit Tests (Strep,
    Mono, Chlamydia)
Drug Level Screening
Theophylline, Dilantin,
    Phenobarbital, Tegretol
Chemistry
Bilirubin, Cholesterol, Glucose

*The indications and justifications for the various lab tests listed are beyond the scope of this chapter.

---

who perform the test.[4,5] A limited number of people should perform all lab work and some practices may require the employment of certified lab personnel. The risk of error increases in offices where all medical personnel perform lab tests. By limiting the number of people involved and insisting on adequate training and supervision on each piece of equipment, test accuracy and reproducibility can be better assured. Every office should have a physician director who oversees the lab and its personnel. He/she should be familiar with all tests being performed in the lab, quality controls, the working of all equipment, and the appropriate procedure to follow should there be difficulty with specific tests. Day-to-day pressures may tempt pediatricians to delegate more responsibility to laboratory personnel, especially certified medical technologists. However, even medical technologists need supervision from an involved physician.

Physicians have a responsibility to ensure the safety of their personnel as well. A strict protocol concerning the handling and disposal of blood and body fluids must be followed.[6] All personnel should be instructed in the proper techniques for handling specimens. Hazardous waste disposal should carefully adhere to state and federal regulations; consult with your local health department for details.

Quality control

There should be no clinically significant difference between lab tests performed in the private office and those of a large hospital lab. This quality can only be assured by following carefully planned protocols. Every office should have a procedure manual in which the technique for performing every test is discussed.[7] This manual should include information about safety guidelines, the method of collecting and disposing of specimens, the type of equipment used, the timing of certain tests (such as drug levels), and the names of outside labs for more sophisticated testing. In offices with automated machines, clear descriptions of instrument maintenance, daily standardization procedures, and methods of performing positive and negative controls should also be in the manual. In addition to daily controls, proficiency testing should be performed on

each machine at regular intervals. Proficiency testing programs are available from several sources. The results of this testing should be carefully documented in a separate log book.

Governmental laboratory regulations

Meticulous attention to detail and careful recordkeeping will assure the highest quality service for pediatric patients. Federal and state regulatory agencies are becoming more interested in monitoring private laboratories.

As presently written, the draft rules for the Clinical Lab Improvement Amendments of 1988 (CLIA 88)[8] would require federal regulatory oversight for all physician office laboratories. The regulations are only in the developmental stage at this writing. They will probably define labs in three categories (waiver, level I, and level II). Significantly increased costs and additional paperwork for documentation will result if the office lab does not qualify for the waiver level. Rigid personnel requirements may preclude office-based testing for certain procedures.

Several states have or will have similar regulations in place which will impact on the office laboratories. It is essential to know the federal and state regulations to ensure that current operations are in compliance and before expanding any laboratory services.

Screening tests

The decision over which screening tests should be done on each patient and at what intervals is difficult. Standardized testing for all patients is critically important. For example, some practices now screen all children for cholesterol. If such screening is done, there should be a detailed office protocol which deals with the level requiring therapy, levels requiring follow-up testing, the schedule for reassessment and the educational materials regarding nutrition and exercise, etc, which should be provided to the patient.[9]

Reporting of laboratory results

Just as pertinent history and positive physical exam findings are important to document in the patients' charts, so, too, is documentation of laboratory work. A copy of the results of the lab work should be entered into the chart. It is often suggested that a second copy be entered in a log book in the laboratory. Any tests sent to an outside lab could also be listed in the separate log book with the following information: patient's name, test draw, date test sent, date results received, and the actual test results. This duplicate copy in the lab will allow the physician access to the results if the chart is misplaced.

X-ray/diagnostic services

Those considering adding x-ray to the practice should recognize that the purchase of x-ray equipment may be a convenience, but it may not be cost effective. The medical and legal ramifications of taking and interpreting x-rays also must be carefully considered. The decision to implement in-office x-ray utilization involves aspects beyond the scope of this manual. A few basic issues are touched on below.

The need for x-ray availability may be a consideration in certain clinic settings, such as rural areas, inner city and suburban clinics removed from hospital-based facilities. The availability of on-site x-ray to make the diagnosis of minor fractures, such as distal radius fracture or fractured clavicle, may certainly improve patient compliance, expedite appropriate therapy, and improve physician time utilization. X-ray can be a profit center; in a clinic setting, however, the prime motive should always be to provide necessary needed services. Considerations include:

Cost of equipment

X-ray equipment is very expensive compared to other capital clinic outlays. Consider the cost of extra space, utilities, housekeeping, storage facilities, a filing system for old films, and ongoing maintenance costs. The cost of borrowing money for such a large capital outlay may also be of concern.

Quality care issues

Personnel

The days of on-the-job training for x-ray technologists are long past and certainly at this time, qualified and licensed x-ray technologists should be employed. Hiring such a person will add costs for labor and ongoing education.

Procedures and maintenance

There will be a need for regular updates and periodic safety checks on equipment. Radiation presents safety problems. A quality care manual and a procedure manual should be developed and monitored.

Reading of films

Proper documentation in the chart, availability of a radiology overread, the need for proper reports, and the mechanics of relaying information back to the physician and then to the patient must be considered.

State regulations

Most states regulate such facilities. Before purchasing and making a decision to buy x-ray equipment, review regulations with proper licensing authorities.

Developing on-site x-ray facilities is a major decision. Taking and interpreting x-rays entails medical and legal considerations that must be considered.

Office-based medication dispensing

Many pediatricians dispensing medications from their offices have found this practice to be accepted enthusiastically by patients. The Academy statement of January 1989[10] indicated that office medication dispensing is acceptable and appropriate as long as the best interests of the patients are served and there are no state regulations prohibiting it. Each practicing doctor will have to make his own decision on this complicated issue, based on predicted patient enthusiasm, possible alienation of local pharmacists, cost-benefit analysis, and concerns over liability.

References

1. Pysher TJ, Daly JA. The pediatric office laboratory. A look at recent trends. *Pediatr Clin North Am.* 1989;36:1
2. Belsey RE, Baer DM, Statland BE, et al. *The Physician's Office Laboratory.* Oradell, NJ: Medical Economics Books; 1986
3. Sander KM. Formulas help determine costs of in-office lab tests. *Am Med News.* Dec 11, 1987:13
4. Gwyther RE, Kirkham-Liff BL. Laboratory testing in the offices of family physicians. *Am J Med Technol.* 1982;48:697
5. Schoen I, Thomas GD, Lange S. The quality of performance in physician office laboratories. *Am J Clin Path.* 1971;55:163
6. Ng RH. Quality performance in the physician's office. *Med Clin North Am.* 1987;71:677
7. Laessig RH, Ehrmeyer SE, Hassemer DJ. Quality control and quality assurance. *Clin Lab Med.* 1986;6:317
8. Notice of Proposed Rule-Making on Clinical Laboratory Improvement Amendments of 1988: Medicare, Medicaid and CLIA Programs (42 CFR 405). *Also see:* Public Health Service Act (42 USC 263a) Clinical Laboratory Improvement Amendments of 1988
9. Groner J. Screening for hypercholesterolemia. *Adv Pediatr.* 1982;29:455
10. American Academy of Pediatrics, Committee on Practice and Ambulatory Medicine. Office-Based Medication Dispensing in Pediatric Practice. *Pediatrics.* 1989;83:143

Checklist

✓ Is your office laboratory in a central location?
✓ Have you performed a cost analysis prior to acquisition?
✓ Are your lab personnel trained in all aspects of lab work?
✓ Is quality control being followed and carefully documented?
✓ Are results recorded in the lab and/or in the chart?
✓ Do you have a laboratory procedure manual?
✓ Is there a doctor in charge of all laboratory functions?
✓ Have you established waste disposal and safety guidelines, procedures, and policies?
✓ Have you researched federal and state laboratory regulations before purchasing new equipment?
✓ Have you considered dispensing medications in your office?

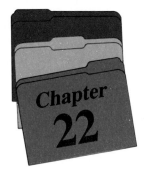

Adolescents and Young Adults

A practice can be expanded to provide more services for adolescents and young adults. This chapter discusses why and how this age-group should be cared for by pediatricians, including:
- physical facilities
- appointments
- confidentiality and consent
- reimbursement
- professional and patient education
- cut-off policies for aging patients

Expanding a practice to include more adolescents and young adults can be both professionally and personally rewarding. It can offer continuity of care to a population and help to fill an unmet community health care need.

The decision to incorporate older patients in a practice will depend on many factors, including (1) community need; (2) present or future practice characteristics; (3) availability; (4) professional preparation and experience; and (5) (perhaps most important) the pediatrician's degree of ease and comfort with patients of this age. There are no insurmountable impediments to expanding the practice to include patients in this age-group if the pediatrician has the desire, the time, and the commitment to do so.

In 1972, the Academy established the pediatric care age range as a period beginning before birth and continuing until the patient is 21 years old.[1] Historically, pediatricians have taken the lead in adolescent health care training, research, and more recently, continuing medical education. Pediatricians are considered the development specialists of medicine and are innately orientated to the dynamics of adolescent maturation.

Pediatricians who have been in practice for a number of years and have had no formal adolescent health care training are experienced in areas of care with younger children which will easily carry over to the older age-group. Many skills not developed during formal training can be acquired easily

through continuing medical education or professional interaction with consultants. The pediatrician does not have to be all things to all adolescents concerning their health care. Even those who practice adolescent medicine as a subspecialty cannot attain expertise in every area of health that pertains to adolescents. Providing care to the limit of professional comfort and incorporating the dimension of case management will be extremely beneficial to the adolescents in the practice.

Adolescents in the practice

Each pediatrician should evaluate current policies regarding the scope of adolescent services, including those concerned with age limits for accepting new and terminating the care of established patients (so-called "new or old patient cut-offs"). These policies have been found to vary considerably (from 12 to 21 years old and older), when they are codified at all.[2] In group practices, some degree of consensus should be reached concerning the extent of adolescent services to be provided and the ages of patients to be served. Regardless of the size or type of practice, there is a definite need to communicate new policies to the office staff, patient families, and professional colleagues. (See Figure 22-1.) Staff attitudes and normal concerns related to controversial types of care (eg, reproductive health care) may need to be

discussed, and educational resources should be provided.

Also, listen to the staff regarding anticipated practical problems in caring for adolescents, and try to generate options for solutions. Problems can occur in the area of facilities and equipment, scheduling, compensation, and public information. The staff needs to reflect the pediatrician's interest in serving older patients and in showing the flexibility and affability necessary to make teens feel welcome.

Physical facilities

The office does not need to be "teen" oriented, but the decor also should not say, "infants and children only." A separate adolescent reception area has many advantages, but it is not a necessity. If space allows, a low planter or aquarium can serve as a divider. Even a small area of waiting space to which older patients can be directed at the time they sign in is helpful, if it has age-appropriate furnishings and reading materials. This creates an initial impression that the adolescent will not be treated "like a kid." Regardless of the reception area limitations, most adolescents value the quality of the office encounter far more than the reception area ambience.

Ideally, there should be separate consultation and examination rooms. Such an arrangement can facilitate the opportunity for the physician to spend some time alone with the adolescent patient,

JOHN J. SMITH, MD, FAAP, FSAM

Pediatrics, Adolescent care

800 Main Street, Anytown 30056
(201) 663-9479

Dear Mr. and Mrs. Jones:

Now that Amy is ten years old and is entering adolescence, there are some things I would like to bring to your attention that are important to ensure the positive continuity of care.

As you are aware, in addition to the physical and sexual changes that are or will soon be taking place, there are significant changes in attitudes and feelings at this age.

During Amy's future visits to the office, I will address her reasons for the visit, and I will explain the treatment plan to her. It is most important that she understand that I regard her as my patient and respect her feelings, wishes, and concerns. As an integral part of this new relationship, we all must be aware of the confidential nature of our interactions. There will be some things that Amy will feel comfortable talking about only to me. I very much appreciate your understanding of the effectiveness of this new adolescent/doctor relationship and I think that Amy will appreciate it as well.

Another goal of this special relationship is to make Amy aware of the importance of her own role in accepting some of the responsibility for her health care. If there are any questions or problems you would like to discuss, I will be delighted to meet with you.

I enjoy treating your children and look forward to many more years of continuing medical care. It is important that we make your adolescent feel at ease. I know we all will continue to be proud of our budding adult as we watch Amy grow.

Fondly,

John J. Smith

John J. Smith, MD, FAAP, FSAM

Figure 22-1: Sample letter for patients entering adolescent care.

a requirement now considered a standard and important component of adolescent health care. The consultation room would contain a desk or similar writing surface, and comfortable seating for the pediatrician, the patient, and at least one other person. The examination room should contain an adult-sized table which can accommodate gynecologic stirrups, a procedure light, a mobile stool for the doctor, and a stationary chair for one other person (parent/friend/chaperone). Somewhere in close proximity, there should be adequate storage space and equipment for measuring height, weight, and vital signs. A single room can be designed and equipped to accomplish both consultation and examination functions provided it contains a writing area, seating for at least three people, and equipment necessary to accomplish complete physical examinations.

Furniture placement creates an important impression. If seating for the adolescent is at the side of the pediatrician's writing area rather than across from it, a barrier is removed and eye contact is more likely; it also is easier to observe body language.

Privacy is essential for adolescents of both sexes when disrobing prior to and dressing after the examination. It is best for the health care provider to leave the room during these times. If that is not possible, these functions should be performed behind an adequate screen or curtain. During the examination it is important to protect the patient's dignity (and modesty!) by utilizing some combination of gowns, sheets and towels to cover body parts which are not being examined. Remember, teenage boys are just as self-conscious about their bodies as are teenage girls.

Appointment scheduling procedures

Time allocation for adolescent appointments varies with the purpose of the visit as it does with other patients. (See Appointments: Scheduling for Patient Care, Chapter 7.) The module appointment system is as adaptable to this age-group as to younger patients. The duration of the office encounter for acute illness is remarkably similar for all ages. Health maintenance visits for adolescents may be somewhat longer than those for younger children, however, because of problems specific to adolescents. The number of modules provided for the various types of adolescent visits will depend on the pediatrician's practice philosophy, but a realistic amount of time should be allocated on the schedule. Adolescent patients do not require urgent care as frequently as younger patients, but there are times when they should have a same-day appointment for nonurgent care. Even visits for sports preparticipation examinations are viewed as "emergencies" when the patient is not permitted to practice until the examination is completed. The complexity of an unanticipated problem may demand additional time, and a return appointment is usually practicable, well accepted, and appreciated.

Adolescents have many demands on their time. In addition to school (which takes much of each day), there may be sports, extracurricular activities, and employment. The staff should be aware of these demands when scheduling appointments, and total visit time should be kept as short as practical.

Special hours

Separate office hours may be useful in creating an ambience of the pediatric practice committing itself to the special needs of teenagers. Whether or not this is practical depends upon facilities and staff. If these special hours reduce time lost from school, extracurricular activities, and work, then they have definite value to the patient.

Adolescents will, at times, have concerns they do not wish to share with the appointment secretary or nurse. Office staff should be sensitive to these concerns. Adolescents need to know that they can ask to speak directly to the pediatrician. Little of the pediatrician's time is usually required, and a potentially "sticky" situation can be promptly and properly handled. Experience shows that most adolescents do not abuse telephone access.

Confidentiality and consent

A major problem in caring for adolescents is that of maintaining parental trust and support while respecting the adolescent's confidentiality and consent. The transition to adolescent care makes it imperative that the pediatrician begin to relate primarily to the patient and secondarily to parents. As Cohen[3] so well stated, "Unfortunately, some pediatricians view this shift in emphasis as an assault on the family and thus adolescent medicine is often cast in the role of anti-family. This could not be further from the truth. To support and interact with a teenager, especially one in trouble, is the ultimate in family support and integral to the nurturing of a stable family unit."

In this context, the conduct of the office encounter becomes extremely important. The adolescent and his or her parents may need to discuss certain issues apart from one another. Private discussion is less awkward if at least part of the visit is conducted with the patient alone. This is well accepted by most parents, even welcomed by them. It affords an opportunity for a freer flow of health issues and, frequently, more decisive management. A discussion of consent and confidentiality is far beyond the scope of this book, but these subjects have been covered elsewhere.[4,5] The pediatrician should thoroughly review the statutes pertaining to treatment of minors for the state in which the practice is located.

The office visit

As just discussed, the adolescent patient needs to experience increasing independence in his or her health care, just as in matters of family, friends, and school. A provision that at least part of the early adolescent's office

visit take place independent of either parent is a significant step in this direction. The feeling that "I am going to the doctor" rather than "my mother is taking me" cannot be underestimated.

Office policy regarding autonomous adolescent visits should be consistent yet flexible. Some patients are ready at 12 years, others earlier, or slightly later. Sex, ethnicity, and psychosocial development are all factors to consider in making this clinical evaluation. The child's and parent's wishes should be respected.

Genital examination

Examination of the genitalia is often stressful, particularly for the female adolescent. Those in the early years often prefer to have their mother present. Those who are older generally do not, but may ask if a friend may remain in the examining room. Whatever increases the patient's level of comfort should be encouraged.

Whether or not a support person is present, it is both useful and prudent to have a staff member/chaperone present. This provides procedural support and obviates any perception of examiner impropriety.

The issue of the pelvic examination continues to be a barrier to pediatricians treating adolescents. Inadequate training and experience coupled with inherent emotional barriers appear to be the real obstacles in the gynecologic care of adolescents by pediatricians. This is unfortunate, but it should not be a deterrent to general adolescent care. The services of an empathic gynecologist may fulfill this need.

Access to effective support resources

The pediatrician may need to collaborate and consult with physicians in other specialties as well as other professionals to meet the needs of some adolescent patients. The same consultants who assist with younger children can often be used in the care of adolescents, but an interest in adolescent problems and some affinity for this age-group are important. Gynecologists, orthopedists, psychiatrists, and some internal medicine subspecialists are among the most helpful consultants. Other potential resources include effective psychologic and counseling services, crisis-oriented organizations, (eg, chemical depen-

dency, rape) social services, public health, school health, and reproductive health care services. However, because both medical and nonmedical resources in many communities are overburdened, there is a risk that patient care may become fragmented and less effective than it should be. This means that, in most instances, case management must remain with the pediatrician.

Hospital privileges

Hospital privileges should not exclude care of adolescent and young adult patients. Most hospitals do not use hard and fast age criteria for privileges, but stress demonstrated proficiency. Explore the need for nonpediatric privileges, which might allow more latitude in the ages of patients hospitalized. An example would be limited psychiatric privileges on an open ward, if available.

Reimbursement considerations

Office-based pediatricians derive income from fees charged for direct as well as ancillary services such as immunizations and laboratory services. Certain adolescent services will be more time consuming than similar services for younger patients. The 16-year-old patient with multiple health concerns and worried parents will take more time than the healthy 2-month-old infant's health supervision visit. There is ample precedent for inclusion of time requirements in your office fee structure. A review of the patient charge sheet or encounter form (See Charging for Services, Chapter 14) will identify areas which require modification. The AMA's *Current Procedural Terminology* manual (CPT-4), which describes useful billing codes, including those for health supervision of patients 12 years and older and for counseling/conference services, can be helpful. The *Pediatric Procedural Terminology* manual, available through the Academy, can be used in tandem with CPT-4.[6]

Problems with realistic third party reimbursement, both public and private, continue to multiply. The Academy is actively engaged in efforts at both the national and state levels to ameliorate inequities.

Resource Guide for Care of Adolescents in Pediatric Practice

Professional Information Sources: General

Felice ME. Adolescent Medicine. *Primary Care.* 1987;14:1

Hofmann AD, Graydanus DE. *Adolescent Medicine.* 2nd ed. East Norwalk, CT: Appleton & Lange; 1989

Litt IF: Adolescent Medicine. *Pediatr Clin North Am.* 1980;27:1

Long TJ, Fitzpatrick SB, Reese JM, and Felice ME. Basic Issues in Adolescent Medicine. *Curr Probl Pediatr.* Oct 1984;14

Marks A, Fisher M. Health Assessment and Screening During Adolescence. *Pediatrics.* 1987;80(suppl):1

Morrissey JM, Hofmann AD, Thorpe JC. *Consent and Confidentiality in the Health Care of Children and Adolescents: A Legal Guide.* New York, NY: New York Free Press; 1986

Neinstein LS. *Adolescent Health Care. A Practical Guide.* Baltimore, MD: Williams and Wilkins Publishing; 1990

Orr DP, and Ingersoll GM. Adolescent Development: A Biopsychosocial Review. *Curr Probl Pediatr.* Aug 1988;18

Professional Information Sources: Specialized

American Academy of Pediatrics, Committee on Substance Abuse. *Substance Abuse: A Guide for Health Professionals.* Elk Grove Village IL: American Academy of Pediatrics; 1988 (Complimentary copy to each AAP member upon request.)

Blum RW. *Chronic Illness and Disabilities in Childhood and Adolescence.* Orlando, FL: Grune & Stratton; 1984

Copeland KC, Brookman RR, Rauh JL. *Assessment of Pubertal Development.* Columbus, OH: Ross Laboratories; 1986 (PREP support materials available from local Ross representatives)

Emans SJH, Goldstein DP. *Pediatric and Adolescent Gynecology.* 3rd ed. Boston, MA: Little, Brown & Co; 1990

Kreipe RE, Comerci GD. *Assessment of Weight Loss in the Adolescent.* Columbus, OH: Ross Laboratories; 1988 (PREP Support materials available from local Ross representatives)

Lavery JP, SanFilippo JS. *Pediatric and Adolescent Obstetrics and Gynecology.* New York, NY: Springer-Verlag; 1985

Lederle Laboratories. Adolescent Wellness Program. (Monographs, videotapes, and pamphlets on drug and alcohol abuse, depression and suicide, and adolescent sexuality available from local Lederle representatives.)

McAnarney ER. *Premature Adolescent Pregnancy and Parenthood.* New York, NY: Grune & Stratton; 1983

Rogers PD. Chemical Dependency. *Pediatr Clin North Am.* 1987;34:275

Strasburger VC. Adolescent Gynecology. *Pediatr Clin North Am.* 1989;36:471

Strasburger VC. *Basic Adolescent Gynecology. An Office Guide.* Baltimore: Urban and Schwarzenberg;1990

Strasburger VC, Greydanus DE. The At-Risk Adolescent. *Adolescent Medicine State-of-the-Art Reviews.* 1990;1:1

General Health Books for Adolescents and Families

(Consider these for reception areas and examining rooms)

Bell R, Wildflower LZ. *Talking With Your Teenager. A Book for Parents.* New York, NY: Random House; 1983

Gross LH. *The Parent's Guide to Teenagers.* New York, NY: MacMillan; 1981

Lauton B, Freese AS. *The Healthy Adolescent: A Parent's Manual.* New York, NY: Charles Scribner; 1981

McCoy K, Wibbelsman C. *Growing and Changing, A Handbook for Preteens.* New York, NY: Perigee; 1986

McCoy K, Wibbelsman C. *The Teenage Body Book.* New York, NY: Pocket Books; 1986

Rosenbaum A. *The Young People's Yellow Pages. A National Sourcebook For Youth.* New York, NY: Perigee; 1983

Schowalter JE, Anyan WR. *The Family Handbook of Adolescence.* New York, NY: Alfred Knopf; 1979

Simon N. *Don't Worry, You're Normal: A Teenager's Guide to Self-Health.* New York, NY: Thomas Crowell; 1982

Winship E. *Reaching Your Teenager.* New York, NY: Houghton-Mifflin;1983

Resources for Education Materials

(Request current catalogs for exact titles, prices, bulk rates; many provide free sample copies; federal sources permit reproduction of materials.)

American College of Obstetricians and Gynecologists, 409 12th Street SW, Washington, DC 20024-2188
American Social Health Association, PO 13827, Research Triangle Park, NC 27709
Center for Early Adolescence, Suite 223, Carr Mill Mall, Carrboro, NC 27510
Channing L. Bete Co, Inc, 200 State Rd, South Deerfield, MA 01373-0200
DIN Publications, PO 27568, Tempe, AZ 85285
Family Life Information Exchange, PO 10716, Rockville, MD 20850
National Cancer Institute, Building 31, Room 10A24, 9000 Rockville Pike, Bethesda, MD 20892

National Clearinghouse for Alcohol and Drug Information, PO 2345, Rockville, MD 20852
National Clearinghouse for Mental Health Information, 5600 Fishers Ln, Rockville, MD 20857
National PTA, 700 Rush St, Chicago, IL 60611-2571
Network Publications/ETR Associates, PO 1830, Santa Cruz, CA 95061-1830
Planned Parenthood Federation of America, 810 7th Ave, New York, NY 10019
Sex Information and Education Council of the United States, 130 W 42nd St, Suite 2500, New York, NY 10003
The Wisconsin Clearinghouse, PO 1468, Madison, WI 53701

Additional Sources of Information

Local/state office of American Cancer Society, American Heart Association, American Lung Association, American Red Cross, March of Dimes, Planned Parenthood, etc
Representatives for pharmaceutical industries including Lederle; Mead Johnson; Merck, Sharp, & Dome; Ortho; Ross; Searle; Syntex; Wyeth

Information and names of consultants in adolescent medicine in your state are available from Society for Adolescent Medicine, 19401 East 40 Highway, Suite 120, Independence, MO 64055
Information about the *Journal of Adolescent Health Care* is available from Elsevier Science Publishing Co Inc, 655 Avenue of the Americas, New York, NY 10010

Education

Printed educational resources are virtually limitless. The Academy has many publications for and about adolescents.[7] The Section on Adolescent Health, open to all members, publishes a newsletter and sponsors a program at the Academy's Annual Meeting. The McNeil newsletter, *Adolescent Health Update,* and as well as a Hanley Belfus, Inc publication titled, *Adolescent Medicine: State-of-the-Art Reviews,* both published in conjunction with the Academy's Section on Adolescent Health, are excellent resources.

The AAP Committee on Adolescence has compiled a resource list for health professionals titled "Sex Education: A Bibliography of Educational Materials for Children, Adolescents, and their Families," which is updated regularly. The Society for Adolescent Medicine (19401 East 40 Highway, Suite 120, Independence, MO 64055) publishes the *Journal of Adolescent*

Health Care. In addition to excellent scientific articles, this journal has a section called "Resources in Brief" which contains reviews of publications for health professionals, adolescents, and their families. Additional educational materials are available from the American Cancer Society, the American Lung Association, pharmaceutical suppliers and other commercial entities. Any pediatrician can establish a comprehensive "package" of educational materials. (See Patient Education Materials, Chapter 26.)

Provide free pamphlets to patients in examining rooms and reception areas. Brochures might cover such relevant issues as menstruation, breast or testicular self-examination, and alcohol or other substance abuse. Patients like to read while waiting and will take home pamphlets that interest them. The pediatrician also might use these pamphlets for anticipatory guidance. (See Resource Guide for Care of Adolescents in Pediatric Practice, Figure 22-2.)

Health questionnaires

Health questionnaires facilitate routine health supervision visits, problem visits, and consultations, regardless of patient age. There is no one best format. Length and scope depend upon what the pediatrician wishes to achieve. It is not difficult to construct a practice-specific questionnaire.

A questionnaire for parents (Figures 22-3) can set the agenda for the visit and identify parental concerns and expectations. The form may be completed before the encounter if mailed in advance. It can also be completed in the office while the patient is being readied.

The patient questionnaire is essentially a health inventory/systems review. It may have varying degrees of complexity and sensitivity. The form can be unisex (Figure 22-4) or gender specific. It, too, should be completed by the adolescent independent of the parent. Confidentiality needs to be extended in ordinary circumstances. Sensitive responses dictate that parents

Parent's Adolescent Questionnaire

NAME_____ DATE _____

This form is to be completed by the parent. This medical information is confidential. Your answers to this questionnaire will help us to better understand and care for your teenager.

		1.	How does he/she relate to his/her parents?_____
		2.	How does she/he relate to siblings?_____
Yes	No	3.	Does he/she accomplish assigned chores reasonably?
Yes	No	4.	Does he/she hold a part-time job?
Yes	No	5.	Does he/she spend most of his/her free time with other teenagers?
Yes	No	6.	Is he/she popular with his/her peers?
No	Yes	7.	Is there any aspect of sex education and/or behavior you would like us to (or not to) discuss with the patient?_____
No	Yes	8.	Is he/she absent more than 2 days of school each month (over 15/yr.)?
		9.	How is he/she performing in school? do you know his/her G.P.A?
			_____
No	Yes	10.	Has he/she ever spoken about the possibility of dropping out of school? Have you ever been advised by the school authorities of conduct problems in school?
Yes	No	11.	Is he/she usually a happy person?
No	Yes	12.	Do you have to discipline him/her frequently?
No	Yes	13.	Has he/she been introduced to the use of alcohol at home or outside the home?
No	Yes	14.	To your knowledge has he/she tried any drugs?
No	Yes	15.	Do you know if the patient is sexually active?
No	Yes	16.	Has he/she been in trouble with the law?
No	Yes	17.	Are you having any marital problems?
No	Yes	18.	Is there any contemplation of separation or divorce?
No	Yes	19.	Is your family under any serious stress?
No	Yes	20.	Do you have hassles with your teenager over homework, curfew, privileges, dating or other areas? (please indicate area).
			_____
Yes	No	21.	Do you think your teenager is developing a good self-image?
Yes	No	22.	Do you participate as a family in church or other religious activity?
Yes	No	23.	Do you approve of his/her friends and do they spend time in your home?
Yes	No	24.	What does the patient plan to do after high school?_____
			_____
Yes	No	25.	Does he/she communicate with you and/or your husband/wife regarding concerns, frustrations and bad feelings? If not, do you know with whom he/she does communicate these problems?_____
			_____
		26.	Is there anything else about your teenager's behavior you would like to discuss?

Please circle any topics you would like to discuss with us:

School problems   Peer relations   Family/marital problems   Sexual development

Contraception   Veneral disease   Developmental problems   Parent-child conflicts

Figure 22-2: Sample parent questionnaire. This questionnaire is completed by the adolescent's parents before care is initiated. The pediatrician follows up on problem areas identified.

Personal Health Review

Date_____ Name_____ Birth Date_____

Age_____ School Grade_____

This is an important part of your medical evaluation. Perhaps it will be easier for you to tell your problems this way. All information will be kept CONFIDENTIAL and will be REVIEWED with you.

Please fill in this form completely. Circle "Yes" or "No".

1. Do you believe that you have a health problem?   Yes No
2. Are you concerned about your height?   Yes No
3. Are you worried about your weight?   Yes No
4. Are you having skin problems?   Yes No
5. Are you unhappy about your appearance?   Yes No
6. Do you have any eye trouble or wear glasses?   Yes No
7. Have you had ear trouble or hearing loss?   Yes No
8. Are you having tooth or gum trouble?   Yes No
9. Have you ever been seriously ill?   Yes No
10. Have you ever been hospitalized, had an operation, or a
    serious injury? Which?_____   Yes No
11. Are you allergic to anything? What?_____   Yes No
12. Do you have more than occasional headaches?   Yes No
13. Do you have more than occasional stomach aches?   Yes No
14. (GIRLS) Do you have any menstruation problem?   Yes No
15. Do you tire easily?   Yes No
16. Do you get short of breath or wheeze?   Yes No
17. Do you have backaches, sore bones, or painful joints?   Yes No
    Which?_____
18. Is it hard to fall asleep or sleep restfully?   Yes No
19. Do you get easily upset?   Yes No
20. Have you ever repeated a school grade or failed a subject?   Yes No
21. Do you and your parents disagree frequently?   Yes No
22. Do you have any questions regarding cigarettes, alcohol, or drugs? Yes No
23. Would you like information concerning any sexual matter?   Yes No
24. Are there any other questions or personal concerns you would
    like to discuss?   Yes No

We wish to see you alone for most of your health care. We also encourage you to call for advice, or for future clinic appointments, and hope that you will feel free to discuss things that trouble you.

Figure 22-3: Unisex adolescent health inventory. This questionnaire is completed by adolescents prior to the first visit. The pediatrician follows up on problem responses.

Young Adult Questionnaire

Date_____ Name_____ Age_____ School Grade_____

This information is Your CONFIDENTIAL Information. The Questionnaire is to be used during your personal conference.

Please take time to carefully answer each question "Yes" or "No".

1.	Do you get along well with your parents?	Yes	No
2.	Do you get along well with your brothers & sisters?	Yes	No
3.	Do you have any assigned chores at home?	Yes	No
4.	Do you have a part-time job?	Yes	No
5.	Do you spend a lot of your free time with other teenagers?	Yes	No
6.	Do you have a real close friend?	Yes	No
7.	Do you have any questions about sex you would like to discuss?	No	Yes
8.	Do you miss more than 2 days of school each month?	No	Yes
9.	Are you doing all right in school?	Yes	No
10.	Are you thinking about dropping out of school?	No	Yes
11.	Is life in general going OK for you?	Yes	No
12.	Are your parents fair about discipline?	Yes	No
13.	Have you been in trouble with the law?	No	Yes
14.	Do your parents get along well with each other?	Yes	No
15.	Is there any contemplation of separation or divorce?	No	Yes
16.	Is your family under any serious stress?	No	Yes
17.	Do you have hassles with your parents over privileges, homework, curfew, dating or other areas?	No	Yes
18.	Do you feel you are the same type of person as your contemporaries?	Yes	No
19.	Do you participate in church or other religious observance?	Yes	No
20.	Do you like to have your friends visit in your home?	Yes	No
21.	Do you do any volunteer or community service?	Yes	No

22. Things I do that make my Mother and Father
    Happy
    Upset_____

23. Some things my parents do that upset me_____
    _____

24. When my parents are upset with me they_____
    _____

25. For my age my maturity is: Physically – behind, average, advanced
                                  Sexually   – behind, average, advanced
                                  Emotionally – behind, average, advanced

26. What do you plan to do when you graduate from high school?
    _____

27. Do you talk over your problems, concerns, frustrations, and
    bad feelings with someone?   Yes   No

28. Are there any other areas you would like to discuss?

29. Have you ever felt like or thought about doing harm to
    yourself or ever contemplated suicide?   Yes   No

Please circle below if you wish to discuss any of the following:

Masturbation   Drugs   Growth & Development Problems Obesity Peer Pressures

Parent-child conflicts   Plans for future careers   Changes I would like

Sexual development   Menstruation   Contraception   Veneral Disease   Pregnancy

Figure 22-4: Sample adolescent questionnaire.

and patients may wish to complete these forms in private.

At first glance, the use of questionnaires would appear to be time consuming. On the contrary, their use should conserve time by focusing on the important issues and identifying others which are critical to the adolescent's well-being.

Community outreach

Assess the need for community services for such problems as institutionalized youth, chemical dependency, school-aged parents, teen athletics, and school or college health. Pediatricians who feel comfortable working in any of these or similar areas can derive considerable personal satisfaction, although financial remuneration is limited.

Marketing and public information

Pediatricians who wish to establish a practice for the care of adolescents or continue to care for their young patients through the teen years must use marketing tools to educate families about the scope of pediatric practice. Many parents perceive their pediatrician as someone who cares for infants and children, and are likely to ask, "How much longer will you be caring for us?" Pediatricians who wish to see adolescents and young adults should make that clear in practice information materials, and discuss age or event cut-off policies openly with adolescents and their parents. Let them know they are welcome in the practice for as long as they reasonably wish to remain.

When a patient leaves the practice

Adolescents and young adults ultimately "outgrow" pediatric health care services. The transfer to adult care frequently follows a relationship between the pediatrician, patient, and family of many years' duration and one in which there may be genuine mutual affection.

How this "break time" transition is made will, to a large extent, determine the continuity of future care, influence the quality of ongoing services, and enhance patient acceptance and satisfaction. A suggested approach might include the following steps:

1. Define cut-off policies for the practice, allowing for some flexibility and discretion (eg, ages 16, 18, or 21, entry into college or work, marriage, pregnancy).
2. Discuss these policies with older patients at some nonurgent time well before the cut-off time.
3. Recommend another physician(s) to assume care.
4. Initiate transfer of pertinent medical information with a cover letter of introduction to the new physician.
5. Assure the patient of availability for health care until the transfer is completed.

References

1. American Academy of Pediatrics, Council on Child and Adolescent Health. Age limits of pediatrics. *Pediatrics*. 1988;81:736
2. Resnick MD. Use of age cut-off policies for adolescents in pediatric practice: Report of Upper Midwest Regional Physician Survey. *Pediatrics*. 1983;72:420
3. Cohen MI. Commentary – Adolescent health: Concerns for the eighties. *Pediatrics in Review*. 1982;4:1
4. Hofmann AD. A rational policy toward consent and confidentiality in adolescent health care. *J Adolesc Health Care*. 1980;1:9
5. Moore RS, Hofmann AD. AAP Conference on Consent and Confidentiality in Adolescent Health Care. Evanston, IL: American Academy of Pediatrics. March 1982
6. American Academy of Pediatrics, Committee on Practice and Ambulatory Medicine. *Pediatric Procedural Terminology*. Elk Grove Village, IL.: American Academy of Pediatrics; 1987
7. American Academy of Pediatrics. *Publications Catalog*. Elk Grove Village, IL: American Academy of Pediatrics; Annual

Checklist

✓ Do you have a strong interest in this age-group? Are you comfortable with this age-group? Can you establish rapport easily with members of this age-group?
✓ Are your office staff and associates comfortable with this age-group?
✓ What is your present age limit policy? How would you modify it to care for more patients in this age-group?
✓ Is your office suitable for or adaptable to this age-group?
✓ Will changes be needed in fee schedules? In appointment scheduling? In office hours?
✓ Do your present hospital privileges allow for hospitalization of this age-group?
✓ Have you considered the issues of confidentiality and consent?
✓ What consultative and community services will you require? Are you thoroughly acquainted with them?
✓ Have you considered more involvement in community-related activities for this age-group?
✓ Do you have a plan for informing patients, their parents, and colleagues of your expanded role in adolescent health care?

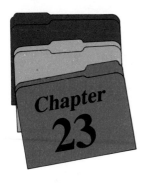

Chapter
23

Allied Health Professionals

Allied Health Professionals are discussed in this chapter from the following perspectives:
- **types of providers**
- **determination of need**
- **utilization and introduction to the practice**
- **responsibility and liability**

"Allied Health Professionals" (AHPs) are professional and technical personnel who interact with physicians. Some of these roles allow for clinical patient care. The first subgroup of AHPs, known as "Nonphysician Providers," consists of individuals who deliver direct primary patient care, usually under physician supervision. It includes pediatric nurse practitioners, child health associates and pediatric physician assistants. The second subgroup includes such AHPs as behavioral specialists, health educators, nutritionists, occupational therapists, physical therapists, psychologists, social workers, and speech therapists.

The AHP nonphysician provider concept is relatively new. Formal education and certification for pediatric nurse practitioners began in mid-1965.[1] Medicine has changed rapidly in the interim; the pediatrician of the 1990s has a very different role from a pediatrician of that era. The ability to delegate tasks and share clinical care has expanded considerably. Newborn and hospital sick care has decreased significantly, while school problems, allergic conditions, and general parent and child counseling have dramatically increased.

These changes reflect social evolution. The increase in adolescent pregnancies, alcohol, tobacco, and other substance abuse, and problems associated with more children in day care are but a few examples of new demands for services. Today, 35% of pediatric office visits are for well child care, 14% for otitis media, 10% for pharyngitis, 8% for pneumonia, and 6% for upper respiratory tract infections.[2] The 1980 Graduate Medical Education National Advisory Committee (GMENAC) report anticipated an expanding role for AHPs. Currently about 5%-7% of pediatric visits are delegated to nonphysician providers.[3]

In these two decades of experience with nonphysician providers, physician and patient satisfaction has been extremely high and liability issues minimal. Still, data shows that the employment of non-physician providers in pediatric offices has stabilized.[4] In the clinic and office setting, nonphysician provider utilization has been limited by fears about professional liability, concern about inability to assist with after-hour coverage, uncertainty of finances, or lack of physician time to supervise. More recently part-time and consultative nonphysician provider relationships have become more common. Many nonphysician providers now serve in hospitals, governmental and HMO positions. Allied health professional of all types now offer valuable resources and personnel in both urban and rural communities. Searching out these local professionals and creating working relationships could enable today's pediatricians to enhance the effectiveness of the office practice.

Need

It is essential to critically assess the need for assistance from allied health professionals, especially if paid employment is being considered. Generally, nonphysician providers are employed to help deal with an increasing patient load. Therefore, the pediatrician should carefully determine how many extra patients would be needed to support a nonphysician provider. The specific duties of each type of allied health professional for whom employment is being considered should be clearly defined. Any allied health professional whose supervision requirements increase the pediatrician's work load without adding any specific benefit to the practice will not enhance practice quality. Allied health professionals should free-up physician time and allow the pediatrician to devote more time to patients who require physician expertise.

Other considerations

The personalities of the allied health professional and the physician must be professionally compatible, since there will be some similarities in the relationship to that of taking in a new associate. A harmonious relationship provides the context for parents to accept and trust the allied health professional, and also affects the parent-physician-child relationship.

Allied health professionals, especially nonphysician providers, can be expensive practice additions. Overhead allocations must be made. Salary cost, especially for an experienced full-time AHP, should be weighed carefully. Freeing-up physician time may be worth the cost, but the pediatrician should realize that the benefits of working with a pediatric nurse practitioner, while genuine, are often not economical. Since nonphysician providers have become more established and professional, physicians can expect requirements for salary increases, paid educational leave, books, and journals, and even profit sharing. Requirements for hospital privileges for nonphysician providers are becoming more complex. Credentialing, supervision and proof of liability coverage are all becoming areas of concern to hospitals.

Often, a part-time pediatrician can be hired for a similar salary. There are advantages to this alternative: a part-time physician can practice independently, (which eliminates AHP supervisory tasks) and provide night call relief.

Many third party organizations do not reimburse for allied health activity. Prior to any employment contract, it is important to discuss reimbursement with third party organizations. Some governmental programs allow allied health care provider billing. Others require that every patient be seen by a physician, in addition to any AHP services.

The role of AHPs

Allied health professionals have both educational and therapeutic roles. Pediatric nurse practitioners can assist greatly in prenatal and neonatal counselling, as well as general routine and sick child care. In many pediatric offices, the physician and the nonphysician providers alternate well child visits, which gives parents additional contact points and enhances continuity for the family. Nonphysician providers with counseling skills excel at telephone management; patients who view their concerns as a waste of physician time are often more comfortable with them. Many states do not allow nonphysician providers to write prescriptions, but if permitted, they can provide this service.

Many allied health professionals write and/or edit office educational material. More pediatricians are using office newsletters to communicate with patients, and various allied health professionals can contribute significantly to these projects. Some alternatives to full-time employment of allied health care providers include utilizing AHPs for leading parent group sessions in the office, case management with physicians, developing specific programs, and conducting inservice seminars on new concepts of improved patient care. A nutritionist, for example, can help office nurses understand cholesterol evaluation and control. After training, the nurses can teach parents the specifics. Difficult situations can be referred to or be managed by the nutritionist. The pediatrician can oversee the program, including lipid testing interpretation, compliance, and outcome.

Types of Allied Health Providers

NONPHYSICIAN PROVIDERS

Pediatric Nurse Practitioners (PNPs)

Some pediatricians employ PNPs to make independent health assessments, to provide health maintenance exams, and to treat illnesses via office protocol. These individuals are registered nurses with additional specific training. The original 1 year certificate programs have essentially been replaced by 1 to 2 year master's programs. Certification by the National Certificate Board of Pediatric Nurse Practitioners and Nurses or the American Nurses' Association is documentation of their skills and knowledge. Each state has specific guidelines concerning licensure, prescriptive privileges, and scope of practice. These are often stated in the Nurse Practice Act, but other laws may apply. Specific guidelines can be obtained from the state Bureau of Examination and Licensure.

Child Health Associates (CHAs)

Trained only at the University of Colorado School of Medicine, this 5-year preprofessional and master's degree program is essentially that of a children's physician assistant. The certification is similar to that of pediatric nurse practitioners. States other than Colorado may not recognize this certificate, and may require them to function as a nurse associate. Any pediatrician planning to work with a CHA should be cognizant of state laws and regulations regarding their potential role within the practice.

OTHER ALLIED HEALTH PROFESSIONALS

Pediatricians have found social workers, psychologists, nutritionists, developmentalists, speech therapists, health educators, occupational therapists, public health and school nurses, and physical and rehabilitational therapists to be excellent sources of information and expertise. This group of allied health professionals can be utilized in the office either in an employment situation or on a specific case management basis. They are especially helpful in a rural situation, most often part-time. State, county, and school district allied health professionals are excellent referral sources. Pediatricians can also find expertise in their own practice. Mothers and fathers with professional backgrounds may volunteer for special projects or patient problems. Before deciding to work with a practice volunteer, careful research into state licensing or registration and supervision requirements is necessary.

Supervision

Whatever the allied health professional's role, the physician must provide supervision. Supervision can vary from availability by telephone or close proximity to prospective chart reviews of each patient.

For nonphysician providers, more intensive supervision is required. Specific treatment protocols can provide both the nonphysician practitioner and the physician with the confidence that guidelines are being met. Protocols are commercially available for a variety of topics, or they can be individually prepared. Quality assurance reviews are necessary; guidelines make this chore easier and more specific. State regulations must be followed. Regularly scheduled conferences are important to explore new areas and review problems.

The physician's supervisory responsibilities can be time consuming. Documentation is essential, especially where required by third party or state regulations. An integrated office chart allows efficient reviews. Cosigning AHP notes may also be worthwhile. Some states formally dictate that physicians cannot supervise more than one or two nonphysician providers.

Liability issues

Nonphysician providers are not generally associated with enhanced liability, but their malpractice rates are rising significantly in some states. Hospital bylaws often require direct physician supervision; the pediatrician should discuss employment of a nonphysician provider with his or her malpractice carrier.

The physician who employs a nonphysician provider accepts responsibility for his or her activities. The pediatrician must conduct regular chart reviews, conferences, and consultations. Protocols are helpful. A good way to document supervisory activities when nonphysician providers handle telephone responsibilities is by initialing the telephone log after review.

Recruitment and introduction of new providers

Advertisements in professional journals and newspapers, letters to training institutions, and personal contacts are common recruitment tools. If the allied health professional is a "first" in the practice, it is important to educate patients and office staff. Shared visits and personal introductions for the first several weeks are helpful. Community newspapers may be interested in featuring this new trend. Adding the new staff member to office stationary, signs, and other printed material promotes acceptance. The physician's demonstrated confidence and trust is readily shared by patients.

An allied health professional employed in a clinical setting can offer improved patient care, and became a key person in building lifelong, mutually satisfying interprofessional relationships.

References

1. Burnett RD, Bell LS. Projecting pediatric practice patterns. *Pediatrics*. 1978;62 (supplement):625-680
2. Hoekelmen RA, Starfield B, McCormick M, et al. A profile of pediatric practice in the United States. *Am J Dis Child*. 1983;137
3. *The Report of the Graduate Medical Education National Advisory Committee*. Hyattsville, MD: Health Resources Administration; September 1980. US Department of Health and Human Services publication HRA 81-656, Volume VI
4. Chapman DD, Matlin NM. Issues in pediatric manpower impacting children's access to primary care in the 21st century. In: *Educating Pediatricians to Provide Access to Primary Care*. Hyattsville, MD: Bureau of Maternal and Child Health and Resources Development; June 1989. US Department of Health and Human Services grant no HRSA MCJ-009094-03-0

Bibliography

American Academy of Pediatrics, Committee on Medical Liability. *An Introduction to Medical Liability for Pediatricians*. 4th ed. Elk Grove Village, IL: American Academy of Pediatrics; 1989

Chapman DD, Hodgman, Johnson RL, Matlin NM. Replacing the work of pediatric residents: strategies and issues. *Pediatrics*. 1990;85:1109-1111. Commentaries.

Council on Long Range Planning and Development. *The Future of Pediatrics*. Chicago, IL: American Medical Association; 1987

Honigfeld LS, Perloff J, Barzansky B. Replacing the work of pediatric residents: strategies and issues. *Pediatrics*. 1990;85:969-976

Checklist

✓ Does your practice meet the demands for services?
✓ Are you capable of delegating health care tasks traditionally in the domain of the pediatrician?
✓ Do state statutes and hospital bylaws provide for activities of an allied health professional?
✓ Is professional liability insurance available for the allied health professional?
✓ Have you considered the issue of off-hour coverage?

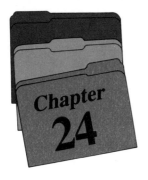

Time Management

Chapter 24

Time is a precious commodity for the pediatrician, his staff and the patients they serve. This chapter explores factors that frustrate and methods to maintain a consistent time management system:
- planning ahead for the efficient use of time
- structuring the office day
- delegating to save time
- minimizing interruptions
- use of special time savers

Proper time management allows the pediatrician to direct and control professional and personal activities. Some challenges are unique to the specialty; some solutions are limited by context. But in any practice situation, an affirmative approach to time management can yield multiple benefits.

Office location

Practice location is extremely important. Proximity to patients is the first consideration; hospital access is also crucial.

Pediatricians usually follow their obstetrical colleagues to the hospitals they use. While the area may support more than one obstetric or pediatric unit, staff privileges may mandate other time-consuming responsibilities, such as emergency room coverage and committee work. For these reasons, only as many hospitals as are needed to support the practice should be utilized. Group practice models may find it possible to provide cross-coverage for morning or evening rounds, which makes multiple staff privileges more reasonable. Cross newborn coverage with other pediatricians in closer proximity is another option.

Driving time is another factor. Time is money and not all travel is cost effective. Is travel from home to each hospital and from one hospital to another a good use of professional time? Weigh the role of travel time in the event of an emergency or the need to attend at a newborn delivery.

Time periods

The day can be broken down into definable parts. For purposes of discussion the day might be separated into:
- Morning
- Lunch Break
- Afternoon
- Evening
- After-hours

Morning

There are two time periods in the morning for most of us, a flexible one and a more structured one. The flexible period may start with exercise, a breakfast with family or peers, an early morning meeting, and/or, more traditionally, hospital rounds. This period is more controllable than the rest of the day and should be safeguarded.

Hospital patients warrant special consideration. When the pediatrician arrives to see nursery charges, babies should be available for examination and the mother should not be in the shower. Parents of children on the pediatric ward should be encouraged to stay overnight. When this is not possible, they should be informed of the time that you generally arrive at the hospital for morning rounds. Phone numbers must be available for those who cannot be present.

Morning office hours signal the structured part of the day. An effective appointment system is critical. (See Appointments: Scheduling for Patient Care, Chapter 7.) It is wise to call patients the day or evening before a scheduled appointment to remind parents of the day and time they are expected. "No shows" will be minimized and appointment errors can be corrected. Mail reminders are less effective.

The office visit should be a relatively controlled event. The pediatrician should make every effort to be punctual. Studies have shown that patients become upset when they have to wait for more than 20-30 minutes in their doctor's office. Promptness is interpreted by parents as caring. Repeated failure to stay on schedule can, for some, be reason enough to change doctors.

Questions to consider when evaluating professional time management

- Do you and your staff get started on time?
- Do you delegate non-physician tasks?
- Does your staff notify you when sick children need to be seen out of turn?
- Are patients properly prepared before you enter the examining room?
- Do you save nonurgent administrative tasks for low-volume days or do you schedule time for administrative tasks?
- Do you use preprinted forms whenever possible?
- Are printed materials for patients readily accessible?
- Is there consistency in the layout of the examining rooms?
- Do you insist on an agenda for all meetings?
- Do you dictate all of your office records?
- Are you interrupted or is your day extended by telephone calls that could be handled by someone else?
- Are interruptions – telephone or otherwise – minimized?

Staying on time requires meticulous office organization. Rooms must be cleaned and well stocked throughout the day. Each practitioner requires at least three examining rooms. Nurses or assistants should be trained to collect and chart preliminary data prior to the pediatric interview. History and standard measurements, (eg, height, weight, head circumference, speech screening, hearing and vision testing) can be carried out and charted before the patient is seen by the pediatrician. The patient should be appropriately disrobed and ready when the doctor enters the examining room. Laboratory work can be done by appropriately trained staff. Finally, the traffic pattern in the office must be conducive to expeditious billing and collection activity.

Lunch break

Time should be made available late in the morning and during the lunch break to return phone messages and complete other unfinished morning business. Occasional meetings can be scheduled during the lunch break, but there should be some pause in your schedule to allow you and your staff to unwind and relax. The road to "burn out" is traveled by some who fail to plan for a bit of respite. The lunch break might also be used for professional or pleasure reading. A brief nap for some can serve to recharge the batteries for the afternoon.

Afternoon

The afternoon is generally approached in the same manner as the morning. Time should be set aside for phone calls, paperwork and correspondence. Many feel that late afternoon is ideal for scheduling longer patient consultations, including prenatal visits, as well as more difficult medical problems and adolescent patients.

Counterpoint

Although late afternoon is a traditional time for longer consults, some pediatricians prefer early morning or lunch time appointments. Whatever the time slot, uninterrupted consultation periods should be designated in the appointment schedule. It is important to select certain times during the day to minimize disruption of patient flow.

Interruptions

Interruptions during office hours are common in a pediatric office. The pediatrician who deals with them effectively can greatly enhance office efficiency.

Emergencies do occur. Cesarean sections, seizures, and trauma occurring during office hours will disrupt the day's schedule. Lacerations, head injuries, and fractures require immediate attention. Office staff should be taught to deal efficiently with emergencies. Each practice should adopt procedures to limit inconvenience to other patients. Office staff training should specify triage guidelines. Rescheduling and reshuffling requires pediatric guidance, but contingency plans should be in place. Parents can more readily accept inconvenience if they know that the doctor has been delayed by an emergency.

When a complex social problem requiring more than a brief office visit is discovered during a routine examination, a consultation should be scheduled to pursue it properly. The patient or parent will most often appreciate your explanation that additional time is required to examine the matter appropriately.

Calls from sales persons, stockbrokers, and insurance agents can effectively be limited to a designated time of the day. Many of these can be screened by the office manager.

The pediatrician should seek opportunities to delegate. An appropriately trained nurse or receptionist can meet with pharmaceutical and medical supply representatives. Your polite "cameo" appearance assures visitors that you will follow through. Standing orders and telephone guidelines enable trained staff to manage most incoming telephone calls concerning growth and development, minor illnesses, and feeding problems. Set aside time to review all calls, at least at the end of the day. (See the Office Telephone, Chapter 8.)

Extended hours

Evening and weekend office hours are valued by the majority of American mothers employed outside of the home. Patients appreciate your availability, and practice income improves with extended hours. The advent of urgent care centers in many communities has made patients increasingly reluctant to

wait until the next day with even relatively minor problems. Some group practices have rotated an evening shift into the schedule.

After-hours

After-hours has always been the bane of the pediatrician's existence. Sharing call and group practice serve to ease the pressure. Expanded office hours will also limit after-hours telephone interruptions.

Time out of the office

Pediatricians must be ever-mindful that a sound personal and family life are the basis for professional success.

Many pediatricians take an afternoon or day off each week for personal business, physical exercise, hobbies, family time, or practice planning. This time is a solid investment in your practice. Of course, appropriate coverage or backup should be arranged. For maximum efficiency, vacation and continuing education time should be scheduled well in advance. Patients will understand time out of the office if there is advance explanation, but have little empathy when asked to cancel an appointment on short notice.

Other time-savers

The chapter on medical record-keeping points out that dictating (as opposed to writing chart entries) conserves time. Dictation is at least six times faster than writing. It is more complete, more legible, and more efficient. The pediatrician spends more time with patients and less with paperwork. Dictation requires some investment in personnel and equipment. With improved efficiency, reports and correspondence that previously took hours can be accomplished in minutes. Dictation should, when possible, be done at the conclusion of the visit. If it waits until the end of a time period, the record is not as accurate and the time advantage could be lost.

Patient education materials to cover information discussed during anticipatory guidance also saves time. Some pediatricians prepare their own, while many obtain them from the Academy, pharmaceutical companies and community agencies. (See Patient Education Materials, Chapter 26.) Favorite books on child care can be loaned or suggested at appropriate times in the health supervision schedule.

The contented practitioner is efficient and well-organized. Careful planning is required to establish a positive, productive practice environment.

Time management techniques

Some time management techniques physicians find to be effective in lowering stress are:

1. Keep a log of your work and outside activities over a 3-day period. Rate your satisfaction with and the priority of each activity. List the major time-wasters. Develop strategies to modify, eliminate or delegate low priority activities and the major time wasters.

2. Plan ahead: Planning both your work and outside activities today means a more relaxed tomorrow.

3. Remember the 80/20 rule: we spend 80% of our time doing activities that accomplish only 20% of the total job results.

4. Keep a daily short-term goal list. Do tough, difficult tasks first, not last.

5. When you have a tight schedule, write down things you will not do.

6. Delegate tasks for which the time needed to complete the work is long in relation to the time to instruct and supervise.

7. Avoid reverse delegation: follow-up on tasks that you have delegated.

8. The waste basket: one of the best places to delegate.

9. Touch paper only once.

10. Schedule time for interruptions for the inevitable fires that must be put out.

11. Plan meetings: have a purpose, an agenda and limit its length.

12. Cut back on activities that are not compatible with your mission and goals.

13. Set goals for changing how you spend your time. Change one thing at a time and ask others to support your changes.

14. Prioritize work and outside activities. Don't let low priority tasks get in the way, no matter how demanding others can be.

The definition of time management is the act of controlling events. We can gain control by selecting the events which have priority and determining the time that we spend with each. (Also see Taking the Stress Out of Stress, Chapter 32.)

Checklist

✓ Do you see your first patient on time?
✓ Do you delegate many nonphysician tasks to your office staff?
✓ Are patients properly prepared before you enter the examining room?
✓ Do you and your staff agree about what constitutes appropriate interruptions?
✓ Can you get to your hospital(s) quickly?

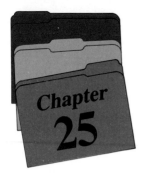

Patient Compliance

Promoting Adherence to Therapeutic Recommendations

The pediatrician needs to be aware that parent/patient noncompliance is a persistent reality. Compliance is influenced by many factors discussed in this chapter, including:
- **patient education**
- **satisfaction with the physician-patient encounter**
- **monetary considerations**
- **clarity and feasibility of instructions**
- **physician encouragement of subsequent self-management**

The pediatrician must always think about the possibility of noncompliance because patients follow medical instructions far less often than most of us would like to believe.[1,2] Several studies have determined that 10%-80% of patients complete a 10-day course of penicillin prescribed for streptococcal pharyngitis or otitis media.[1,3] The poorest compliance was noted in clinic populations, but studies in other practice settings revealed rates as low as 55%.[3,4] More recent reviews of compliance with other medication schedules or with recommended health-related behaviors have confirmed these findings. For example, in one study less than half the parents used car seats or belts for their children after being urged to do so by their pediatrician.[5]

Compliance is a complex issue, further complicated by pediatric expectations that most patients are compliant. Studies find that pediatricians rarely predict accurately who will follow medical recommendations versus who will not.[6]

Wide variations in the percent of patients who follow professional instructions have been reported in various adherence studies. These differences are poorly understood, although a recent review by Becker[6] attempted to analyze some of the confounding elements. Two factors play a major role in the differences: (1) the socioeconomic status of the population, and (2) the quality of the interaction between the health care provider and the patient or parent. Dr Becker found that satisfaction with the encounter was more likely to be associated with greater adherence.[6-8] An explanation to the parent or patient about why completing a course of mediation is important, accompanied by specific instructions, can influence adherence considerably.

Another unexpected finding in adherence research is that knowledge about desirable health behaviors seldom results in actual behavioral change.[9] For example, obese patients or their parents frequently are well versed in the caloric content of foods, but their weight charts show little proof of practical application. Multiple studies have shown that knowledge alone is rarely sufficient to change patient behavior.[7]

The impact of nonadherence

Nonadherence to a recommended medical regimen may go undetected because initial therapy (not the full course prescribed) is effective, or the problem resolves spontaneously. However, unrecognized noncompliance may result in needless changes in therapy, unnecessary diagnostic studies, or a vicious cycle of pediatrician-parent antagonism as the patient appears not to respond to the prescribed therapy.[7] This is why the pediatrician should be aware of possible compliance problems and be prepared to deal with them pragmatically.[10] Evidence or suspicion of nonadherence to a recommended medical regimen as well as any attempted corrective action should be documented in the medical record for liability purposes.

Failure to follow medical advice

Why do some patients or parents fail to follow medical advice? There are no simple explanations. It is quite evident that health-related behavior is often motivated by attitudes and beliefs that operate independent of information and objective evidence of the illness or the prescribed therapy. Key factors include whether the parent cares about health, agrees with the diagnosis, perceives the condition as serious or not, believes the proposed medication will work, fears side effects, or feels capable of ameliorating the condition by personal behaviors.[2,6,7,11,12]

The pediatrician can improve patient or parent adherence to recommended therapeutic regimens by use of some of the suggestions discussed below.[6,7,9,14-16]

Maximize the quality of the pediatrician/patient interaction

Adherence is higher when the parent is satisfied with the visit, sees the pediatrician as friendly, and believes the pediatrician understands and has responded to the complaint.[10] Parent satisfaction with the office visit is enhanced when the pediatrician elicits and respects the parent's concerns, answers each and every question, provides responsive information regarding the child's condition and progress, demonstrates sincere concern and sympathy, and terminates the office encounter in an unhurried, courteous fashion.

Provide written reinforcement of verbal instructions

The written material should be simple, concise, and free of medical jargon. Aim for text consistent with an elementary grade reading level.[17] There are computer programs available which can convert the reading level.

Simplify the treatment plan

Reduce daily medication administrations to as few as possible, synchronize medications, and tailor the medication schedule to the patient's regular daily routine and parent work schedule.

Be sure the family can afford the medication

Keep current with the estimated cost range of medications in your community and give this information to the parent. Prescribe generic medications whenever appropriate, and discourage purchase of ineffective over-the-counter medications as often as possible.

Make certain parents, other care givers, and family members are able and willing to support, assist, and encourage the patient to follow the therapeutic regimen

For those patients who are recent immigrants and who may not completely understand the English language, the pediatrician can improve compliance by providing written instructions which can be read by other family members at home. Other methods include calling the other parent (who often has a stronger grasp of the language) at work to go over the instructions; and making a follow-up phone call to the home the next day to be sure the appropriate regimen is being followed.

Consider arranging home visits in appropriate situations

The Visiting Nurse Association can be asked to look in on a child with a chronic illness. These visitors can help enhance adherence by assuring acquisition of the medication, making certain the parent understands the regimen and how to use any special dispensers such as nebulizers, and by making helpful suggestions (eg, having the parent post medication dosage reminders in conspicuous places). They also can provide feedback to the pediatrician about special problems compromising the therapeutic plan.

Anticipate the possibility of nonadherence

Where appropriate, obtain a compliance-oriented history and make appropriate changes in therapeutic strategy.

In suspected problem situations, use an objective test of medication adherence and provide feedback to parents and patients about the results

Measuring the amount of penicillin in the child's urine, or performing an assessment during the follow-up visit of the amount of unused medication still remaining in the bottle, are quick, objective assessments.

Conclusion

Nonadherence to recommended therapy is a common problem and must be anticipated. In many cases, identification of the problem and thoughtful selection of the appropriate approach will rectify the problem.

References

1. Becker MH, Drachman RH, Kirscht JP. Predicting mothers' compliance with pediatric medical regimens. *J Pediat*. 1972;81:843
2. Becker MH, Drachman RH, Kirscht JP. A new approach to explaining sick-role behavior in low income populations. *Am J Public Health*. 1974;64:205
3. Williams RL, Maiman LA, Broadbent DN, et al. Educational strategies to improve compliance with an antibiotic regimen. *AJDC*. 1986; 140:216-220
4. Cramer JA, Mattson RH, Prevesy ML et al. How often is medication taken as prescribed? A novel assessment technique. *JAMA*. 1989; 261:3273-3277
5. Tietge NS, Bender SJ, Scutchfield FD. Influence of teaching techniques on infant car seat use. *Pat Ed and Counsel*. 1987;9:167-175
6. Becker MH. Patient adherence to prescribed therapies. *Medical Care*. 1985;25:539-555
7. Maiman LA, Becker MH. The clinician's role in patient compliance. *Trends Pharm Sci*. 1980;1:457
8. Cameron R, Best JA. Promoting adherence to health behavior change interventions: Recent findings from behavioral research. *Pat Ed and Counsel*. 1987;10:139-154
9. Haynes RB, Wang E, Da Mota Gomes M. A critical review of interventions to improve compliance with prescribed medications. *Pat Ed and Counsel*. 1987;10:155-166
10. Francis V, Korsch BM, Morris NJ. Gaps in doctor-patient communication. *N Engl J Med*. 1969;280:535
11. Becker MH, ed. *The Health Belief Model and Personal Health Behavior*. A Health Educ. Monograph. 1974;2:324
12. Clark NM, Rosenstock IM, Hassan H, et al. The effect of health beliefs and feelings of self efficacy on self management behavior of children with chronic disease. *Pat Ed and Counsel*. 1988;11:131-139
13. Becker MH, Nathanson CA, Drachman RH, Kirscht JP. Mothers' health beliefs and childrens' clinic visits: A prospective study. *J Comm Health*. 1977;3:125
14. Perrin EC, Shapiro E. Health locus of control beliefs of healthy children, children with a chronic physical illness and their mothers. *J Pediatr*. 1985;107:627-633
15. Stewart M. The validity of an interview to assess a patients' drug taking. *Am J Prev Med*. 1987;3:95-100
16. Lima J, Nazarian L, Charney E, Lahti C. Compliance with short-term antimicrobial therapy: Some techniques that help. *Pediatrics*. 1976;57:383
17. Flesch R. *The Art of Readable Writing*. 25th ed. New York, NY: Harper-Row; 1974

Checklist

✓ Are you aware of noncompliance in your practice?
✓ Do you ask about previous experience with the treatment plan?
✓ Do you give preprinted or written instructions to reinforce verbal instructions?
✓ Is your treatment plan simple enough to be followed easily?
✓ Can the family afford the medication or treatment plan?
✓ Do you appear to exit the examination room hastily and leave the patient or parent with unanswered questions or doubts about your instructions?

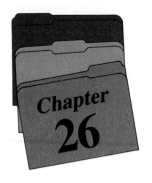

Patient Education Materials

Magazines, books, and pamphlets are basic elements of pediatric office decor. (Indeed, the proliferation of modern teaching aids can make the waiting room look more like a crowded, cluttered family room!) The pediatrician and office staff should work to develop a professional, effective, and cost conscious patient education program. Its basic element include:

- value
- acquisition
- preparation
- presentation

A comprehensive patient education program includes prevention, health promotion, and active patient/parent participation. It supports healthier life-styles and parental responsibility in managing acute and chronic health problems. A good health education program will:

- Provide a knowledge base to prompt healthier life-styles.
- Affect health behaviors as well as knowledge.
- Empower parents as health care advocates, and encourage their proper partnership role in managing acute and chronic illness.
- Enhance patient compliance and satisfaction.
- Help to structure a more marketable, efficient, and cost-effective practice.

Parents rely on their pediatrician to provide the best and most up-to-date information. Undoubtedly, much can be accomplished during an office visit or phone call, but time constraints limit these encounters. Written material, whether taken home or read in the office, serves as a very useful educational supplement. Whatever advances are to be expected in the field of audio-visual education, written material will likely continue to be the least expensive and most accessible medium for teaching and updating parents on current health care issues. Options for the pediatrician include searching for the most appropriate material, presenting this material in a variety of different media or creating original material that best reflects the pediatrician's personal views.

This chapter will discuss the value, acquisition, preparation, and proper presentation of educational material. The best patient education material serves as a supplement to the verbal communication between a parent/patient and their pediatrician. Good written or audio-visual material can serve as a powerful substitute, a good time-saver and a self-teacher.

Quality materials provide a knowledge base

Child development, behavior, safety, and related pediatric concerns are multifaceted. The pediatrician cannot expect to cover all areas in personal consultation. Parents look to friends, relatives, and the media for answers. They often need help to interpret and apply information, and select good material. The pediatric office can act as a resource center.

Patient education materials are an effective way to improve health care outcomes. For example, the new diabetic patient and family need intensive education to be able to manage the child's disease at home. Age-appropriate material that explains a disease and its treatment can result in fewer complications and a better outcome for the patient.

The pediatrician who provides well-screened resources for distribution, makes them available on a loan basis, and/or creates a list of materials for purchase, communicates personal concern

and an educational orientation. The pediatrician who develops material independently can give parents insight into his or her philosophy. Parents may not always agree with you, but they will likely respect your willingness to present carefully developed opinions. Many will be more likely to raise specific concerns for your personal input.

Patient education empowers parents as health care advocates

Quality printed material enables parents to obtain information about the management of simple problems or illnesses without feeling uncomfortable about inconveniencing their pediatrician. This will encourage confidence and independent thinking. Simple written instructions or good pamphlets regarding illness management and well-child care become greatly appreciated and well-worn references.

The Federal Education of the Handicapped Amendments of 1986 (PL 99-457, 20 USC 1400) empower family members to act as case managers for their special needs child. This legislation requires that parents become more informed and involved in the care of their handicapped child. The pediatrician caring for children with special needs will become increasingly involved in helping the parent become an informed case manager.

Good resources enhance patient compliance and satisfaction

In a busy pediatric office, a patient and his/her parent may receive information from several different personnel. When a child is sick the parent is stressed,

Resource Guide

Academy Child Care Guidebook Series

This series of three child care guidebooks will provide parents with reliable information about raising healthy children.

Now Available

Caring for Your Baby and Child: Birth to Age Five
This first book in the series has 31 chapters and over 1,500 illustrations. Topics covered include preparing for a new baby, part-time care for children, emergencies, physical problems, behavioral problems, developmental disabilities, and family issues.

Caring for Your Adolescent
This book discusses parenting philosophies; teenage physical, psychological, educational, and social growth and development; acne; substance abuse; and sexuality, among other topics.

Available in April 1992

Caring for Your Child: Ages 6-12
This guidebook will offer helpful information on such topics as nutrition, fitness, family and friends, school and community issues, emergency situations, common illnesses, psychosocial and behavioral problems, chronic diseases, and handicapping conditions. It is scheduled for publication in April 1992.

For more information about these guidebooks, contact the AAP Division of Public Education, 141 Northwest Point Blvd, PO Box 927, Elk Grove Village, IL 60009-0927, 800/433-9016.

Resource Guide for Office Educational Materials

Office Magazines for Parents

American Baby. Published by Cahners Pub Co, 475 Park Ave S, New York, NY 10016.

Beginnings. Published by Health Team Interactive Communications, 246 5th Ave, New York, NY 10001.

Exceptional Parent. Published by Pay-Ed Corporation, 1170 Commonwealth St, Boston, MA 02134.

HealthLink Waiting Room Television. Produced by the American Academy of Pediatrics and Lifetime Medical Television. Write the American Academy of Pediatrics, 141 Northwest Point Blvd, PO Box 927, Elk Grove Village, IL 60009-0927.

Healthy Kids. Published by the American Academy of Pediatrics and Cahners Publishing Co. Write the American Academy of Pediatrics, 141 Northwest Point Blvd, PO Box 927, Elk Grove Village, IL 60009-0927.

Parenting. Published by Parenting Magazine Partners, 501 2nd St, San Francisco, CA 94167.

Working Mother. Published by Working Women, McCalls Group, 230 Park Ave, New York, NY 10169.

Booklets, Pamphlets, Posters, and Videos

Most health organizations and government health departments provide educational materials at nominal or no cost. Listed below are specific groups whose materials have been found to be useful.

American Academy of Pediatrics. Extensive assortment for a small charge on numerous topics, all of which are listed in the Academy's Publications Catalog. Also available, TIPP (The Injury Prevention Program) and AAP policy statements. Call 800/433-9016 for ordering and information.

American College of Obstetrics-Gynecology. Material on sexuality. ACOG Distribution Center, PO 91180, Washington, DC, 20090-1180. Telephone 800/762-2264

Mead-Johnson. Materials for parents of infants and young children, including a New Arrivals Kit at no charge. Contact representative.

Network Publications. Pamphlets on birth control. PO 1830, Santa Cruz, CA 95061. Telephone 408/438-4060

Whittle Communications. Parenting Advisor is an attractive frame poster and free supply of pamphlets changed periodically by company. Has advertising. 505 Market St, Knoxville, TN 37902. Telephone 800/251-5002

Personnel Products Company. Material on fitness. Van Liew Ave, Milltown, NJ 08850. Telephone 908/524-0500.

Ross Laboratories. Free material (some multilingual) on numerous topics, including nutrition, safety, and particularly young child development and care. Also prepackaged material for ease of distribution. Contact representative.

US Public Health Service. Material on AIDS. Telephone 202/245-6067.

Wyeth-Ayers Laboratories. Materials about infants and young children. Contact representative.

Books for Reading in the Office or Short-term Lending

Brazelton TB. *Infants and Mothers.* New York, NY: Delacorte PF; 1969.

Brazelton TB. *On Becoming a Family.* New York, NY: Dell Publishing Co, Inc; 1981.

Caplan F. *The First Twelve Months of Life.* New York, NY: Grosset & Dunlap, Inc, The Putnam Publishing Group; 1973.

Chess S. *Your Child is a Person: A Psychological Approach to Parenthood Without Guilt.* New York, NY: Penguin Books; 1977.

Eiger M and Olds. *The Complete Book of Breastfeeding.* New York, NY: Bantam Books; 1986.

Ferber R. *Solve Your Child's Sleep Problems.* New York, NY: Simon and Schuster Publishing; 1986.

Freiberg S. *The Magic Years: Understanding and Handling the Problems of Early Childhood.* New York, NY: Scribner's; 1984.

Greenspan S. *First Feelings.* New York, NY: Penguin Books; 1986.

Rakowitz E and Rubin G. *Living With Your New Baby.* New York, NY: Berkley Publishing Group; 1986.

White B. *The First Three Years of Life.* New York, NY: Avon Books; 1984.

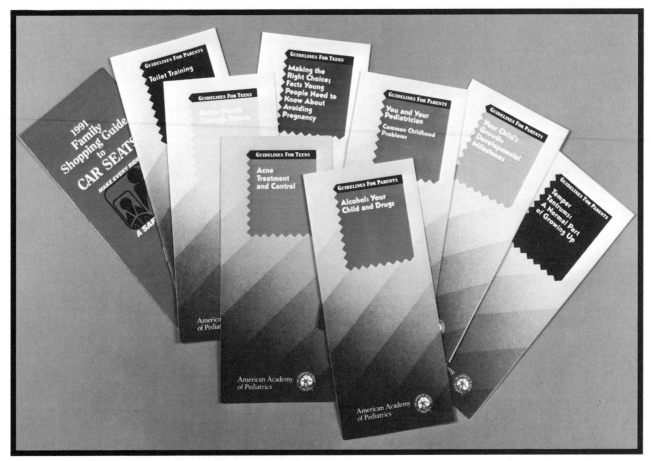

Figure 26-1: American Academy of Pediatrics patient education brochures. The pediatrician either hands these to parents at appropriate times, or they are placed on display racks for parents to take.

and may have difficulty retaining detailed instruction. Written instruction is very helpful, and assures that directions can be followed. The likelihood of misunderstanding is diminished, which improves patient compliance and limits the number of repeat visits or after-hours calls. A written instruction policy may improve health care outcome and could resolve potential medical-legal questions about patient communications.

Quality material tastefully displayed is always noted and appreciated, not only by patients in the practice, but also others in the community who have contact with your patients. This increased satisfaction will attract more families to your practice.

Systematic patient education facilitates a more marketable and cost-effective practice

Some pediatric offices have employed health educators to provide and expand patient education opportunities. This can be a critical time-saver for the busy pediatrician. The health educator or other employee might visit new mothers in the hospital, participate in prenatal classes, or develop patient education brochures. Alternatively, employment of appropriate office staff to manage these time-intensive activities may be a cost-effective efficiency for many pediatricians.

Cost, space and maintenance should be considered when developing a patient education program. A comprehensive program need not be costly. Patient educational materials require space and equipment, such as file cabinets and display racks. Appropriate display is important; the best literature or audiovisual film will be of no help to the patient if it is not used.

Age-appropriate guidance materials can also be placed in the chart prior to scheduled visits to facilitate distribution. Pediatric offices are full of very good information tools that have become outdated, sometimes even before they are given out to the public.

Ongoing review for timeliness and accuracy is important.

Acquisition of material

Printed material may be acquired from a variety of sources including nonprofit disease-oriented organizations, professional organizations, and for-profit businesses. The AAP, for a small but reasonable charge, provides high quality material for display and distribution. (See "Resource Guide for Office Educational Materials" on the preceding page.) All AAP materials are thoroughly reviewed to ensure that information is consistent with Academy policy and generally accepted standards of pediatric health care.

Academy brochures are well-written and timely. A large variety of topics are covered, spanning infancy through adolescence. (See Figures 26-1 and 26-2.) The AAP also is a good source

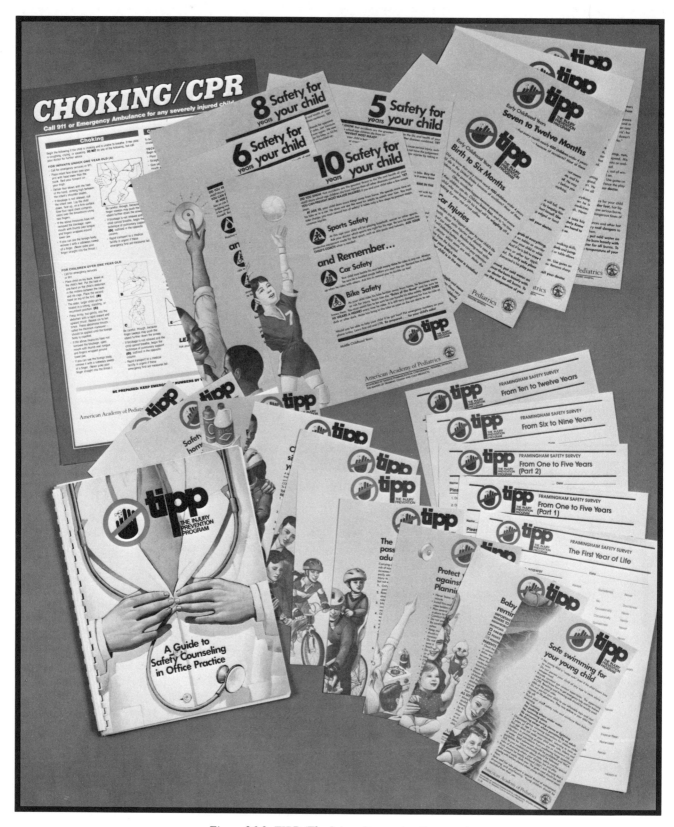

Figure 26-2: TIPP (The Injury Prevention Program) materials from the American Academy of Pediatrics. These are reviewed with parents as part of health supervision.

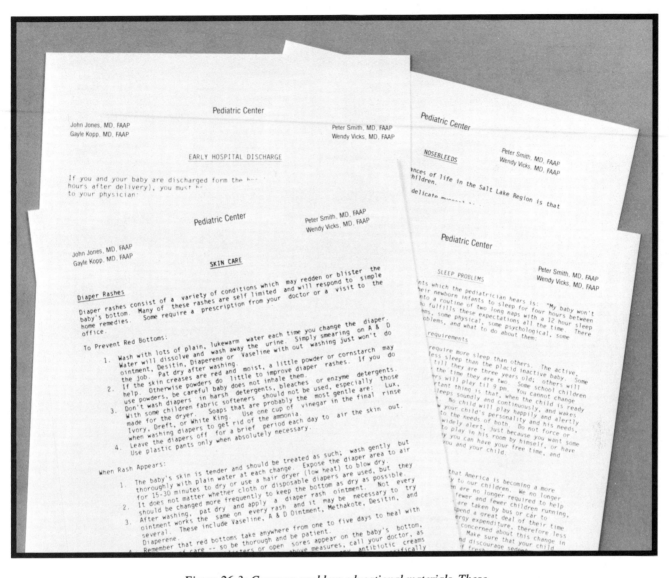

Figure 26-3: Common problem educational materials. These are color coded for easy identification and are handed to parents at the appropriate times.

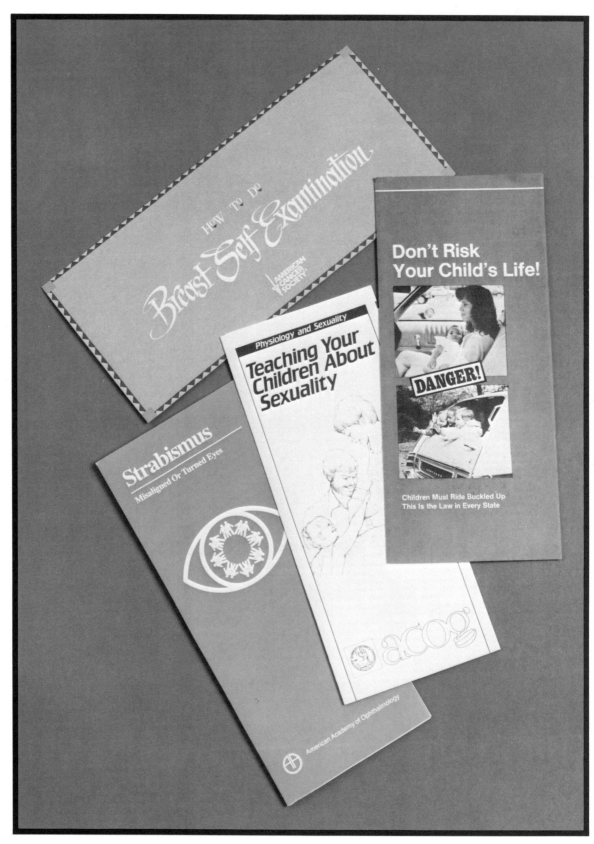

Figure 26-4: Other problem-oriented patient education materials. These are available from a variety of sources.

for posters and videos. Many of the videos are independently produced, but all have been reviewed and approved for technical accuracy. Video programs can be shown in the office or provided as loaners to parents. Many are accompanied by printed support materials.

The Academy also publishes a series of age-specific magazines called *Healthy Kids,* which are provided free of charge to members. Each issue covers a wide range of topics. The magazines can be personalized to include the pediatrician's name, address, phone number, and office hours. They are designed to be personally distributed to parents for leisure reading. Reception room television also is provided free of charge by the Academy. Participants receive complimentary videodisc machines, along with monthly videodiscs on a full-spectrum of topics, newsletters, and brochures.

Official AAP policy statements are an authority that can help strengthen your discussion with families. These are available from the Academy's Publications Department. A catalog is published annually.

National and state disease-oriented organizations are a great resource for the pediatrician's office. (See Figure 26-4.) Many organizations, such as the American Lung Association, American Heart Association, and March of Dimes provide excellent brochures at little or no cost. They may also provide speakers or videos for group meetings.

Other sources of information include state and county health departments, state highway safety commissions, special education services, and medical school libraries.

Pharmaceutical companies are another resource. This information should be carefully reviewed to ensure that it is appropriate, unbiased and accurate.

There are numerous magazines available gratis from publishers listed in the Resource Guide. They contain articles specifically written for parents, which should be reviewed by office staff. Feature stories and news articles from local or national newspapers can be clipped and displayed; sometimes they contain accurate, useful health information.

Developing materials independently

Few pediatricians have received formal instruction in structured patient education, but the fundamentals are a part of their natural knowledge base. Patient education is rewarding and motivating for both pediatrician and staff. Creating your own educational material can be time consuming, but the rewards are clear. There is no better way to promote your practice and yourself, and help your patients.

Few parents will criticize less than perfect grammar if the information is helpful and clearly written, although the advice or assistance of a writer or editor can be beneficial in preparation of booklets and pamphlets. (Keep in mind that a one time cash outlay for these services will produce copy usable for many years.) Remember to proofread all copy carefully before it is printed. Consider obtaining a copyright for all original materials to protect your work from plagiarism.

Pediatricians apprehensive about preparing their own printed materials can begin slowly by producing two of three guidance or safety sheets, then "graduate" to more complicated instructions, pamphlets, or booklets.

There is no need to be an expert on everything. Begin with one topic and write about it. It may be a booklet describing your practice. Or if you feel strongly about child behavior, it can address a particular issue, such as toilet training. Commit this view to paper and distribute it in the office. Or if you want to go further, and many pediatricians have, create a monthly or bimonthly newsletter that contains your views. Consider including guest writers, events, special programs, or telephone numbers for self-help groups (but include only those of which you have knowledge). Providing such a community service can only enhance your reputation as a quality physician and citizen.

Many pediatricians have taken the time to create a brochure describing their practice. Such an introduction to the practice provides basic information about procedures and office policies. (See Printing for the Pediatrician, Chapter 11.)

Presentation of material

Patient information should be appropriately accessible. All printed educational material that leaves your office should carry your preprinted label to identify the practice. The label should be clearly visible, and include a telephone number. Displays should be attractive, tasteful, and professional. Listed below are some pointers to avoid the clutter of pamphlet, poster, and magazine overkill.

Bulletin board

Organize your office waiting room walls with bulletin boards. Title each board for a particular purpose, then post relevant articles, newsletters, or posters. For example: a board for parents of infants, one for parents of toddlers, one for adolescents, and one for general safety issues. Reserve one board for community or practice-related activities, such as lectures, movies, or available tapes for lending. Consider a formica-covered piece of pressed wood, rather than a classic cork bulletin board, to avoid tacks and pins.

Display racks

Organize pamphlets and booklets in a similar fashion, either in the waiting room or examining room or both. Well-designed display racks with titles help direct parents and patients to the right sources.

Magazines

Magazines will eventually be scattered everywhere. It is unavoidable. Just make them available on tables and try to encourage your staff to periodically restack them as neatly as possible and throw away the ones that are outdated. Have age-appropriate magazines in the reception area and in each examining room.

Special material

It is a good idea to prepackage a selection of booklets and pamphlets for personal distribution to parents of children at certain developmental points, or with special needs. These might include packages for new parents, parents of toddlers, asthmatics or diabetics, or a selection of safety information. Some pharmaceutical companies provide such packages, which, if screened, are a welcome resource.

Staff help

No educational program of any sort, can be successful without a concerned and supportive office staff. Unless your staff is willing to direct people to what they need, to pay attention to replacing what is missing, to help update and change material, and, in general, to be alert to the needs and concerns of parents and children, your patients will not get the help that you want them to have. Spend some time talking to your staff about their importance to you and the families that you serve.

Conclusion

Educating patients and parents is certainly only one part of a pediatric practice. But it is a part that constantly touches on the success of all other parts. Pediatricians can never stop teaching: that is the nature of the field. Whether explaining an illness or discussing the logic of toddler stubbornness, pediatricians probably spend more time communicating and teaching than any other specialists. A good educational program helps make the job easier and reinforces the knowledge base. Patients and parents appreciate these efforts, and will better comply with a treatment approach they understand. A pediatrician who is a good educator and encourages questions builds mutually rewarding, potentially lifelong relationships with patients and their families.

Bibliography

Greenberg LW. Build your practice with patient education. *Contemporary Pediatrics*. 1989;6:85-106

Checklist

✓ Is your name, address, and telephone number displayed prominently on all printed materials?

✓ Have you investigated the many sources of educational aids?

✓ Are brochures, magazines, and other resources displayed attractively and accessibly?

✓ Do you seek opportunities to reinforce patient education by recommending or distributing materials in the course of office visits?

✓ Do you periodically revise and update your inventory?

✓ Have you considered developing a brochure to introduce new families to the practice?

✓ Have you thought about developing independent educational materials, or even a periodic newsletter?

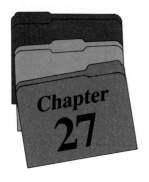

Improving the Quality of Office Practice

Chapter 27

Quality improvement (QI) is a new approach to a classic concept. Modern quality improvement examines the physician-patient relationship, and asks, "Whom do I wish to serve, and what do they need from me?" QI seeks to improve quality of care by analyzing and amending the processes by which these needs are met.

The search for improvement is second nature to the pediatrician. From the earliest moments of medical training the message is clear: "The art is long." We are schooled to educate ourselves continually, to remain up to date on the latest clinical knowledge, and to be our own harshest critics. Regulatory processes and formal organizations have imposed review procedures which are sometimes cumbersome and even abrasive, but their intent underscores a basic motivation toward continuous improvement that is in the marrow of the true pediatrician.

In recent years, health care organizations have begun to realize that the classic traditions of quality assurance in medical care are not the only methods for addressing the quality of practice. Over the past 3 decades, industries outside health care have developed some useful methods for improving quality, many of which are readily adapted for use by physicians. These methods now constitute a body of management sciences that can help to determine how best to organize work in support of optimal human performances.[1]

Key concepts

Three terms are especially useful in discussing modern quality improvement methods: "process," "customer," and "supplier."[2-5]

A **process** is a sequence of steps through which something is transformed into something else more valuable. In manufacturing, processes are concrete. Perhaps two components are made and then combined into a working piece of electronic gear. Perhaps the process assembles a car or changes one chemical into another. In service industries, and especially in health care, processes are less concrete, but they exist nonetheless. In the process of *patient registration,* information is obtained, assembled, and moved from place to place to make it accessible for later use. In the process of *prescribing medicine,* the intention of the physician is transformed into a working written prescription, and then into a container of medicine given to the patient. The clinical process of *taking a history* transforms disparate facts into a story with meaning, and the process of *referral* converts the questions of the referring doctor into information for the consultant, an appointment for the patient, and a recommendation for management.

Almost any such productive sequence can be drawn as a series of steps transforming one thing into another, or moving something from place to place or time to time. Conceptualizing medical care in terms of processes can greatly assist quality improvement efforts.

Those served by a process are called **customers** in this way of thinking. In fact, the process exists to serve customers. That is its purpose. Closer examination reveals not one but two types of customers in this context. Some are not part of the process itself; they are *external customers.* In the dispensing of medication, for the most part, the patient who will receive the medicine container is an external customer. Other people work *inside* the process, and are called *internal customers.* They are served by others within the process. The pharmacist, for example, is an *internal customer* for the physician in the prescription process. Such an internal customer depends on others in the process in order to function properly. If the physician makes an error in writing the prescription, the pharmacist's efforts are frustrated.

For every customer, there is a **supplier,** usually more than one, who also can be *internal* to the process or *external.* If the pharmacist is the internal customer of the physician, the physician is, by definition, the internal supplier for the pharmacist. External suppliers give the process what it needs; for example, those who print prescription blanks may be external suppliers to the prescription process.

In quality management, the word "quality" is defined as meeting the needs of customers. The quality of a process is its ability to provide what the customer needs. The quality of a process depends on the smooth functioning of customer-supplier relationships. For that reason, customers and suppliers within processes need to understand each other as well as they practically can. Suppliers must know what customers need; customers must understand what suppliers can and cannot do for them.

This is the central focus of modern ideas of quality improvement: *To improve quality, one must improve the processes through which the needs of customers are met.*[6] The idea is very simple; implementation is often complex.

Translating modern quality improvement for office practice

Modern quality improvement methods translate readily to medicine but that translation requires a leap of imagination. There is little doubt that modern companies outside health care have achieved enormous improvements in

QUALITY OF OFFICE PRACTICE – 159

quality, productivity, and efficiency by putting a few basic principles into everyday practice. One need only look to the number of foreign cars on American roads to realize that other societies adopted some important ideas about quality long before the American automobile industry, which waited until it was almost too late to learn some of the same lessons.

But what does building a car have to do with the office practice of pediatrics? Here are a few simple ideas, rooted in quality improvement methods but presented in office practice terms:

Know your customers and their needs

In modern quality improvement (QI), getting close to your customer is the essential first step. The process begins with self-examination. In medical terms the physician might ask, "Whom do I wish to serve, and what do they need from me?"

Is the child your customer? Of course. What does the child need? What delights children in the office? How do you know? Make a list of the probable needs of those key customers in all of the dimensions that they (and you) care about. In each case, ask yourself how you know that what you do meets that need, and how you could find out with more certainty.

The parents are customers, too. What do they need? How do you know? Really progressive companies put lots of energy into asking their customers for definitions of quality. In health care, that might mean ending patient encounters with some question like this: "If you could spare one more minute, would you mind telling me your impressions of what happened today in my office? What was the best thing my staff or I did for you? What would you have liked to be different?" Of course, the patient or parent may not be able to comment on the particular drug you prescribed or the diagnosis you reached, but they may comment with great precision on many other important aspects of your care. If you listen carefully, you may find out a great deal about where you are achieving your own goals, and where you are unintentionally falling short. You may discover that you have some misimpressions about what your customers actually want and need.

Think, also, about other customers – other people who depend on you and whom you wish to serve. What about the pharmacist? What about the nurses on the pediatric ward? Or the school guidance counselor? A quality improvement approach would suggest that you touch base with them and ask how you might help them better. Ask the ward nurse, "Is there anything I could do differently to make it easier for you to help my patients?"

Fancier methods for listening to customers include formal questionnaires, special group meetings of customers with open-ended conversation (focus groups), and special surveys which seek the help of customers in designing new programs or services. Health services research journals can be helpful in this regard.

One form of "listening to customers" peculiar to health care is the use of *health status measurement* to assess the health, symptoms, and functioning of the patient or family.[7-9] In recent years, excellent short questionnaires have been designed by researchers, allowing almost anyone to assess function or symptom levels in quantitative terms, and, theoretically at least, to follow improvement or deterioration precisely.

Such health status measurement tools have not yet reached common use in practice, but some are ready to use; for example, there are the simple "Dartmouth COOP Charts," which allow the patient to select a cartoon that represents current symptom levels.[10] Pediatric and adolescent charts are being developed.

Suppose you are uncertain about which of two antibiotics produces more rapid resolution of ear infections. The systematic use of a very simple outcome measurement (eg, symptoms reported by the mother after 2 days of treatment) might just hold the answer if used in a small, clever design. Such "clinical research" is not at all beyond the means of a small group practice, or even a single doctor who wants badly to know the answer. Systematic data collection and analysis are almost always better than anecdotal review.

Identify and diagram the processes you use

You work all day in processes, even if you do not call them by that name. Processes are the established sequences by which you get your work done. Improv-

ing quality means improving those processes. The more reliable, streamlined, simple, and uniform they are, the better will you be able to control the quality of your help to patients. Unless your office is already very special, you and your patients may currently be paying a high price in the deficiencies of those processes; their embedded waste, duplication, complexity, and unpredictability produce frustrations every day for both you and your patients.

You can begin by simply listing the processes you use. The list will be long; when you really get going you may be able to identify as many as fifty or one hundred processes in your office alone. Here are some that you probably use now:
- Registering patients
- Preparing examination rooms
- Preparing the patient for examination
- Taking a history of the chief complaint
- Stocking equipment
- Scheduling patients
- Checking on inpatients
- Maintaining office records
- Finding office records
- Writing letters
- Selecting continuing medical education courses
- Writing prescriptions
- Ordering x-rays
- Teaching parents about asthma
- Teaching children about bicycle safety

There are many more. Each process has a **purpose,** that is, an intended output. It is supposed to get something done. Each also has **customers** and **suppliers,** both *internal* and *external*. Your quality improvement efforts will be directed toward these processes one at a time; you must define each one, perhaps graph it out in a series of logical and actual boxes, and be clear about its purpose in operational terms (that is, in terms you might measure if you wished).

Setting out this list of processes is a first step toward an agenda for improvement. You cannot work on them all at once. Which will you tackle first? Perhaps it should be the ones that your customers say are most important to them. Or perhaps it should be one which you suspect involves a lot of waste. Make a sensible choice. There will be lots of time to work on the processes you choose. The key is to get started. Simple, proven methods for illustrating processes ("process flow diagrams") are easily learned and can help a great deal in understanding and simplifying processes.[2,5,11]

Identify costs of poor quality

When processes fail, (by being wasteful, complex, unreliable, or redundant) costs can mount quickly. These troubled times are not ones in which extra costs can be easily tolerated. Ask yourself this question: "If this process ran perfectly every time, what would be saved in terms of dollars, time, and other things my customers and I care about?" Be complete in your listing. This assessment of total costs may lead you to begin work urgently on some other processes.

Overall, in clinical practice, the same questions about total cost must become familiar and lead to action. A good rule: Do for your patients clinically what is known, with reasonable certainty, to help them – nothing less, but nothing more. The burden of proof must now be on the person who suggests that a medical resource should be used, not on someone who questions its value.[12,14]

Identify and talk with your suppliers

Whom do you rely on to get your work done? They are your suppliers. Sometimes they may seem unwilling or unable to help, but apparent unwillingness may represent a failure to understand your needs. Thinking in QI terms means making certain that: (a) your suppliers know that they *are* your suppliers; (b) your suppliers know your needs and expectations; and (c) you know your suppliers' constraints and needs. Little of this can be achieved without direct and open dialogue. Eventually, you should aim to have this discussion with every key supplier: "This is what I need from you; what do you need from me?"

Who are your suppliers? Only you can know. They probably include your office staff, equipment vendors, nurses, other doctors, school personnel, repairmen, and pharmacists, among many others. Talk with them. The time you spend now will be returned later in more effective processes and more delighted customers. As with customers, you can use many different methods to listen to suppliers: questionnaires, group meetings, and phone chats.

Search for benchmarks inside and outside health care

One of the key distinctions between a good company and a world class company is the commitment to "benchmarking." Benchmarking is the search for ideas and standards of performance outside of one's own organization.[15] Do you wish to improve the smoothness and reliability of your patient registration process? Study how registration is done in a world-class hotel. Do you want to improve your office records? Ask ten other pediatricians in your region to show you their record systems. Do you want to improve your taking of clinical histories? Ask some doctors you admire if you could sit in on their history-taking for a few hours, and study the differences.

The process of benchmarking can be great fun. Looking outside health care for analogies and lessons can reveal surprises and wonderful new ideas. Where in the world could you learn something you could use to improve an office process? Airlines? Schools? Clockmakers? Baseball managers? Let your mind wander, make some phone calls, and enjoy your journey of discovery.

Try to make processes predictable

The best processes are totally reliable; they run exactly as they have been designed, every time. Unpredictability introduces cost, waste, frustration, and error. In improving processes, the goal is to make them increasingly reliable – continually reducing unintended variation.

Of course, the art of medicine involves the intended, conscious customizing of care to the real needs of the individual patient. "Reliability of process" does not necessarily mean "standardization of practice." If the patient needs an unusual antibiotic or a unusual dose, use it, of course. But a reliable prescription process would be one in which *if* you intended that the patient receive amoxicillin in a certain dose and quantity by a certain time, *that* is *exactly* what happens, every time.

How do processes become reliable? By removing undesired sources of variation. The basic idea of process improvement is to understand where undesired variation comes from, and then to eliminate it.[5]

The enterprise of reducing variation is easier if you are clear about how you want the processes to run in the first place. If you see eight routine cases of otitis media in a day, do you really wish to vary randomly in treatment? Probably not. You operate with an implicit road map for treating otitis media. Why not write it down and try to stick to it, at least until you find a better one? If you practice in a group, make your processes more reliable by agreeing on them; you pay a price for "individualizing" practices when there is little reason to do so. The price is in the extra work, complexity, and redundancy your suppliers and customers experience because you do things different ways.

Learn to identify complexity and variation as an enemy of quality. The good pilot develops a sound routine for landing an airplane. A group of good pilots agrees on a routine so that the tower does not risk error with adjustment to every individual pilot. Good doctoring should involve clear statements of intended practice, and reliable, professional implementation of those intentions.

Measure, measure, measure

Nothing supports quality improvement better than information. Not the kind of useless, rote information that too many reporting systems require of the hospital and practitioner today, but rather the kind of information that you stay up late at night to comb out of a set of data. If you are going to be serious about improvement, invest in data and enjoy it.

What data? Feedback from patients and other customers. Diagrams of the processes you use, drawn by you and others in the processes to uncover unneeded misunderstandings and complexities. Data on the health status of your patients. Data on the processes themselves: waiting times for appointments, waiting times in your waiting rooms, frequency of lost records, reasons for lost records, turnaround times for laboratory tests, clarity of consultants' reports, length of stay in hospitals, and so on. The data you need will depend on the questions you are asking about the processes you are trying to improve. Collect information that will help you understand when and why processes become unreliable. Does the process vary because of special circumstances that you need to control? Or does it vary randomly? Is the process changing over time, or is it stable? Books on quality improvement provide clever and simple ways to collect and study such simple data. Collecting the data should become part of your daily work. You can improve processes if you have the knowledge to do so; without knowledge, your efforts may only make them worse.

Suppose you want to improve the way you refer patients to orthopedists. Diagram the referral process. Ask orthopedists what they need in a referral. Identify some key characteristics of the process; maybe they include "completeness of information," legibility," "timeliness of referral," and "sound instructions to the patient." Measure how well each of these is achieved for each referral over time. Find the "failed" referrals, and ask how each failed. Develop a list of causes of referral failure, and redesign the process to remove the most common cause of failure. This, in real steps, is the sequence of design, data collection, and redesign that can lead to continuous improvement of processes. You can use it anywhere.

The most sophisticated office-based data systems for the future may be those that measure and track patient health status. If the measurement of health status becomes routine and standard in your practice, you may then begin to design small local studies to improve what you and your patients care the most about: health status outcomes.

Draw graphs and charts

The best data are useless until someone understands what they mean. This means finding some sort of display format that makes the lessons leap out at us, converting "data" to "information."[16] Charts and graphs can help a lot. Even simple ones can show us things we easily miss in long lists or tables. Here are a few types of graphs and charts that are both simple and powerful:

Histograms
Charts using bars to show frequency, such as a histogram of waiting times according to time of day;

Scatterplots
Charts displaying two variables on a plane, such as a graph of height by weight. These can show a relationship, or lack of one, between the two variables;

Run charts
Graphs of a key variable over time, such as pharmacy error rates over a series of weeks;

Pareto charts
Ordered histograms, showing the most frequent event on the left, the next most frequent next, and so one. For example, one might show the causes of missed appointments in such an ordered chart.

Train your office staff in simple quality control methods

Anyone can learn to collect and analyze data on processes, or to draw a simple process flow diagram. Anyone can talk with customers about their needs, or with suppliers about their requirements. In an office oriented toward QI, the office staff learns to think in terms of process, customers, suppliers, measurement and improvement, just as the physicians have. QI involves everyone, and formal training and supervision make the techniques familiar and useful to everyone. Not only are your office staff key customers and suppliers for you, they are your best partners in improvement. Create a team and lead it.

Experiment

Try out new methods. QI thinking encourages frequent, friendly experimentation as a mode of learning about how to improve. If you cannot decide between two registration procedures, use one this week and the other next week, and measure, measure, measure. The same thinking can be applied responsibly to clinical practices (not the truly experimental therapies that require human subjects review, but the irksome, familiar controversies in which Common Therapy A competes with Common Therapy B, without a clear victor in the absence of systematic study). The only rule of experimentation in QI thinking is that it must be systematic enough to learn from. Variation without study is wasteful and perhaps even irresponsible. Variation with study holds the seeds of learning and improvement. Let your changes be guided by knowledge, and your innovations proven by study.

Following these ten rules of quality improvement is not guaranteed to remove all of your frustrations, nor will it take a rocky vessel immediately into calm waters. But they will let you begin the enterprise. The voyage is long; it may last your professional lifetime. But it will eventually pay enormous returns in satisfaction for you, efficiency for

your practice, and reliable, supportive care for your patients.

References

1. Berwick DM. Continuous improvement as an ideal in health care. *New Eng J Med*. 1989;320:53-56
2. Laffel G, Blumenthal D. The case for using industrial quality management science in health care organizations. *JAMA*. 1989;262:2869-2873
3. Walton M. *The Deming Management Method*. New York, NY: Dodd, Mead & Co; 1986
4. Juran JM, Gryna FM, eds. *Juran's Quality Control Handbook*. 4th ed. New York, NY: McGraw-Hill Publishing Co; 1988
5. Scholtes P. *The Team Handbook*. Madison, WI: Joiner Associates; 1988
6. Deming WE. *Out of the Crisis*. Cambridge, MA: MIT Center for Applied Engineering Studies; 1986
7. Lewis CC, Pantell RH, Kieckhefer GM. Assessment of children's health status: field test of new approaches. *Med Care*. 1989;27 (Supplement):S54-S65.
8. Nelson EC, Berwick DM. The measurement of health status in clinical practice. *Med Care*. 1989;27 (Supplement):S77-S90
9. Stewart AL, Greenfield S, Hays RD, et al. Functional status and well-being of patients with chronic conditions: results from the Medical Outcome Study. *JAMA*. 1989;262:907-913
10. Nelson EC, Wasson JH, Kirk JW, et al. Assessment of function in routine clinical practice: description of the COOP chart method and preliminary findings. *J Chron Dis*. 1987:40 (Supplement):55S-63S
11. Berwick DM, Godfrey AB, Roessner J. *Curing Health Care*. San Francisco, CA: Jossey-Bass Publishers;1990
12. Brook RH, Lohr KN. Efficacy, effectiveness, variations, and quality: boundary-crossing research. *Med Care*. 1985;23:710-720
13. Chassin MR, Brook RH, Park RE, et al. Variations in the use of medical and surgical services by the Medicare population. *New Engl J Med* 1986;314:285-290
14. Eddy DM. Variations in physician practice: the role of uncertainty. *Health Affairs*. 1984;3:74-89
15. Camp RC. *Benchmarking: The Search for Industry Best Practices that Lead to Superior Performance*. Milwaukee, WI: Quality Press; 1989
16. Plsek P. A primer on quality improvement tools. In: Berwick DM, Godfrey AB, Roessner J. *Curing Health Care*. San Francisco, CA: Jossey-Bass Publisher; 1990:177-219

Checklist

✓ Do you know your patients' needs?
✓ Do you have a system to evaluate processes you use, ie, patient registration and patient scheduling?
✓ Do the processes you use fulfill their purposes?
✓ Do you identify and talk with your suppliers?
✓ Do you look to "benchmarks" inside and outside of medicine to improve QI?
✓ Do you use graphs and charts to convert "data" to "information?"
✓ Do you have a method to measure the effect of new office procedures?

Section IV

Special Issues

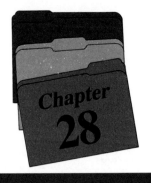

Chapter 28

Professional Courtesy

Full professional courtesy may be archaic and extremely disadvantageous to the pediatrician. This chapter will discuss:
- **background**
- **advantages/disadvantages**
- **reasons for adoption or discontinuation**
- **appropriateness in today's practice**

The extension of professional courtesy to colleagues is a long-standing but rarely discussed tradition in medicine. The pediatrician has few or no guidelines to use in making a decision about professional courtesy and may wonder about its propriety. This chapter will describe alternatives to the traditional form of full professional courtesy and will discuss the philosophy behind charging physicians for professional care.

History

The historical precedent for the philosophy of professional courtesy can be found in many early medical writings. In the 1800s, medicine was formally organized in the United States under the American Medical Association. A code of ethics adopted at the first meeting of this new organization, revised and interpreted through the years, offered general philosophical guidelines for professional courtesy. It was generally accepted that: (1) the physician should not be embarrassed to accept a fee for services if the recipient of services insists on payment; (2) if the recipient of services has insurance which provides benefits for medical or surgical care, the physician who renders the services can accept the insurance benefits without violating professional courtesy practices; (3) if services are provided to other physicians or their families on a frequent or long-term basis, an adjusted fee may be charged so an unreasonable burden is not placed on the physician providing service; and (4) professional courtesy should always be given to physicians who are in financial hardship and to their dependent family members.[1] As of 1989, the American Medical Association no longer had a policy on professional courtesy, leaving the decision to

offer professional courtesy to the discretion of each physician.

Dissent to the concept of full professional courtesy has evolved through the years because of the realities of practice: it takes time to see patients, it costs money to see patients, it is frequently inconvenient to see courtesy patients, and often one physician seems to see a large proportion of the community's professional families.

Psychiatrists and analysts[2,3] were the first to discontinue professional courtesy. Physicians in other specialties have begun to consider whether or not the practice of professional courtesy should be continued, and many of them also are discontinuing it or never beginning it.

Counterpoint

Before reaching a decision on professional courtesy, it would be wise to check what is being done by other physicians in the area, perhaps through the local medical society. If professional courtesy is routinely extended in the community and the pediatrician does not continue this practice, difficulties and "backlash" from the medical community may occur.

Disadvantages

Several disadvantages are inherent in the care of physicians and their families:
- Families may be slow, or even reluctant, to seek health care.[4-8]
- Many feel it is an imposition or that they should be able to care for their own medical problems.
- A parent-physician or patient-physician may have special but hidden

anxieties because of his or her medical knowledge.
- The treating physician may rely on the patient-physician for part or all of the diagnosis and treatment.
- Self-referral and self-treatment are common.
- History taking may occur in the hospital corridor or at cocktail parties.[5]
- There are gaps and variations in record keeping.
- The treating physician may treat both anxiously and more cautiously if he or she feels under scrutiny.
- The patient-physician may feel unable to complain about care or be reluctant to change physicians.

In general, both the treating and the patient-physician are more likely to behave in ways contrary to the behaviors prescribed by traditional roles.[7] Carey and Sibinga[8] state that treating families of physician friends carries with it the additional disadvantages of unrealistic expectations and hidden motivations, trouble keeping social and medical relationships separate, and difficulty by both parties in handling dissatisfaction. Auerback,[9] writing the first comprehensive report on professional courtesy in 1962, concluded that it may be a barrier to good medical treatment, causing delay in seeking medical help and producing negative feelings on the part of the patient-physician and treating physician.

Consideration

It is a compliment, and perhaps a privilege, to be chosen to provide care to a physician's family. This care has, in the past, frequently been provided at no charge because of a long-established precedent. But because professional courtesy appears to interfere with the appropriate utilization of medical care and results in less than optimal attention, it may have outlived its usefulness.

The central concept of the physician-patient relationship, regardless of who the patient is, should be a special sense of caring. Pediatrics, perhaps more than any other specialty, requires frequent communication and visits between physician and patient and extensive use of the telephone. If because of professional courtesy physician-parents and their spouses may be deterred from using pediatric services appropriately, they may not receive optimal care.

Pediatricians can continue to provide care to physicians' families by offering complete professional courtesy, partial professional courtesy (eg, discounted fee), or no fee other than acceptance of third party payments as payment-in-full for professional care. The latter arrangement is most common today because physicians frequently have good insurance coverage, either in the traditional form or in a managed care program.

Whatever the choice, pediatricians should have a policy which should be clearly stated to the physician's family as they enter the practice or, if a change is necessary, to families already established in the practice.

Before a policy is established, the pediatrician should understand the attitude in the pediatric community toward this delicate subject, as well as the general physician's attitude toward professional courtesy (see Counterpoint). Once a policy is established, it is difficult to change. See Figure 28-1 for an example of a letter which can be modified to explain any of the above options.

Dear Dr

It is our privilege to provide to your children what we feel is the best pediatric care available.

In these troubled economic times, when our expenses, as yours, have increased so drastically, we find ourselves in a difficult situation.

With the influx of so many families to our area, the volume of pediatric responsibility has increased considerably.

Sheer economic demands and pressures give us no choice but to discontinue professional courtesy on a "no fee" basis, but we will offer a 20% discount.

This policy has been followed for some time in many areas of our country, to the mutual satisfaction of all concerned.

We realize this is a delicate subject to introduce, but this will enable us to provide your family with the professional time and attention required.

We hope that this policy will enable you to avail yourselves of our service without reticence and eliminate an often expressed reluctance to call on us.

Figure 28-1: Sample letter for discontinuing professional courtesy to families of physicians.

References

1. American Medical Association. *Judicial Council Opinions and Reports.* 1977 ed. Chicago, IL: American Medical Association; 1977:26
2. Schur M. *Freud: Living and Dying.* New York, NY: International Universities Press; 1972:408-409
3. Menninger K. *Theory of Psychoanalytic Technique.* New York, NY: Basic Books; 1958:9
4. Sharpe JD, Smith WW. Physician, heal thyself: Comparison of findings in periodic health examination of physicians and executives. *JAMA.* 1962;182:234
5. Kennell JH, Boaz WD. The physician's children as patients. *Pediatrics.* 1962;30:100
6. White RB, Lindt H. Psychological hazards in treating physical disorders of medical colleagues. *Dis Nerv Syst.* 1963;24:304
7. Franklin RW, Goolishian HA, White RB. Psychological hazards involved in treatment of medical colleagues. *Dis Nerv Syst.* 1965;26:731
8. Carey WB, Sibinga MS. Should pediatricians provide medical care for their friends' children? *Pediatrics.* 1968;42:106
9. Auerback A. The psychiatrist looks at professional courtesy. *Amer J Psych.* 1962;119:520

Bibliography

Bass LW, Wolfson JH. Professional courtesy. *Pediatrics.* 1980; 65:751

Bass LW, Wolfson JH. Professional courtesy is obsolete. *New Engl J Med.* 1978;299:772

Bass LW, Wolfson JH. *The Style and Management of a Pediatric Practice.* Pittsburgh: University of Pittsburgh Press; 1977

Paxton HT. Drawing your boundaries for professional courtesy. *Med Econ.* March 3, 1989

Spock B. Should not physicians' families be allowed the comfort of paying for medical care? *Pediatrics.* 1962;30:109

Checklist

✓ Are you aware that there is nothing binding about offering professional courtesy to your colleagues' families?
✓ Would failure to offer professional courtesy result in community backlash?
✓ If you're not planning to offer or plan to discontinue professional courtesy, have you considered an explanatory letter to help avoid any misunderstandings?

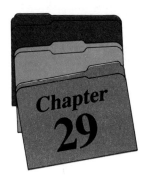

Chapter 29

Professional and Community Relations

A pediatrician's interaction with the community and professional colleagues can significantly affect the quality of services provided by the practice. Areas which are addressed in this chapter include:

- community participation
- public relations
- relations with physicians and other health care professionals
- school interactions

Pediatricians should be sensitive to the needs of the community and how those needs relate to his or her practice. Community service, working with schools, interacting with news media, and establishing dialogue with political figures, are ways to build bridges. Sound professional relationships enable a practice to thrive. The pediatrician must work well with physicians and other health care professionals in order to provide patients with the best possible care.

Community participation

Community activity sends a message of caring about the community. Volunteering for service on nonprofit charity boards generates good will and builds a network of peers in community leadership. Bike-a-thons, marathons, telethons, and little league sponsorship are also good ways to participate. Physician volunteers are welcome additions to school boards, United Way, Big Brother, Big Sister, or other similar civic organizations. A pediatrician might conduct physical exams for needy children at the request of a charitable organization. Most schools need a team physician, who is most often greatly respected and appreciated.

Over the past 10 years, the public's use of day care facilities has increased dramatically. A pediatrician can provide insight, guidance, and advice as a volunteer medical director. The risk of liability may increase, and malpractice carriers should be consulted before undertaking any of these activities. But benefits far exceed risk in most communities.

Pediatricians who successfully establish communication within local school organizations can provide a great service by working directly with educators and giving guidance.

Public relations

The pediatrician who offers to act as a resource for radio, television, and print media counters misinformation and raises health awareness. Weekly or monthly magazine and newspaper editors often welcome articles on health or other issues relating to children.

An effective media expert must be flexible, and occasionally willing to accommodate inconvenience. The Academy's Division of Public Relations is available to assist members who would like to become local spokespersons. (See Community News Media, Chapter 30.) Some local pediatric societies also sponsor spokespersons. The AAP spokesperson network can supply accurate, current information for news releases or interviews.

Ongoing discourse with federal, state, and local legislators enables the physician to express views on important issues in child health care, and reinforces his or her position as a child advocate. Physicians, acting individually or as a group, can have a significant impact. Pediatricians should become familiar with local and state legislators, and make a point of meeting with them. Become an active member of your AAP chapter and volunteer to assist with statewide initiatives on behalf of children.

Professional relations

Intraprofessional relationships are equally important. Pediatricians work within the medical community as consultants, referral sources, and peers in the practice of medicine. The pediatrician should develop a working list of suitable health care providers who would welcome referrals. Evaluate and, when possible, visit each one before making any referrals. This list should include medical and surgical subspecialists, internists, and family physicians (for parents who ask your advice), dentists, psychologists, psychiatrists, home medical service specialists, podiatrists, occupational therapists, physical therapists, educational facilities, and speech and language therapists. Patients greatly appreciate referral to another high quality health care provider. Good communication between the pediatrician and other health professionals assures optimal care.

The pediatrician can also act as a resource for parents seeking day care, swimming, sports, music, and preschool programs, as well as other activities of interest around the community. *As with any recommendation, the pediatrician should know first-hand that the service or facility has been professionally evaluated.*

The pediatrician should be familiar with local and state health and human services authorities, with contact persons in each. Knowledge of these services will allow the pediatrician to refer the appropriate patient to the appropriate agency.

The pediatrician's relationship with other primary care physicians is bolstered by a good reputation for quality care and a good working relationship with colleagues. Family practice physicians may not know how often a pediatrician is asked for a "good family doctor." Certainly, healthy relationships are built on referring to quality family practice physicians. On the other hand, patients who have been referred for consultation are to be encouraged to return to their family practitioner to maintain a good working relationship. Finally, when seeing a patient for a second opinion, never criticize the other physician's treatment.

Common courtesy would dictate that it is just good manners to place your own phone calls to other physicians. While asking someone else to place the call may save a few seconds, that consideration cannot compensate for the irritation at the other end.

In establishing relationships with obstetricians it is obvious that the pediatrician needs to be sensitive and responsive to their needs. A stand-by Cesarean section in the middle of busy office hours may be inconvenient, but such responsiveness does not go unnoticed. Any problems which develop in the newborn period should be transmitted to the obstetrician directly and followed up with a letter or phone call detailing treatment and outcome. Assuming a healthy newborn without problems, a letter thanking the OB for the referral is always appreciated.

Relationships with the medical community include those with local hospitals. Both the physician and the hospital are in the business of providing quality health care; good communication enables each to help the other. The physician new in practice can build a professional network and assist the hospital by serving on hospital committees. Many new physicians receive financial and/or organizational assistance from the local hospital, which benefits both parties. This assistance should be accepted only after frank discussion of mutual and individual goals.

Volunteer staff physicians at teaching institutions enhance their reputations within the medical community. Teaching nurses, medical students, and residents encourages tomorrow's referrals from today's medical and nursing students. This is probably one of the best investments in developing an enviable reputation. Didactic lectures, third

The pediatrician often consults for other physicians about specific patients. In a 1983 article, Goldman and Rudd discussed the "10 Commandments for Effective Consultations." Although written specifically for internists, the "10 commandments" could apply to any consulting physician.

10 Commandments for Effective Consultations[1]

The consultant should:
1. Determine the question that is being asked
2. Establish the urgency of consultation
3. Gather primary data
4. Communicate as briefly as appropriate
5. Make specific recommendations
6. Provide contingency plans
7. Understand his role in the process
8. Offer educational information
9. Communicate recommendations directly to the requesting physician
10. Provide appropriate follow up

Reprinted from the Archives of Internal Medicine. *1983; 143:1753-1755. Copyright 1983, American Medical Association.*

party rounds, conferences, or direct hands-on patient teaching in the office or at the hospital are worthwhile interactions. They also provide continuing medical education and stimulation for the pediatrician.

A local pediatric society could be formed to share expenses for practice management consultation, analysis of new insurance programs, or marketing and advertisement for the general good of the group. A group such as this could identify significant pediatric issues and act as an educational resource for hospitals, HMOs, PPOs, Medicaid, and insurance companies. Pediatricians participating in this type of arrangement should consult with an attorney regarding antitrust constraints.

Schools

Pediatricians can make a pivotal contribution to school boards and parent/teacher associations. Pediatric consultants must be aware of public laws influencing the education of children. On October 8, 1986, President Ronald Reagan signed Public Law 99-457, the Education of the Handicapped Amendments of 1986 (20 USC 1400). It requires early intervention services and preschool programs for infants, toddlers, and preschoolers with handicaps.

PL 99-457 includes a discretionary program for states seeking to provide comprehensive inter-agency services for young children with disabilities (birth through age 2) and their families by the year 1991. The practice of pediatrics involves the identification of children with handicapping conditions or who may be at risk at developing them. Appropriate pediatric case management will lead to good community involvement. The pediatrician who acts as an advocate for these patients in a constructive, non-adversarial manner serves the institution and demonstrates expertise.

In many communities, schools are the primary focus of activity from preschool and day care through elementary and secondary education. These community centers often seek information and guidance on about health issues, growth and development, and the effect of new legislation. Opportunities to serve will arise as a matter of practicing pediatrics.

Pediatricians new to the area will want to become familiar with schools, day care, mother's day out programs, preschool situations, and other community educational resources. Physicians should make time to attend school board and Parent Teacher Association meetings, visit local school campuses, volunteer to guest lecture, and attend athletic events.

Educational institutions need current information about sports injuries, appropriate conditioning of athletes, fad diets and nutritional supplements, and weight restrictions for athletic and drill team participation. Pediatricians who perform preparticipation physicals and should be aware of the local school or coaching philosophy. Those who counsel sports teams should stay current with information and research developed and substantiated by the AAP Committee on Adolescence or Committee on Sports Medicine. Given today's litigious society, great care must be exercised in providing any professional advice.

Pediatricians are well advised to pursue community service opportunities. They lend variety to the daily routine of pediatrics, and provide valuable service to youth and the schools.

Conclusion

Service provided to the community and professional colleagues can greatly enhance a pediatrician's practice, pleasures, and education. In establishing good relations within the professional community, the pediatrician can develop a reputation as a caring and conscientious physician. By working within the community as an advocate for children's needs, the pediatrician can be a potent moving force for positive accomplishments. Establishing this positive image is probably the best "marketing" technique that a pediatrician can develop.

Reference

1. Goldman L, Rudd A. Ten Commandments for Effective Consultations. *Intern Med*. 1983;143:1753-1755

Bibliography

Burgoon JK, Buller DD, Woodall WG. *Non-verbal Communication – Unspoken Dialogue*. 1st ed. New York, NY: Harper & Row; 1989

Hickson ML, Stacks DW. *Non-verbal Communication – Studies in Application*. 2nd ed. Dubuque, IA: William C. Brown Pubs;1989

Checklist

✓ Have you identified community health resources?
✓ Do you maintain a referral list of suitable health care providers?
✓ Do you place your own telephone calls to other physicians?
✓ Are you a volunteer in any community programs?
✓ Would you be willing to act as a resource to the media on pediatric health issues?

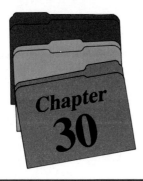

Chapter 30

Community News Media

Advice for dealing with the news media is discussed in this chapter, including:
- **proper response to media inquiries**
- **initiating media contact**
- **full utilization of various forms of news media**

This chapter will emphasize the need for the pediatrician to use the mass media to accomplish one or more of these objectives: (1) inform the public of medical opinion about appropriate news developments and preventive health measures; (2) gain support for community activities; (3) gain personal recognition.

Events which may not be of interest to the media may nevertheless provide valuable opportunities for public education. Activities which garner credibility and recognition for both a sponsoring organization and participating individuals include health fairs, speakers' bureaus, and informal community meetings. Although some of these activities also will have news appeal, their inherent value lies in direct access to the public, and the fact that the content of your message can be controlled.

Handling media inquiries

Professional contacts and activity in a well-known organization may lead to media requests for a particular pediatrician whose expertise or interest areas are known in the community. Some tips for handling inquiries follow.

- Provide information in lay terms, and either respond promptly or refer the reporter to another source for additional or more specialized information if necessary. Ask the reporter's deadline at the outset to allow enough time to gather the necessary information.
- Do not try to prevent a reporter from doing a story, or argue over what is newsworthy. Withholding information leads to inaccurate or unbalanced public education. Take advantage of the opportunity to contribute to a story.
- The person being interviewed is "on the record," so do not expect "off the record" considerations. There is no

such thing as "off the record." If you don't want to be quoted, don't say it.
- Don't ask to review a story before it appears; however, offer to verify facts. In that way quotes can be checked to be sure they were used in context. Also be aware that the reporter's story is edited, (usually by a "city editor") and that the reporter does not write the headline.
- Before consenting to be interviewed – whether by print or broadcast media – clarify several points: Who is the audience? Is it one-on-one with an interviewer or will this be a panel? What opposing points of view might be represented by other panelists or the interviewer? Regarding format, is there a chance to make a clear statement explaining key points apart from any free-wheeling discussion with other panelists? Does the interviewer plan to limit discussion to defined areas? How long will it last?
- Anticipate questions, especially the hostile or negative ones, and prepare succinct replies. Determine how to include and emphasize important points. Practicing with someone who plays the "devil's advocate" may help.
- If the interview is to be a broadcast, review the ground rules for format with the interviewer. During the interview, be brief but complete when answering questions. Decide two or three main points you wish to get across. State the facts at the beginning of the interview and restate them at the end of the broadcast. Avoid technical language. If on television, look at the interviewer, not the camera. On television or in person, facial expression and body movements are part of the message. Speak slowly and distinctly, especially if being interviewed for radio, because the message must be conveyed by voice alone. If several questions are asked, identify which

question is being answered. When representing an organization, make clear which answers are personal opinion and which are official opinions of the organization.

Initiating media contact

Knowing the proper way to initiate contact with the media or seek publicity requires judgment about which vehicle to use.

- To respond to a newspaper article or editorial – whether to correct information or to add salient points – write a three or four paragraph letter to the editor or contribute a longer article to the "op-ed" page. (This is the page opposite the editorial page reserved primarily for syndicated columnists but which, in some papers, also carries contributions from non-professional writers.) In an op-ed article, complex multi-factor issues can be analyzed, such as health care costs. A letter to the editor permits dealing with only one or two points. There is less opportunity to respond to radio or television news coverage or commentaries, but many stations now accept editorial replies to station management editorials.
- To gain editorial support for positions covered in the news and about which there may be differing public opinion, call or write the editorial page staff at various newspapers or the editorial director of radio or television stations to arrange an "editorial board" meeting. Also ask if particular reporters, such as the medical writer, can be included in the interview. Be prepared to document all statements.
- Another technique to help personalize a message and perhaps cover more than one topic is to write

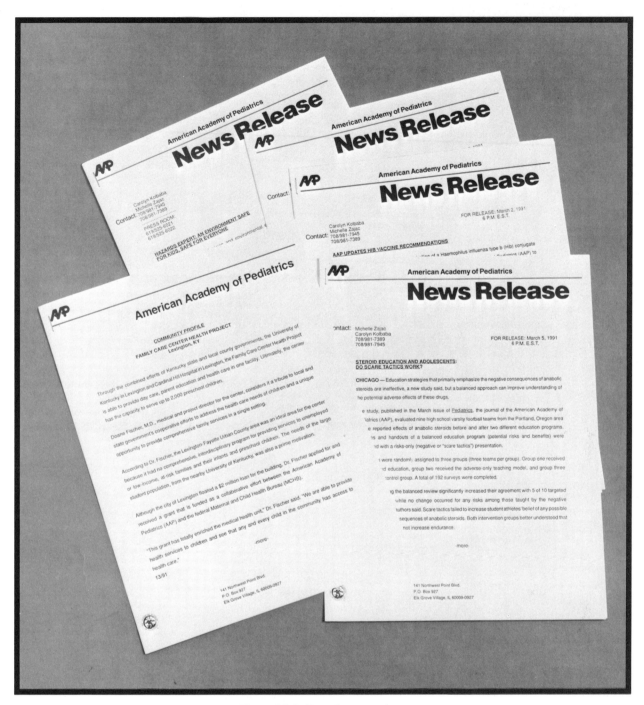

Figure 30-1: Sample news release.

a letter to a radio or television station requesting an interview. If necessary, obtain the name of the producer of a program to whom the letter should be addressed by calling the station. Alternatively one may talk to the program director about an appropriate program for the subject. The letter, suggesting at least one topic and a particular guest, should include some attention-getting facts or questions that can be covered in an interview. Follow the letter with a phone call to the producer a week or two after he or she should have received it. Express interest in learning the station's programming needs. Sometimes the timing is not right, but follow up later if the producer suggests it.

- Occasionally, contacts result in an invitation for a pediatrician who has a good writing style or broadcast personality to prepare a regular health tips column for a weekly newspaper or conduct a regular television or radio program. The pediatrician may suggest a column or program, but be sure to offer an outline of the format, topics, and possible guests you propose. For a large television or radio station, contact the program director or the general manager. Be flexible on the show's production; the station's assigned producer will exert some control. Do not try to inject a personal position on controversial subjects unless you are specifically asked to do so; stick to public health advice.

- To convey useful information on which the public can act, offer news releases to local newspapers or spot scripts to television and radio stations. Stations use these announcements as a service gesture to the community and to help fulfill community service requirements of the Federal Communications Commission. To get air time, public service announcements must be in the format the station uses – 10, 20, 30, or 60 seconds long, a script or tape, perhaps a slide accompanying a script for television. They must be of a genuine service nature, and be given to the proper person at each station. Make personal contact with the public service director or the station manager before preparing the script and at least 2 weeks before it is to air. Public service announcements can be aired at any time. Unlike advertising, which is purchased for certain time periods or programs, these announcements are used at the station's discretion. Consider the average listener of each station and distribute scripts to stations accordingly. Remember to write the script for a speaking person.

Conclusion

Practice constructive communication. Communications strategies which anticipate and act on opportunities for public education are more effective in gaining recognition and acceptance for the pediatrician than merely reacting through the media to a problem or crisis. Continuously listening to and communicating with different individuals can help avert problems. The public needs sufficient information on medical issues, medical care costs, and the quality of care available. The pediatrician is an "expert" with the knowledge – perhaps even the responsibility – to provide this information. Know and use the major points you want to emphasize.

Checklist

✓ Are you responding to media inquiries appropriately and effectively?
✓ Are you using the media thoughtfully and effectively?
✓ Do you make yourself available for media inquiries?
✓ Do you call attention to health care issues?
✓ Are you careful to write and speak with clarity so the public can understand you as well as the issues?

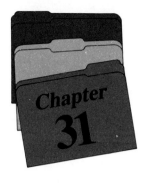

Chapter 31

Retirement

This chapter considers the many facets of retirement planning, and addresses the end of practice as an evolutionary phase of professional life. Content will raise and respond to such questions as:
- **should you retire?**
- **are you ready to retire?**
- **when should you start to plan?**
- **do you have financial security?**
- **have you prepared your practice for retirement?**

Our culture identifies people with their work. Our professional status signifies success and we identify ourselves as pediatricians. Given the time and effort required to become a physician, it is not surprising that we consider our vocation to validate our self-worth.

The concept that "work equals worth" affects how we deal with retirement. The end of practice can be approached as an opportunity for further growth and enjoyment, the end of personal importance, or a time of confused adjustment. Physician retirement is most often a voluntary step, taken after lengthy consideration. Retirement planning includes adapting to a new life-style, which implies myriad considerations that should be addressed long before leaving practice.

Should you retire?

Retiring from practice is most often elective, although many group practices require it. Age is rarely the sole factor in the decision. If you are healthy, enjoy your work, stay current, and contribute your share to the group, there is no need to retire, assuming that your colleagues agree with your assessment. Many pediatricians narrow the scope of practice as they become older, either because they are more interested in certain conditions or because they feel they are not competent in the entire field. Referrals to other members of the group who are more proficient in specialty care, such as diabetes or adolescence, are easily made and accepted by patients and parents.

Many pediatricians want to retire and joyously plan for it. A few set a certain age for leaving practice and know what they want in the future, but the majority do not face the possibility until circumstances make it necessary. Some pediatricians tire of the regulatory hassles, litigation and managerial problems, and view retirement as a solution. Others may feel practice no longer provides the challenge and satisfaction it once did and long for change. Most of us would rather retire *to* something than *from* something.

Partial retirement

Partial retirement (phasing down) may seem attractive with advancing age if there is a desire to work less – and assume less practice responsibility. This may lead into full retirement. This approach can be effective, but it is fraught with problems. If one member contributes less income to group practice, while practice liability insurance and other mutual expenses remain constant, it may be impossible to take in a new member, who would work full-time and generate more income. That situation can irritate younger members, who believe they are contributing more and receiving less, and conflicts often arise in personal relationships. Ill will also results if the retiring member of a group believes he or she is unfairly treated. It is wise for a group practice to reconsider retirement policies periodically, because practices evolve and situations change over the years.

In the group practice setting, each group sets its own policy. The 1978 Age Discrimination in Employment Act[1] says that an employer cannot force a person to retire before the age of 70. But no law requires an employer to allow elderly employees to work fewer hours if they so choose.

The needs of the group and group continuity are paramount. Successful plans match decreasing hours and call schedules with appropriate salary reduction to facilitate the group priority of continued full service to patients and community. Additional pediatricians may be necessary to fill any void, especially if the on-call schedule is part of the change. The salary reduction should not be so prohibitive as to prevent phasing down, if the group allows this accommodation. At the same time, the reduction should be sufficient to discourage a large proportion of early retirees, which would play havoc with scheduling and continuity of care.

A dollar value determination should be placed on the parts of the practice that ensure not only income, but group viability and group vitality. A value should be assigned to night call, weekend call, holidays, management responsibility etc. Values for elimination of night and weekend call may in some cases result in a reduction of income up to 50% that can sometimes allow the group to hire a full or part-time replacement. Then, when a pediatrician group member elects to phase down, the menu is in place, along with the enumeration of practice benefits. The person making changes can pick and choose freely with total group support.

Voluntary phasing down is not for everyone. It may not be practical in every type of group setting. But as we continue to live longer, healthier lives and as the laws continue to change to accommodate the elderly, phasing down promises to become a more popular option among group practice physicians.

Considerations before retirement

If retirement is voluntary, financial position is usually the major consideration. Leaving practice may have to be postponed a few years if present or future financial obligations are high. Unanticipated circumstances can disrupt even the best long-term financial retirement plans.

In truth, few doctors know their current cost of living expenses or future retirement income. They are very often ill-equipped to project the effect of retirement income on life-style goals.

Many factors affect what might become a successful retirement. Divorce, with perhaps two groups of children to support and educate, may make financial security difficult. Aged parents may require supervision and money, or there may be grandchildren to care for and educate.

Health and personal needs are always a major consideration. Careful evaluation of personal, family, and potential future responsibilities is both necessary and important in planning for retirement.

Next, refine your personal definition of retirement life-style. Do you plan to remain in your present home? Do you intend to purchase a second home? Are there major travel plans? Is a part-time job part of the picture? What does your spouse want or expect from your retirement years? The answers to each of these questions shape the nature of your retirement and how it will be financed. Many difficulties can be prevented with careful self-examination and planning.

Retirement has psychological effects, and we all cope with change differently. Ending a significant life-phase is traumatic; the psychic stress is eased by realistic evaluation of the future. Retirement rarely affects only the individual. In most instances it involves a spouse and other family members as well.

Retirement can be a time of growth and enjoyment. Alternatively, it can signal a decline in self-respect for those who feel that they are no longer needed and have ceased to contribute to society, as evidenced by the fact that they are no longer earning income. Retirement for some physicians represents only an escape from problems viewed as intolerable, which is a poor

---

The First Step to Retirement

Advice was once given to a retiring colleague who said he was uncertain about leaving the work and office that had meant so much to him: "On that last day, stay until everyone else has left. Then walk around, look in every room and remember the joys and sorrows, the successes, mistakes, and failures you had in caring for children in those rooms and with the parents you came to know. Then stand in your own office, alone and quiet. Think of all you have done for many years, and finally walk out of the office, close the door, and look to the future, whatever it is. You can't go back, but you will always have many wonderful memories." That is the first step into retirement.

---

orientation for new beginnings. Nevertheless, there is usually a temporary sense of deep personal loss that must be addressed. This can make it difficult to direct one's attention and energies toward the future.

Finances

Financial security is the primary concern in retirement planning, and it requires a structured program. Most of us will begin to plan for that goal early in our practice careers, because inflation multiplies costs each year ($10,000 in 1970 was worth only $3,500 of buying power in 1986). A good financial plan must grow faster than inflation. Compounding yields and reinvestment of dividends, (especially in a tax-deferred program) can provide for tremendous growth possibilities. For instance, $2,000 invested each year in an IRA at 8% will be worth $372,200 in 35 years.

Competent physicians are not always shrewd investors. Investment strategies require skill and business experience. It is wise to consult an appropriate financial advisor to plan retirement finances. (See Professional Advisors, Chapter 17.) Choose your advisors carefully and wisely, because your financial future is at stake. Evaluate your investment personality. How much risk can you live with? How

much time can you give to managing your assets? What are your investment goals? All of these will affect your investment strategy.

It is good policy to include estate planning as part of retirement considerations. Do you have a will? Is a living trust for you, or will a testamentary trust be better? Should it be revocable or irrevocable? Choose a lawyer who is knowledgeable about estate planning and in whom you have confidence. This is important, because estate taxes can change financial resources dramatically for a surviving spouse if plans are not carefully made.

What will your financial needs be in retirement? It may be too early to be precise, but it is never to early to think ahead. Factors to be considered include housing, health expenses, insurance, income and estate taxes, leisure activities, travel, food, and clothing.

It is unlikely that there will be major changes in the way a couple lives unless there are large, unexpected expenses. Therefore income after retirement is extremely important. Work with your financial advisor to maintain a cash flow worksheet, a list of income needs in retirement, and a calculation of your net worth, which should be updated at least annually. Sources of income may include social security, pension plans (corporate or Keogh), IRA accounts, personal investments, part-time employment, and annuities.

Social security payments are available to everyone who has been employed or self-employed. If you have been employed by a corporation, social security deposits should have been deducted from your salary and a contribution should have been made by your employer. If you have been in solo or partnership practice, your annual contributions to social security would be made as a self-employed individual. In planning for retirement, one should write to the local social security office and inquire as to the number of quarters for which contributions have been made. Anyone born after 1928 must have paid social security taxes for 40 quarters (10 full years) to quality for retirement benefits. For a person born before 1928, payments for 29 to 39 weeks are necessary. It is important to be sure that you have enough quarters of payment for maximum benefits while still in practice.

Another source of income is a corporate or individual pension plan. Investigate the stability of your pension plan and its investment strategy. Invest the maximum possible in tax-deferred pension during the years of practice. The pension contribution and the gains accrued can be withdrawn in retirement years when income taxes may be in a lower bracket. Remember that the government places a severe penalty on withdrawal from a pension fund before the age of 59½ years, or after age 70½. Enlist the help of your accountant to set a schedule for withdrawal.

Whether in a corporate practice or partnership, the terms of your retirement benefits should be carefully spelled out in the employment contracts or partnership agreements. It is too late to make financial arrangements with the practice at the time of retirement. The retiring doctor is at a serious disadvantage with late decisions on terms. Spell it out when you form a partnership or join a corporate practice. Retiring can be amicable if details are specified in advance in writing. Contracts and retirement policies should be reviewed frequently and changes made by mutual agreement, especially if a new member joins the group.

Personal investments are another source of income in retirement. Each of us must consider our investment philosophy and realize that it will change as we get closer to retirement.

Plan wisely, and do not hesitate to ask for help from a financial advisor, your bank and/or your attorney. Remember that once retired, it is almost impossible to make up a financial loss with new income.

As a source of income, as well as a psychological boost in retired years, consider part-time employment or an income-producing career change. Hobbies alone cannot provide satisfaction to one who has had a busy, service-oriented professional life. A useful, post-retirement involvement is often a step to a happy retirement. Possibilities include hospital clinics or teaching activities, medical administration, insurance examinations, peer review organizations, locum tenens opportunities, volunteer medical activities in underserved areas of the world, clinical participation in needy areas of this country (urban and rural), and consultant relationships with prepaid medical plans or child-oriented industries. Care must be taken with any of the post-retirement activities so one is not jeopardizing his professional liability insurance "tail." Be sure to get advice on this point.

Exiting the practice

The actual process of leaving a practice varies with the practice arrangement. While solo practice retirement can be time consuming, partnership and corporate retirement terms are ordinarily spelled out in the initial agreement.

Many solo practitioners take in an associate in anticipation of a retirement date, and arrange a buy-out. It is always wise to bring in the associate early enough to introduce patients, arrange hospital privileges, and orient him or her to community practice patterns. It is very important to have a written contract with the associate with all details specified in advance.

If one will be closing a solo practice without bringing in an associate, particular care must be given to the patients' future medical care to avoid the possibility of abandonment.[2] Patient families should be notified, preferably by mail, of the closing of the practice. They should be advised that medical records may be picked up personally or sent to another physician upon request. Some provision must be made for obtaining records after retirement. Copies of the records should be given to the family or sent to another physician, and the original records kept in storage for the extent of the statute of limitations in the retiree's state.

Every attempt should be made to collect accounts receivable before leaving the office because it will be more difficult to do so after leaving. Hospitals, insurance payers, medical organizations, and licensing authorities should be notified of the retirement. Magazines, pharmaceutical companies, and detail men should be informed. Particular help should be offered to employees in finding new employment, in receiving unemployment benefits if applicable, in securing health insurance if there had been a group purchase plan, and in providing letters of recommendation if appropriate. Consideration should be given to the possibility of maintaining emeritus status on hospital staffs and medical societies and in continuing to hold an active medical license. In some states an active license status might involve special assessments, and similarly, hospital staff appointments might result in monetary consequences.

Retiring from a partnership should be less difficult because contractual arrangements should have been specified well in advance. A 1-year notice of elective retirement is not unreasonable. With a busy partnership practice, it may be wise to consider bringing in a

Practice Assets to Consider in Retirement Transactions

Partnership contracts ordinarily specify "buy out" terms, and generally consider purchase of the following assets:

Equipment – hard assets
Valued by age, maintenance required, and obsolescence. The two most frequent valuation methods utilized are book value (original price minus depreciation accumulated) and fair market value (the price that the equipment could obtain in today's market).

Supplies
Administrative, clinical, and drug supplies determined at fair market value.

Owned Real Estate
Straightforward.

Cash on Hand
Proportionate value of cash in checking account, savings account, etc.

Accounts Receivable
Worth less than face value (ie, bad debts, ages of collectibles, possible third-party adjustments, etc).

Covenant not to compete
Including liquidated damage figure if covenant is broken.

Goodwill
One suggested method is to determine average gross receipts per physician and multiply this number by the most current goodwill factor for pediatric medical practices reported in the Goodwill Registry 1991, available from the Health Care Group.

---

new associate and having the retiring partner "slow down" in night and weekend calls.

Retirement from a corporation practice is discussed in detail in the articles of incorporation or bylaws. Retirees may require the services of accountants and lawyers who have worked with the corporation.

It is essential to know medical liability policy requirements for post-practice coverage. The statute of limitations defines a liability "tail" period, which may vary from state to state. Regulations concerning hospital appointments, the continuation or discontinuation of a state medical license, medical society membership, and working relationships with the medical community may affect medical liability status after retirement. It is advisable to discuss retirement plans with your malpractice carrier.

Finally, consider your relationship to the remaining physicians and staff of the practice you are leaving. Medical practice and management concepts change constantly. We may change little with age, but surely medical practice will evolve into new modes of health care delivery. It may be better for the retiree to establish some distance from the practice. This is an individual decision, but in any case, remember that it is no longer "our" practice. Friends and patients will tell us how much we are missed. Do not succumb to the tendency to offer advice.

Adapting to retirement

Retirement raises many questions and often engenders a fear of inactivity. "What will I do with my time?" may be the physician's major concern. Practice has dominated thoughts and energies for years, and leaving practice creates a void that must be filled.

There is a myth that older persons and adolescents have unlimited time. In truth, both age-groups are usually busy. More old people today are capable of leading rewarding, independent lives than ever before.

The myths concerning retirement and old age are balanced by the truths. One truth is that our personalities are exagerated with increasing age. If we have lived a structured life, it will be more rigid. If we have been opinionated,

brusk, arrogant, miserly, wimpish, complaining or demanding, it is likely that these traits will become more evident. We can change, but changing is difficult and must have a high priority among retirement objectives. If we have adjusted to the many changes in our lives with humor and intellectual curiosity, it is likely we can adapt well to the changes of retirement. Just as adolescents require a few years to fit into society, retirees need time to adapt. Those who nurture long-denied interests in nonmedical areas will widen mental horizons and benefit psychologically.

Personal status changes with retirement. Most of us will want to maintain membership in professional peer groups. Sadly, some physicians feel that they have lost affinity for their peers after retirement. It is important to remember that true friendships are based on relationships and not day-to-day activities. Some of us need to interact with people a great deal, while others are contented with a very small circle of friends, but friendships are important for everyone.

Many retirees are tempted to move to another city, perhaps far from their present location. It is valuable to know that moving can be lonely and disappointing; plans should be carefully considered. We have become used to being recognized as doctors; sudden anonymity can be troublesome psychologically and bring a feeling of isolation. The absence of friends, acquaintances and community position can exert a profound effect. On the other hand, mov-

Checklist before leaving practice

Patient notification
Patient records
Medical liability insurance
License renewal or cancellation
Hospital notification
Telephone answering service
Colleague notification
Medical society notice
Social Security notification
Change of address to Post Office
Pension plan notification
DEA to cancel or renew license
Destroy Rx blanks
Employee matters
HMO and PPO notification
Personal insurance
 (eg, office overhead)
Group insurance policies

ing may represent the fulfillment of a long-term dream and the source of much happiness. Most persons suggest that renting a home and living for a few months in the new community can do much to settle the question of a change, especially if it is done on several vacations prior to retirement.

Interpersonal relationships within the family are of great importance and the practice of medicine often tests the commitment of husband and wife. Retirement can greatly alter the bonds of a couple. Consideration must be given to its effects on the spouse, who has valid needs and must also adapt to changes. Again, a lengthy time may be required for both partners to adjust, to find new ways to live together, to change, to embrace a new set of values and objectives, and nurture a close relationship. Retirement can be more difficult for a spouse than for the retiree, but it offers the chance of a better life together.

Retirement and aging go hand in hand. The retiree's debt to society has been paid; age is a season for personal growth and enjoyment. Tournier has said that the major task of aging is to remain as active, sociable and friendly as we can.[3] We must learn to use leisure profitably, develop new interests, and welcome young people and new ideas. We must continue to think and plan, acquire wisdom, and practice gratitude. Our greatest challenge in aging is to find a way to integrate into society and avoid regression, boredom, or even anxiety neuroses.

Some of us feel guilty if we don't work. If the desire to work after retiring from practice is great, it may be impossible to adjust. Many physicians find that a part-time job eases the transition.

Leisure activities can be far more than simple hobbies. Satisfying leisure activities contribute to the meaning of our lives; they are more than time-fillers. Success in retirement depends on continuing, lifelong psychosocial development. As we age, stress emphasizes our faults and virtues. The important things in retirement are those we do freely, those that mean something to us, that widen our horizons and interests and help to counterbalance the effects of our highly specialized professional occupations. Leaving practice, we have a grand opportunity for intellectual and spiritual growth.

We can consider retirement as freedom to explore the many things the world has to offer, and we can continue to enjoy life as we become older. As Thomas Wolfe has said, "You can't go home again."

References

1. The 1978 Age Discrimination in Employment Act, PL 95-478. 42 USC 3001-3013. Also see: Older Americans Act of 1975, PL 94-135, 42 USC 3001; Civil Rights Commission Act of 1978, PL 95-444, 42 USC 1975
2. American Medical Association. *Closing Your Practice*. Chicago, IL: American Medical Association; 1989:7
3. Tournier, P. *Learn to Grow Old*. New York, NY: Harper and Row; 1983.

Retirement Resource Guide

An extensive bibliography, incorporating several articles pertinent to physician retirement, may be obtained by writing the Division of Pediatric Practice, American Academy of Pediatrics, PO Box 927, Elk Grove Village, IL 60009-0927.

Organizations and Corporate Sources of Information

American Association of Retired Persons (AARP)
1909 "K" Street, NW, Washington, DC 20049 (202/872-4700)
   Planning your Retirement PW 3729 (788) D12322
   Think of Your Future, Retirement Planning Workbook #24893
   Money Matters PF 3677 (1186)
   Take Charge of Your Money
   Info Pak, Retirement Planning Programs

American Association of Senior Physicians
1 East Erie Street, Chicago, IL 60611 (312/280-7260)
   Get More Out of Your Years after Age 50

The Health Care Group
140 W Germantown Pike, Suite 200, Plymouth Meeting, PA 19462 (215/828-3888)

Merrill Lynch Consumer Market
NY Sales Office, World Financial Center, South Tower, 4th Floor, New York, NY 10080-6104 (800/338-2814)
   Retirement Builder: Guidebook to Planning Financial Security (Code #10461/1188)
   Defining The Future: Two Views of Retirement Planning (Code #10843)
   Analytical Retirement Planning Services (Code #10638)
   The Distribution Decision Analysis Service: A Guide to Making the Most of Your Lump-Sum Distribution (Code #10767)

Courses on Retirement

Gearing Up For Retirement
American Medical Association, Dept of Practice Management, PO Box 10946, 535 N Dearborn, Chicago, IL 60610, 312/645-5000

Achieving a Successful Retirement
American Association of Senior Physicians, 1 East Erie Street, Chicago, IL 60611, 312/280-7260

Think of Your Future: Retirement Planning Workbook
AARP, 1909 "K" Street NW, Washington, DC 20049, 202/872-4700

Planning for Creative Retirement: Exploring Psychological Considerations
Meninger Clinic, Box 829, Topeka, KS 66601-0829, 800/288-0318

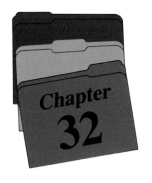

Chapter

32

Taking the Stress Out of Stress

RX for Success in Practice

This chapter examines stress as a phenomenon of professional life. It considers ways the pediatrician can root out its causes and address its management. Topics for consideration include:
- **definitions**
- **causes**
- **"burnout" versus "rustout"**
- **suggestions for coping**

Today's pediatricians face myriad demands and stresses as a result of recent dramatic changes in health care and society as a whole. A 1985 national survey by the Children's National Medical Center in Washington DC, conducted with the support of the American Academy of Pediatrics, found that 81% of responding pediatricians reported feeling moderately to highly stressed in their daily professional activities. The majority of these respondents (85%) also reported feeling very successful and moderately to very satisfied (76%) with their professional lives.[1]

Some of the reasons for the high degree of stress are related to a new environment that is no longer predictable and regular. Many pediatricians report dissatisfaction with the threat of malpractice, the changes in the reimbursement system, the managed care plans and contracts and their effect on patient care and practice income, the competition for patients, the long, irregular and unpredictable hours, the endless telephone calls, and limited time for research and teaching.[1,2]

Many of these changes do not allow pediatricians and their staff to respond automatically to pressures and demands, as was possible a decade ago. We are overloaded on a daily basis with many more events and problems, yet the time for evaluation and decision-making has, if anything, diminished.

We cannot escape the stress that accompanies the many changes in our daily professional lives. The challenge we face is how to take the stress out of stress.

What is stress?

Hans Selye, MD, a pioneer in modern stress research, created widespread attention to the word, "stress," in 1956 with the publication of his book, *The Stress of Life*.[3] Stress, according to Selye, is the nonspecific response of our body to any demand placed upon it. For example, stress can result from a change or threat and can be pleasant or unpleasant. The purpose of the stress response is to protect our body from the external event or demand, and bring our body back to normal both physically and emotionally.

The human body reacts in the same way to emotional stress as it does to physical stress. Until this century, most stress was primarily a physical threat requiring a physical response of "flight or fight." The physical response involves the body producing chemicals for extra strength and energy to respond to the stressor. Today, our stress is different. Modern stress is primarily mental and interpersonal. Yet, our bodies react as they have for millions of years by producing high energy chemicals and a rise in blood pressure and heart rate for "fight or flight"...instead of for low physical energy demands.

Too much stress, whether it is physical or emotional, can be harmful instead of protective. A wide variety of familiar stress symptoms, such as headaches, back pain, high blood pressure, anger, lack of energy, sleeplessness, impaired performance, inability to achieve satisfaction and helplessness, overeating or loss of appetite, drug or alcohol abuse, job burnout, and divorce bear witness to its influence.

The challenge is to develop appropriate responses to the new type of stress we encounter today.

"Burnout" versus "rustout"

We all know colleagues, staff, family, patients, and parents who exhibit many of the symptoms related to excessive stress. Yet, others who experience the same pressures, changes, and demands appear to excel under these same conditions. Why do the same "stressors" result in dysfunctional symptoms in some and not in others?

Stress can be viewed as ally or an enemy. Too little stress can result in boredom or "rustout."[4] On the other hand, too much stress can overload us and impair our performance. How do people find that optimal level between "burnout" and "rustout" and turn stress into an ally?

Of particular interest to these questions is the 20 years of research of Charles Garfield.[5] Garfield, in contrast to most psychological researchers, studied top achievers in the United States in corporations, the professions, government, athletics, arts, and sciences. He developed a common profile of these "peak performers."

Peak performers, contrary to the popular myth, are not Type A personalities. *They are balanced.* They work hard, yet they know how to stop and play and take care of themselves.

Peak performers know how to make stress work for them, not against them. They have the ability to find the optimal level of stress that leads to peak performance instead of burnout. Some of the common characteristics of peak performers are:

- **A Mission.** They have a picture or vision of what they would like to achieve that motivates their actions and those around them. Peak performers develop their missions as a practical way to express their intrinsic values. They know what they really care about and want to accomplish. They commit themselves to that goal, and set about developing the expertise to meet it.
- **Planning.** Peak performers are self-directed planners who set realistic and reachable goals to turn their vision into reality. *Their goals are clear and concise* and are compatible with their mission. Their sense of mission gives them the staying power to overcome the obstacles and achieve their goals.
- **Doing.** The Nike slogan, "Just do it," can be applied to peak performers. They are able to commit appropriate time and resources to achieving their goals. They can distinguish between tasks they must perform perfectly and tasks that require a response or a best possible response under the circumstances without getting bogged down in perfection or details.
- **Effectiveness.** Peak performers have a bottom line orientation whether it is budget, quality, service, or investment. They think in terms of progress and acquiring the skills that are needed to succeed.
- **Skills.** Effectiveness is not an innate quality of peak performers. They have learned to be effective. They learn the skills that are necessary and compatible to achieving their mission. Most report that they have not yet mastered all the skills they would like.
- **Flexibility.** Peak performers expect change and know how to manage it. They view change as an opportunity. They are flexible, and their priority is finding solutions to problems – not blaming others for failures. Peak performers themselves are flexible about their failures. They have little fear of failure, viewing their failures as well as successes as part of the process in achieving their missions.

- **Team Players.** Peak performers are team players. They recognize few tasks or goals can be performed by one person. They are visionaries whose sense of mission motivates others to work as a team to accomplish the task or goal.
- **Self-caring.** True peak performers, while capable of intense effort, protect their physical and mental health. They know their overall fitness increases their effectiveness and that poor health and poor personal relationships can require more energy than the work itself. Peak performers value their work and family relationships and work to resolve problems to maintain healthy relationships. They are committed to their mission and appreciate the pivotal value of healthy bodies, minds, and relationships.

Peak performers, as can be seen, are able to turn stress into an ally and achieve the balance between "burnout" and "rustout." They know who they are, where they are going and how to maintain their perspective to stay on track.

Guidelines for taking the stress out of stress

The next step is to find that balance between "burnout" and "rustout" or too much stress and too little stress. Burnout and rustout often are synonymous with the accelerated life-style in the United States where it is easy to lose touch with our values, skills, styles, relationships, and goals. When we neglect these, we often may begin to feel "stressed out" and controlled by what we do and outside events.

Most importantly, there are a number of steps that we can follow to take the stress out of stress and regain control in our everyday lives. Some of the best strategies to gain control and make stress work for you instead of against you are listed below.[2] Each pediatrician should develop his or her own individual strategic plan that includes stress and time management. This plan is based on a self-assessment of one's unique values, skills, and interpersonal styles. Each individual should be able to list a wide variety of immediate and long-range goals. These will include small things, such as spending a few hours a week teaching, to major

shifts in professional emphasis, such as taking an administrative position in medicine, or leaving practice.

The steps below will help you to develop an individual strategic plan and take the stress out of stress. Each pediatrician finds different strategies to make stress an ally. Your challenge is to find the "combination" that works for you.

Step 1: Reassess your values and skills

The insidious pressure to subordinate one's values and skills to the many new demands and changes taking place in the health care system is a major source of stress working against us. Each pediatrician should answer the questions: Who am I? What are my values, skills, and personality styles? How do others perceive me?

The following questions can help you to examine what is important to you, what is satisfying, and what is dissatisfying and stressful. The purpose is to give a framework for strategies to achieve a balance between "burnout" and "rustout."

What are my values?

A value is a principle or quality we hold as important and is usually expressed in the way we behave. An example of some work values are: pay, security, peer relationships, challenge, good variety of work tasks, a sense of contribution, advancement opportunity, opportunity to supervise others, and good supervision.

Think about what you value most at work and at home. Then, rate your satisfaction with each of these values. In areas where you are dissatisfied, think about steps that you can take to make changes. For example, many pediatricians in general practice express concerns about the everyday routine and lack of challenge. Some report that devoting a few hours each week to teaching, participating in some research or developing a subspecialty for their practice, dramatically increases career satisfaction and reduces stress. Working with local, state, and national pediatric issues, school boards, and boys/girls clubs, can also be of benefit.

What are my skills?

A skill is a developed aptitude or ability to use one's knowledge effectively and competently in a particular task. Your skills are the second most important aspect to consider in taking the stress out of stress, because of the impact they have on your career fit and options.

A good way to assess your skills is to think about a major achievement you have had in your work in the past few years. Next, answer these questions:

- What skills did you use to accomplish the task?
- What do others like about me? What do they dislike?
- How often do you use these skills in your present work?
- How can you build into your work the skills that you use only occasionally?
- What other skills do you enjoy?
- What skills would you like to have that you do not have now? Peak performers, as you recall, do not feel they have all the skills they need and are learning new skills, as necessary, to achieve their mission.

Pediatricians report a wide variety of ways to use under-utilized skills and develop new ones. Those, for example, who are interested in better practice management, can take courses to increase their management and financial skills and assume more of that role in the group practice. Others might do a mini-residency or other CME activity to develop a subspecialty for their group practice, such as in counseling for school problems and learning disorders.

What are my personality styles?
An awareness of one's personality style is important to making stress an ally. You will recall that peak performers recognize the need to have a good team to achieve their goals. Team builders have an awareness of how they interact with others. That awareness enables you to adopt a style that is compatible with and motivating to the colleagues and staff with whom you work. It also allows you to identify a compatible team at work and at home. *There are no right or wrong styles.* Some questions you may ask yourself about your personality style and those around you are:

- What do I like to do with others? Do I like to include them in what I do? Do I like to take charge? Am I warm and close to others or businesslike?
- What do others like about me? What do they dislike?
- What do I want others to do to me? Do I want others to invite me to join them? Do I want others to take charge? Do I want others to be warm or businesslike toward me?

- What is my personality style under normal conditions? What is my personality style under stress?

Now that you have a brief overview of your style, think about colleagues and staff with whom you work: 1) the best, 2) worst. Based on your style and others' styles, identify strategies that will achieve your goals. For example, if you are a take-charge person, seek to surround yourself with others who want someone else to make the decisions and assume the leadership role. Alternatively, some individuals are able to take control, but also to allow others to assume control as the circumstances may require. They can be businesslike or warm and personal when necessary; and include or not include others.

It takes time to assess values, skills, and personality styles. A career planning seminar or other such formal educational program may help you to assess your values and skills to set goals that make stress work for you. Remember it takes time to find what it is important to you. Don't let this process be another source of stress by setting unrealistic expectations.

Step 2: Setting goals

Now, that you have looked at your values, skills, and personality styles, setting short-term and long-term goals is the next step.

When you are setting goals, set some that can be accomplished in the next 2 to 12 months (short-term goals) and that are compatible to the achievement of your long-term goals (1 to 5 years). Goals fall into four categories: work, recreation, relationships and self. Your short- and long-term goals should be developed to build your values, skills, and personality style into everyday activities based on what is realistic. Remember, the purpose of this assessment is not to increase your stress!

Step 3: Achieving goals

"A plan is nothing unless it degenerates into work."[6]

Peter Drucker

A strategy to assess how you best achieve your goals is to think about

goals that you have successfully accomplished. Secondly, think about what you did to achieve them. Think about obstacles and how you overcame them. Then, list some of the most successful strategies you used and apply them to your strategic plan and goals.

Some classic strategies: 1) put your plan and goals in writing with action steps and time lines; 2) communicate them to at least one other person; 3) reevaluate them often. Follow the lead of peak performers, who know that it is necessary to commit time and appropriate resources to accomplish your plan.

Step 4: More strategies to manage stress

Some of the best strategies to manage stress are listed below. Try some or all of them and find what works for you.

1. Stress: "Is it worth dying for?" Robert Eliot, MD, a cardiologist who had a stress-related heart attack at age 41, says: "Rule No 1 is, don't sweat the small stuff. Rule No 2 is, it's all small stuff. And if you can't fight and you can't flee, flow."[7]
2. Physical Exercise: Physical exercise is not only necessary for health and physical development; it also enhances intellectual functioning.
   Peak performers make a commitment to fitness and take care of themselves. One of the best ways to begin to manage stress and get control back into your life is to get your body into shape. You will find that you will have more energy and a better perspective for work, recreation, and relationships. Find the exercise program and the foods you like so your commitment to good health will be long term.
3. Self-Talk: Have you ever thought about what you say to yourself? During most of our waking hours, even when we are with other people, we are talking to ourselves.
   This stress management strategy for conversations we have with ourselves is considered one of the most valuable. How we think can either motivate us or demoralize us and actually create or reduce stress for us.
   A number of factors contribute to the amount of stress we create for ourselves. The way we have learned to respond, past experiences, our process of analysis, what we expect

and believe of ourselves and others. *We can change by eliminating negative conversations with ourselves.*

Some other strategies to improve your self-talk:

- Setting realistic expectations or goals. In your self-talk, do not minimize or overestimate your abilities and behaviors, or those of others. This is a setup to create stress.
- Eliminate stress-creating words from your conversations with yourself. Words such as "if only," "should," "could," "never," "can't," "always," are among those that create stress through producing mistakes in the way we think. "Shoulds, coulds, and if-onlys" are punishing ways of thinking and do not solve the problem. "Never" and "always" imply perfection, which is difficult to attain.
- Use positives. It becomes easy to disregard your own and others' positive attributes and behaviors, especially when you are operating under stressful conditions. When stressed, take a deep breath and talk to yourself using a balance sheet approach. Look at your positive attributes and accomplishments, as well as those of others. You will reduce your stress and be more likely to create solutions instead of problems and achieve your goals.

4. Relationships: Peak performers are team players. They know they need other people to achieve their goals. Identify the people who support and encourage you. Different people provide different types of support such as assistance, intimacy, collegiality or guidance. Look at what you need and ask for their help.

5. Time Management: "I don't have enough time," is a modern refrain. Daily life becomes very stressful when we are expected to perform many more activities than in the past with no additional time. Time management strategies are important. (See Time Management, Chapter 24.)

6. Course Correction: Peak performers recognize that they are going to make mistakes, and look at a mistake as an opportunity to learn. A good technique to reduce stress is to cite when you are likely to go off course in work, health, and family relationships. Use these indicators to keep yourself on course and balanced before you stray very far.

Summary

These stress management techniques suggest strategies to manage the stress created by the many changes occurring in health care and our society today.

A good approach to remember in making stress work for you is: *"Peak performers are made, not born."* [5] Garfield found in his research that peak performers have created strategies to perform extraordinarily well under what to many would be very stressful conditions. As a physician, you have created conditions under which you have performed extraordinarily well under what many regard as very stressful conditions.

In the stresses of daily life, we may sometimes lose our balance and missions can be nearly forgotten. Yet peak performers find opportunities to correct course and restore balance. We cannot escape the stress in our professional lives, but the right strategies can help you take the stress out of stress.

References

1. Jewett LS, Leibowitz Z, Greenberg LW. Counseling Residents in Selecting a Career: Techniques for Residency Training Program Directors. Presented at the Ambulatory Pediatric Association Annual Meeting; May 7, 1986, Session I; Washington, DC
2. Jewett LS, Leibowitz Z. Unpublished data from Career Planning Workshops, 1983-1989
3. Selye H. *The Stress of Life*. New York, NY: McGraw-Hill; 1956
4. Blanchard K, Edington DW, Blanchard M. *The One Minute Manager Gets Fit*. New York, NY: William Morrow and Company; 1966
5. Garfield C. *Peak Performers*. New York, NY: William Morrow and Company; 1986
6. Drucker P. *Management: Task, Responsibilities, and Practices*. New York, NY: Harper and Row; 1973
7. Eliot RS, Breo DL. *Is it worth dying for?* New York, NY: Bantam Books; 1984

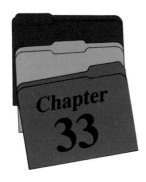

Uniformed Services Pediatrics

Professional characteristics of a pediatric practice in the military medical system are described to illustrate how similar, and yet different, its practice style is.

Many of the principles of practice management in this manual are applicable to pediatricians serving in the uniformed services. This chapter will therefore describe uniformed services pediatrics as a career option, emphasizing its uniqueness, advantages, and disadvantages.

Uniformed services medicine has been described by some as the "world's largest Health Maintenance Organization (HMO)" and indeed bears many similarities without sharing a lot of the problems common to this practice style. Almost 10% (1,700) of the medical students graduating in 1989 were supported in part by the Armed Forces Health Professions Scholarship Program (AFHPSP) and another 160 medical students graduated from the Uniformed Services University of the Health Sciences (USUHS). These new physicians will serve on active duty in the uniformed services after the completion of their training.

The type of pediatric practice these physicians can experience is extremely varied, because military health facilities range from an 800-plus bed tertiary care teaching hospital to small isolated clinics where less than 10 physicians are assigned. Each branch of the service has small clinics where the pediatrician may have a solo practice, medium sized clinics which resemble four to ten member group practices, and large teaching hospital practices with 12 to 30 staff pediatricians and most of the military's subspecialists, who work together to train residents and fellows. Pediatricians also may be assigned as faculty to the USUHS in Bethesda, Maryland.

Many characteristics are common to all the uniformed services:

1. The patients are not charged directly for the services rendered, although trials are being considered to charge a nominal fee for ambulatory visits. All active duty and retired military dependents are eligible for care at any military facility if that facility has the available space and personnel to care for them.

2. The pediatricians are all commissioned officers of the United States military services. Their salaries are equal to the amount paid to any service member of similar rank (which includes nontaxable stipends for housing and food) plus any bonuses or professional pay allocated to physicians.

3. A retirement program is available which can provide up to 50% of base pay for an individual retiring after 20 years of active duty service and up to 75% for a person retiring after 30 years of services.

4. Military pediatricians are members of the military services and they are assigned as required by the needs of the services. Increasing fiscal constraints shared with civilian medicine in this country continually provide new challenges, but have led to much more stability in assignments. Pediatricians also may be assigned duties which are not pediatric in nature, eg, assignment as a general medical officer in the emergency room of a small hospital or clinic. They may also be given additional duties in the administration and/or quality assurance programs of a Medical Treatment Facility (MTF). Each service has requirements for preparation and proficiency in medical wartime skills. Each pediatrician, as well as every other military physician, participates in medical readiness training.

5. Because the patient population is subject to government transfers, it is unusual for a patient to be followed by a single pediatrician from birth through adolescence. However, under new family support programs, children with chronic medical, psychological and educational concerns are being assigned indefinitely to the larger, more completely staffed MTFs, where they can receive subspecialty service as well as better continuity of care.

6. Because the patients are part of an organization, they are subject to the supervision of that organization – the military authorities. This may be a distinct advantage when dealing with victims of child or spouse abuse.

7. There is an opportunity to travel (with someone else planning, arranging, and paying for the move) and to see new areas of the world without the problems involved in setting up a practice in a new community.

8. All branches of the service have training programs and systems to provide various types of fellowship training. The large teaching hospitals have facilities and funds for clinical research studies.

9. Military pediatricians enjoy the freedom to practice optimal medicine unburdened by the pressures often encountered in building and maintaining a practice. Freedom from concern over individual malpractice liability buffers the tendency to practice defensive medicine. While cost containment is as important as in civilian practice, the military pediatrician essentially is freed from concerns regarding the costs of tests, hospitalization, or medicines for patients as well as pressures for early discharge of hospitalized patients.

10. When specialized care for a patient is not available at the local military MTF, the patient can be transferred to another military

facility capable of this care using a sophisticated air evacuation system certainly unparalleled in civilian practice. Military dependents may be referred to civilian physicians in their own offices and to civilian hospitals using local MTF funds or, more commonly, CHAMPUS (Civilian Health and Medical Program of the Uniformed Services) with some cost sharing by the patients. Civilian pediatricians may supplement those working at an MTF by a contractual arrangement or by the more recently developed Health Care Partnerships (a system where civilian physicians see patients at military facilities, billing CHAMPUS a set fee with no cost sharing on the part of the patient).

Although all branches of the military services have much in common, they maintain their uniqueness. The Air Force has many small hospitals as well as many overseas bases. The Army is the largest service and has the greatest variability in opportunities. Small hospitals are available, overseas assignments are possible, and there are more large teaching hospitals than in any other branch of the service. The Navy has many medium-sized hospitals, four large teaching hospitals, and the possibility of assignment to large seaports throughout the world.

The US Public Health Service offers opportunities for assignment to a variety of situations, such as an Indian reservation, a large hospital in a large metropolitan area, the National Institutes of Health, or the Centers for Disease Control. Information about the US Public Health Service may be obtained by writing: Dept of Health and Human Services, US Public Health Service, Recruitment Program, Rm 7A-07, Parklawn Building, 5600 Fishers Lane, Rockville, MD 20857. Or telephone 800/221-9393 (in Virginia 703/734-6855).

Pediatricians interested in learning more about serving in any branch of the service should contact the nearest military recruiter, military treatment facility, or the Army, Navy, or Air Force Surgeon General's Office in the Pentagon at Washington, DC. In addition, most medical schools have a medical school liaison officer assigned by each branch of the military service to interact with the dean's office and the medical students in the AFHPSP. Commissioned officers who wish to explore further military options may write: Physician Placement Officer, CPOD 4-35, Parklawn Boulevard, Rockville, Maryland 20857. Contact by telephone at 800/443-3087.

Checklist

✓ Have you considered the advantages and disadvantages of a career in the armed forces?

✓ Does the opportunity to practice in different parts of the country (or world) appeal to you?

✓ Are you aware that you may have medical assignments involving areas other than pediatrics?

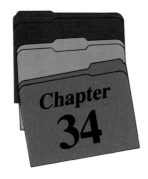

Teaching Practice Management to Pediatric Residents

Chapter 34

Pediatric residents need to be exposed to "private practice." This chapter examines the issue from the academic and private practice perspectives. It outlines methods that can help both the practice and the training program make this system work.

Establishment of a practice management curriculum

Many pediatric residency training programs offer limited opportunities to experience practical aspects of pediatric practice. Most residents select a practice setting for their career after completion of their training. Ideally, training programs should provide a practice management curriculum for residents that allows them to make an informed choice.

Residency programs emphasize the in-hospital, high-tech tertiary care environment – far from the patient needs in the usual practice setting. Although ambulatory experiences are mandated by the Accreditation Council for Graduate Medical Education (ACGME), these traditionally occur in the university hospital with a lower socioeconomic, inner-city population. That patient base has its special problems and needs, and the specific concerns unique to office practice are of lower priority or omitted from the curriculum. Discrepancies between the emphasis of training programs and the care delivered once in actual practice can lead to disillusionment and career dissatisfaction for the pediatrician trained to care for different kinds of pediatric problems than those seen in private practice.

A number of forces can motivate programs to expand their curricula to the office setting. These include economic factors, space limitations, marketing in the community, enhancing primary care to satisfy ACGME requirements, and the prospect of a further shift from inpatient to outpatient care. Medical

centers are feeling the pinch of inefficient patient care systems in their ambulatory departments, and are moving some of their ambulatory care into the community as a result. Training programs also are confronted with space problems, as the number and complexity of ambulatory visits increase. Unintentional competition for patients and space has evolved among trainees and medical students. A training rotation in a private practitioner's office can address some of these problems. Incorporating private practitioners into the curriculum as primary care role models could help to heal the town-gown divisiveness too common in many communities.

The importance of a practice management curriculum is recognized by the ACGME in the special requirements section of the "Essentials of Accredited Residencies in Graduate Medical Education."[1] Office preceptorships may occur for up to 2 months in each of the second and third years of training. Assignments may be in blocks of time or may run concurrently with other responsibilities. Voluntary faculty are designated by the program director and selected for their willingness and ability to teach. The resident is expected to be an active participant in the process, not a passive onlooker. He is expected to maintain office records, manage patients, and accompany the practitioner on hospital visits. These guidelines stop short of mandating a didactic and experiential curriculum in practice management.

Realistically, to appreciate primary care pediatrics as a career goal, the resident must experience life in a practice environment. In the office setting, the practicing pediatrician can serve as

an effective role model, demonstrating his skills as healer, educator, manager, confidant, and advocate. The resident has the opportunity to become familiar with the many facets of practice. He or she can observe and participate in the interactions between doctor and patient/parent, and have access to the office staff, which represents an integral part of the pediatric team.

At least two conditions are necessary to create a primary care experience in a practice environment:

1. The pediatric department chair must be prepared to accept and to actively support inclusion of the practicing pediatrician in the teaching program. The practitioner who assumes an active role in a university teaching program must be judged on the basis of his or her unique contributions.

2. The pediatrician in private practice must not underestimate the value of his or her contributions to the teaching program. Experience in the pediatrician's office should not be a rehash of the discussions of pathophysiology which might take place in the hospital clinic. The pediatrician has much to offer and should feel enthusiastic and remain firmly convinced of the value of the office experience. Pediatricians must be willing to sacrifice time and possibly money.

Establishing goals and objectives

The goals of a program to teach pediatric residents practice management are:

1. Enable residents to understand and appreciate the rewards and liabilities of pediatric practice.

2. Involve practicing pediatricians in the training of pediatric residents within the office setting and medical center.
3. Enable pediatric residents to experience office-based pediatric primary care and to evaluate this area objectively as a career goal.

The objectives of the program are embodied in the curriculum. Practitioners, residents, and the director of the training program should participate in their development. Involvement of practitioners at this stage of planning is essential to tap their experience and to indicate in a concrete fashion the concern and commitment of the university department of pediatrics to the logical development of the program. Content may focus on organizational aspects of private practice as well as the essential elements of primary care. The director of residency training or an individual involved with both residents and community pediatricians should serve as program advocate.

The curriculum should allow the resident to experience and observe all aspects of the office practice with enough flexibility to accommodate different types of practice. This includes handling managerial/business issues, communicating with parents and children, supervising office staff performance, tapping community resources, and continuing medical education. The curriculum should be spelled out in detail and reviewed by all concerned so that expectations of the office practice rotation are clearly delineated for both the practitioner and the resident. The objectives should be realistic and achievable in the allotted time.

Some of the principles of a practice management curriculum can be conveyed in a series of talks which can be incorporated into the residency curriculum. In addition to the practicing pediatrician, other participants may include attorneys, accountants, business consultants, and computer analysts. Program planners should concur on curriculum content for residency training, and how these objectives will be achieved and evaluated.

The organization and presentation of this curriculum (eg, 1 day seminar versus an ongoing series) should be flexible, but ideally should coincide with the time when residents seriously begin thinking about career choices. The content needs to emphasize principles and practice philosophies without delving into the details that may be specific to an individual practice. Personal experiences and actual case scenarios using a problem-solving approach can make the information more real to residents.

Residents working in a pediatric office

All too often, physicians who practice in the community feel isolated. The intellectual stimulation of daily discussion of patients and medical issues that occurred during residency training is missing. Affiliation with a local medical center offers an opportunity to continue contact with other physicians. Although some communities suffer a "town-gown" split, wherein the relationship between physicians in private practice and faculty at the medical center is strained, both parties can profit greatly from an association. Those at the medical center can learn from the experience and practice of the clinical faculty, while practicing physicians can enjoy the intellectual stimulation of collegial interaction.

Traditional roles for community physicians include attending on wards and in outpatient departments. One of the recent innovations in residency training programs that provides an excellent opportunity for clinical faculty is placement of pediatric residents in private offices for their continuity clinic.[2] Residents who participate in such a program gain a very "real-world" experience, learning not only about outpatient medicine, but also about practice management, life-style, and demands of practice.

Community physicians who consider taking a resident into the office must evaluate their interest in teaching, the commitment of time and energy necessary to participate in such a program, the effect on the practice of having residents, and practical issues, such as space, billing, malpractice insurance, and generating a panel of patients for the resident. Some of the major issues are discussed below. Community physicians who have become preceptors have uniformly felt it to be a rewarding experience, both personally and professionally.

Selecting a resident

The relationship between the resident and the private pediatrician is critical. Having a resident join the practice for a few days or weeks, or for 1 to 3 half-days per week, is much like working with a new associate. Pediatricians who wish to participate in this type of teaching program should insist on interviewing the residents, so that they can select one with whom they feel compatible.

Defining expectations

Because the majority of their training takes place in the hospital setting, and because most residents have had little or no experience in a private office, it is important to outline their obligations when they join the practice. Primary among these should be attendance and timeliness. Residents will experience conflict between their hospital duties and their continuity clinics. They must appreciate the demands of private practice and the importance of accommodating patients. It is wise to schedule residents lightly when they are assigned to the intensive care units and following call nights. Residents need to learn to work closely with the receptionist in arranging their schedules, and should be aware that appointments are often made weeks in advance. They should know what to do if an emergency arises that will cause them to be late or to miss their appointed schedule. They should also learn about office routine, such as how telephone calls are managed, and their roles in both seeing patients and responding to calls.

Financial implications

Private physicians precepting a resident are concerned about the financial impact. Teaching takes time, and time means money. Fortunately, in this setting, teaching can be done in a very cost-effective manner. Using the techniques of direct observation and intermittent consultation described below, pediatricians can actually see the same number of patients per half-day when the resident is in the office as when he or she is not. The average resident can generate significant billings for working in the office without necessitating additional office staff. If the private physician does not have to pay any portion of the resident's salary and does not hire any additional personnel, these billings should compensate for the preceptor's teaching time.

Half-Day Scheduling for New Residents

First 3 half-days:	Resident follows/observes preceptor.
Next 7 half-days:	Maximum of 2 patient visits per day, Preceptor observes.
After first 10 days:	No more than 4 patient visits per week (until resident has been there 4 months).
First 4 months:	Two preceptor-observed visits per week, plus 2 visits on their own.
After 6 months with preceptor:	Preceptor and resident evaluate how much resident is capable of doing.
Remainder of year:	Progress to 6 patients on a "consult with preceptor basis," preceptor observing at least 2 visits per month.

Figure 34-1: Sample half day scheduling for new residents.

Malpractice coverage will be handled in various ways, depending on the area of the country and the teaching program. Generally, when the resident is in a supervised setting that is part of an established residency, the program should provide malpractice insurance. If, however, the resident chooses to spend additional hours for which he is compensated by the practice, then the practice will need to provide insurance coverage. This matter should be reviewed with the pediatrician's professional liability insurance carrier.

Scheduling the resident

When the resident first starts in the office, it is prudent to schedule several half-days without seeing patients. The resident should follow the pediatrician, observing the style and content of visits. The pediatrician should explain each component of the patient visit, from why he opens the door slowly (so he won't knock down the 2-year old who is standing on the other side) to what should be included in a 2-month well-child check. The resident should also spend time with the receptionists and nurses to learn how they function and to establish a relationship with them.

After becoming familiar with office routine, the resident should begin to see patients with the pediatrician observing. This can be done efficiently if the preceptor is not scheduled to see patients for the first half hour of office time. The preceptor should continue to sit in on the resident's encounters until he is comfortable that the resident is capable of managing each type of visit independently or with simple consultation. Residents should be scheduled for only two or three patient visits per half-day for the first 2 months in the office. This can gradually be increased as the resident becomes more confident and capable. Figure 34-1 is a sample of a first year resident's and preceptor's schedules and outlines the number of patients a new resident can be expected to see per half-day.

Gathering a panel of patients

One of the concerns expressed by private physicians is whether or not patients will accept the resident. Generally this is not a problem. The preceptor is likely to know which families are open to a new experience. Residents are often free to spend more time with patients, which offers a significant advantage to some families. An explanation of the program for families in the preceptor's practice is helpful. Figure 34-2 displays a brochure that can be kept in the office and given to families to read. A poster with the resident's picture, some personal information, and a narrative describing pediatric specialty training can be placed prominently in the waiting area.

The office receptionists and nurses play a critical role. Those offices that have been most successful in recruiting patients for the resident have instructed their receptionist to introduce the resident as "a physician who is in his subspecialty training in pediatrics and who will be in the office part-time for the next 3 years." The receptionist can offer patients the option of seeing the resident, saying, "Dr X (the preceptor) could see Susan at 4:30, or Dr Y (the resident, whom the receptionist then describes as outlined above) has an opening sooner, and could see her at 1:00. Which would you prefer?"

Another method for building a resident's panel of patients is for the resident to go to the newborn nursery with the preceptor and meet families during the babies' hospital stay. The preceptor can ask the family if they would make an appointment with the resident for the first office visit.

Teaching in the office

When residents and preceptors are paired one-to-one, a unique type of teaching is possible. The value of direct observation cannot be overemphasized. Residents observe their preceptors and learn rapidly about both the process and content of care. When preceptors observe one-to-one, they

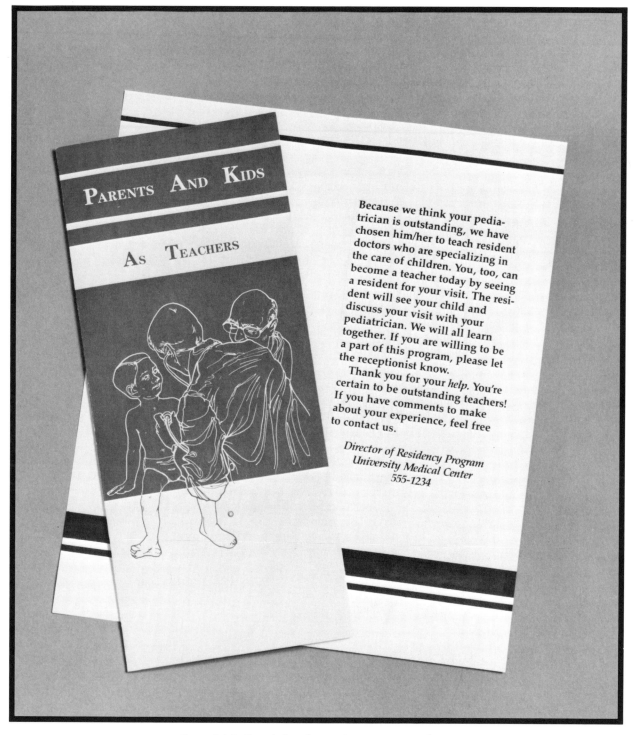

Figure 34-2: Sample brochure informing parents that residents will be coming into the practice as part of their pediatric training.

discover how well the resident interacts with families and with children, and how adequately the physical examination is completed.

Physicians interested in teaching in the office should receive some training. This should be provided by the faculty of the residency training program.

Counterpoint

The question of whether the resident should be an observer or an active participant in this program, particularly the office practice portion, deserves further comment. Some feel that there is less intrusion in the practice if the resident's role is one of observation. Those who advocate this approach state that the resident needs to be exposed to and trained in the day-to-day management of an office rather than focusing on patient care. In addition, teaching in the office places demands on the busy practitioner's time, which are mitigated when the resident observes rather than participates.

There are also arguments advocating the resident's active participation in the office program. For example, patients in a suburban or rural practice setting have different concerns, problems and demographic characteristics than those in the inner city. Residents need to experience first hand what it is like to care for the population with whom they are most likely to work post-training.

Studies about active versus passive learning show that active learners gain more cognitively, retain information longer, and are able to translate theory into practice better than passive learners.[3] Lastly, in programs where residents are responsible for patient care, office revenues do not decrease provided the program is well thought out and organized.

Organization

Incorporating a residency training program in a pediatric office practice requires an investment of time and energy. The pediatrician will want to bear in mind a number of considerations and requirements:

1. In developing a curriculum, the pediatrician should outline all office activities and recall the steps taken in establishing the practice.
2. Each resident should become familiar with the curriculum, so that expectations are clearly delineated.
3. Residents should discuss with the pediatrician the option of actively participating in the practice or closely observing the pediatrician's daily routine (eg, telephone answering, patient care, attending meetings).
4. If the resident sees patients alone, a well-defined plan for supervision should be developed. A few minutes of the pediatrician's time with the family after a resident-conducted visit may help reassure parents about the continuity of their child's care.
5. Office staff should participate and describe their roles and responsibilities to help the resident understand the mechanics of office practice.
6. Consideration should be given to including other health care professionals, eg, pedodontists, pharmacists, and educational psychologists.
7. The office should establish a teaching file or library of pertinent articles, books, and photographs to support the curriculum.
8. In group practices, one individual should assume principal organizational responsibility for the office training program, spending specific time with the resident. All members of the group should be committed to its educational goals.
9. Residents should prepare a written evaluation of the experience and use the curriculum to define what was expected. The pediatrician also should evaluate the resident's performance. Ideally, the evaluations should be discussed face-to-face before completion of the rotation.
10. The pediatrician should make certain that patients are aware of the new training program. In general, patients accept participation of residents in the practice, but information about the program should be given to patients before this change begins.
11. Practitioners and office personnel associated in the teaching program should be offered the opportunity to improve their teaching skills with formal instruction.
12. Instruction of residents takes time and should be a pleasant and positive experience for all concerned.

AAP Curriculum

The AAP has developed a curriculum for teaching practice management to pediatric residents.[4] Residency program directors interested in receiving a copy should contact the Division of Pediatric Practice for details on how to obtain a copy of this curriculum.

Advantages to participating pediatricians

The practice management program provides several benefits for the pediatrician:

1. It fulfills the continuing medical education requirements for Category 3, Medical Teaching, of the Physician's Recognition Award of the American Medical Association.
2. It satisfies the teaching responsibilities required of active staff members of medical centers and center-affiliated hospitals.
3. It provides an opportunity and a stimulus for the reassessment of the practice.
4. It enables practitioners to teach in the setting they know best and adds a dimension to practice, other than service, that can be a stimulant to research and continuing medical education activities.
5. It provides an opportunity for mutual learning and a closer working relationship with residents and the medical center staff.
6. Practitioners have an opportunity to interact with and evaluate the performance of residents, some of whom may be potential partners.
7. The pediatrician has a chance to make a significant impact on the trainee during the critical, formative stage in regard to career choice.
8. Teaching trainees in the office can have a positive influence on patients/parents and practice affiliation with a training program and medical school can be used as a marketing tool.

9. The program enables practitioners to become more involved in the training of residents, both didactically and experientially, ensuring the focus on primary care.

Advantages to the resident

The practice management program also provides several benefits to the resident.

1. It helps the resident understand the role of the pediatrician in the delivery of child health care in different environments, which may be helpful in making decisions about career goals.
2. It allows the resident to become aware of the nonmedical aspects of practice.
3. It enables the resident to experience discussion and feedback from patients in a manner not experienced previously.
4. It enables the resident to view the changing aspects of delivery of pediatric care with less emphasis on illness and more on health supervision.
5. The resident has the opportunity to compare and understand management philosophies (office practice versus medical center) regarding various problems (eg, the febrile infant, the child with tonsillitis).
6. Most importantly, the office experience should enable the resident to formulate a gestalt on the life and work of a pediatrician.

Conclusions

Teaching pediatric residents information and skills on pediatric practice is an essential part of a training program curriculum. Department chairpersons must be positive and firmly supportive, and practitioners must be enthusiastic and firmly convinced of the value of what they have to offer. Practice management programs have been shown to be educationally beneficial and pleasurable experiences for all participants.

Bibliography

Altameier WA III, St. Petery L, Schreklin GL, et al. The demonstration of private practice to pediatric residents through office rotations. *J Med Educ*. 1976;51:138

Berkelhamer JE. Practice management in the general pediatric clinic: Results of a survey of academic departments. *Pediatrics*. 1989;84:98

Greenberg LW. Teaching primary care pediatrics to pediatric residents through an office rotation. *J Med Educ*. 1979; 54:340

Greenberg LW. The role of the practicing pediatrician in resident education. *Pediatrics*. 1980;65:1173

Greenberg LW, Guandolo V. *A Manual for Teaching Residents Office Pediatrics*. Washington, DC: Children's Hospital National Medical Center; 1982

Guandolo VL, Feroll EJ, Mella G, et al. Educational potential in a private pediatric practice. *Clinical proceedings of Children's Hospital National Medical Center*. (special issue) 1983;39:129

Pietroni PO. Community office experience for family medicine residents. *J Med Educ*. 1981;56:43

Reeb KG. Education of residents in the pediatric office. *Pediatr Clin North Am*. 1981;28:601

Schwenk T, Whitman N. *The Physician as Teacher*. Available through the Dept of Family and Preventive Medicine, University of Utah Center for Health Sciences, Salt Lake City, UT 84132

References

1. *1990–1991 Directory of Graduate Medical Education Programs*. Chicago, IL: American Medical Association; 1990.
2. Sargent JR, Osborn LM. Resident training in community pediatricians' offices. *AJDC*. 1990;144:1356-1359
3. Bloom BS. Thought processes in lectures and discussions. *J Gen Educ*. 1954;7:160-169
4. American Academy of Pediatrics, Committee on Practice and Ambulatory Medicine. *Teaching Practice Management to Residents*. Elk Grove Village, IL: American Academy of Pediatrics; 1986.

Checklist

✓ Do pediatric programs in your area include private practice experience?
✓ Is the private practice rotation effective in both clinical and management areas?
✓ Is your office staff involved in preparing for and teaching residents?
✓ Do you have a plan for evaluating the resident's performance?

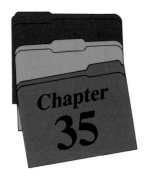

Chapter 35

Membership in the American Academy of Pediatrics

The benefits of membership in and the services offered by the Academy are discussed in this chapter.

Almost 80% of all pediatricians in the United States are members of the American Academy of Pediatrics. Why do so many pediatricians voluntarily give the Academy their time, money, and energy?

First of all, the Academy is unique among medical organizations. Most professional societies are organized to promote their specialty and enhance the business interests of their members. Although these are concerns for the Academy, its focus is much broader.

The Academy's Constitution states: "The Academy pledges its efforts and expertise to a fundamental goal – that all children and youth have the opportunity to grow up safe and strong with faith in the future and in themselves."

Through education, research, advocacy, and organization for action, the Academy has led the way in making professionals, lawmakers, parents, and the public more aware of and responsive to the special health needs of children. The Academy and its members share a strong commitment to improving the health and welfare of our nation's children.

The medical specialty of pediatrics has been shaped by the Academy during the last 60 years. The Academy articulates the goals of pediatrics with a united, clear, and independent voice; without the Academy, pediatrics would not be what it is today. The Academy is firmly established and respected as THE source of information on child health care. Members rely on the Academy for established standards of care and authoritative resources. Academy members know that their support is essential to keeping the future of their specialty in the hands of pediatricians, the foremost authorities on comprehensive health care for infants, children, adolescents, and young adults.

Membership in the Academy has many benefits and privileges. Academy members have instant, affordable access to the resources they need to keep their clinical skills sharp and their practices competitive. The Academy's membership plan is carefully designed to meet the needs of pediatricians at every stage of their careers from residency through retirement.

Membership categories

Resident Fellowship

Pediatricians-in-training at approved residency programs are welcomed in the Academy as Resident Fellows. During this period of intense study and challenge when time and money are scarce, the Academy makes it easy for residents to join their colleagues under the AAP membership umbrella. For a very modest fee Resident Fellows receive a myriad of benefits and services, including a complimentary copy of the *Report of the Committee on Infectious Diseases* (Red Book), and a subscription to *Pediatrics*. Another attractive feature of the Resident Fellow package is the complimentary life and disability income protection insurance free of charge for 1 year and at low group rates in subsequent years.

Additionally, the Academy has secured several corporate grants to provide pediatric residents with essential materials such as *PREP, Guidelines for Health Supervision II,* and *Management of Pediatric Practice II* free of charge. Other special programs for residents include starting in practice workshops, and a grant program for residents in financial distress. The Executive Board of the Academy has created a new Section for Resident Fellows and

Candidate Fellows who are still in training to give this unique group a representative body within the organization of the Academy.

Candidate Fellowship

After residency has been completed, pediatricians pursuing subspecialty training or establishing their careers enjoy Academy membership under the Candidate Fellow classification. Candidate Fellows receive more complimentary publications and pay a slightly higher dues rate than their resident counterparts. Candidate Fellowship is limited to a period of 4 years immediately following completion of the third year of residency training. Candidate Fellows' dues increase gradually each year, but still are significantly less than the full Fellowship fee.

The purpose of Candidate Fellowship is to allow young pediatricians time to take and pass their pediatric boards, a prerequisite to Fellowship, and to continue membership at a dues rate dramatically lower than the full Fellowship fee.

Fellowship

The main category of membership in the Academy is full Fellowship. Pediatricians certified by the American Board of Pediatrics, the Royal College of Physicians and Surgeons of Canada, or La Corporation Professionelle des Medecins du Quebec are eligible to be Academy Fellows with full benefits, services, and privileges including the right to vote on Academy matters. Following Academy custom, they may use the FAAP designation after their name.

Specialty Fellowship

Physicians certified in specialties other than pediatrics who devote at least 50% of their professional activities to the care of pediatric-aged patients are eligible to be Specialty Fellows. Specialty Fellows are entitled to the same membership benefits and services and pay the same dues as Fellows; however, they may hold national office only if additionally certified by one of the approved pediatric boards (eg, the American Board of Pediatrics, the Royal College of Physicians and Surgeons of Canada, or La Corporation Professionelle des Medecins du Quebec).

Emeritus Fellows

Fellow and Specialty Fellows may request Emeritus Fellowship upon reaching the age of 70 or at any age for reasons of health or other circumstances such as retirement. Emeritus Fellows, age 70 and older, pay no annual dues and may receive certain benefits on request or at low fees, but are not eligible to vote or hold Academy office. Emeritus Fellows, under age 70, are charged a $50 administrative fee yearly to cover the costs associated with maintaining their records and providing benefits.

Leave of absence

Fellows and Specialty Fellows in good standing may request a 1-year leave of absence during periods of special need such as temporary disability, parental leave, or unemployment. Members on leave of absence must pay for any benefits and services received and are exempt from the annual membership dues.

Married Fellow program

Married couples who are both Academy Fellows may choose to save money on membership dues by sharing one set of Academy publications and paying one half the dues rate for one spouse. Contact the Division of Member Services for details on this special program.

Other categories of membership in the Academy are Corresponding Fellowship, Honorary Fellowship, Canadian Paediatric Society/American Academy of Pediatrics Dual Fellowship, and Associate Membership.

Pediatricians look at their Academy membership as an investment in their specialty and their career. The benefits of membership are substantive and comprehensive. Perhaps the most important of these is maintaining high standards of competency and professionalism through continuing medical education.

Continuing medical education

The Academy provides a diverse menu of educational programs to satisfy the needs of every member. Since 1979, the Pediatrics Review and Education Program (PREP) has offered a coordinated program of continuing medical education and evaluation for practicing pediatricians. The PREP curriculum is based on educational objectives defined and published in advance each year and includes a Self-Assessment Exercise and a journal, *Pediatrics in Review*. The advantage of PREP is that it allows busy pediatricians to sharpen their clinical skills at their own pace and convenience. The PREP curriculum is also closely coordinated with the Program for Renewal of Certification in Pediatrics (PRCP). For those members preparing for certification renewal, PREP is dedicated to providing materials and resources to assist them with the process. The PREP Self-Assessment program is also available in a computer format (CompuPREP®) for use on IBM and Apple personal computers. The Pediatric *Update* audiocassette tape series is also coordinated with the PREP objectives for those who prefer an alternative learning format.

The Academy holds a major clinical meeting each spring and fall, as well as almost a dozen regional CME courses each year. Documentation of continuing medical education activities is furnished by the Academy. At the AAP annual meetings and spring sessions, a wide choice of topics is offered in the form of plenary sessions, seminars, section scientific programs, and exhibits. Starting in practice workshops and roundtables on practice management and medical liability are also provided. But most of all, these meetings allow pediatricians to meet with colleagues from across the country to forge professional relationships and to discuss pediatrics.

Publications

Regular publications

Pediatrics, the Academy's monthly scientific journal, has a circulation of approximately 50,000 and an international reputation for authoritative pediatric information. Almost all Academy members receive a subscription as part of the membership package.

The Academy's monthly newspaper keeps members current on all aspects of the specialty. Pending legislation, policy statements, practice management advice, and announcements of coming events are covered in *AAP News*.

The *Fellowship Directory* (Blue Book), a listing of all Academy members, is issued annually and distributed free to members. This directory, a helpful referral tool, includes the addresses and phone numbers for AAP members. The Blue Book is indexed alphabetically and by location or section (for subspecialties or special interests). In addition, the directory publishes an index to membership services, rosters of chapter, section, and committee leaders, and AAP Bylaws.

The *Publications Catalog* is a comprehensive listing of all the outstanding materials available from the Academy. It is updated annually and sent free of charge to all members.

Manuals

Pediatricians rely on the Academy for the expert advice provided in a series of manuals for the health care professional. These manuals, internationally recognized standards for care, are provided free or at considerable discounts to Academy members. Manuals or handbooks on topics of general or specific interest to pediatricians are written periodically (and revised when necessary) by Academy committees.

All Academy members receive one complimentary copy of each new edition of the *Report of the Committee on Infectious Diseases* (Red Book). This widely-used manual, first published in 1938, is revised regularly to provide current information and consensus on the effective control of children's communicable diseases.

Guidelines for Perinatal Care (Third Edition) is a multi-disciplinary manual written by the Academy and the American College of Obstetricians and Gynecologists and designed for all personnel involved with the care of pregnant women, fetuses, and neonates. The revised edition provides expanded discussion of preconceptional and antenatal screening, adoption, perinatal infections of both mother and baby, and fetal monitoring. In addition, it features new sections on AIDS, radiation exposure, ethics, fetal therapy, and standard terminology for reporting reproductive health statistics.

Pediatricians-in-training or starting in practice have found *Guidelines for Health Supervision II* an invaluable resource. This updated manual presents guidelines for patient visits from the prenatal visit to age twenty and emphasizes the therapeutic alliance between the pediatrician, the patients, and their families. A pocket-sized bound set of 22 cue cards summarizing each visit accompanies the manual.

Substance Abuse: A Guide for Health Professionals is a self-instructional text offering the latest information on the prevention, early identification, and treatment of substance abuse among young people.

The latest health, safety, and developmental guidelines from the Academy are presented in *Health in Day Care: A Manual for Health Professionals*. Pediatricians find authoritative answers to parents' questions about day care.

Other manuals cover such topics such as nutrition, sports medicine, medical liability and evaluating managed care contracts.

Committees, policy statements, and public education materials

The national committees, a major benefit to members, are a resource for expert guidance and assistance in all areas of pediatrics. The primary responsibility for developing policy statements and manuals rests with more than 30 expert councils, committees and task forces at work in the Academy. Although the committee system frequently is amended to meet new challenges confronting the specialty, the committees tend to be grouped by the general issues they address – psychosocial, technical, and practice.

The committees periodically issue articles, statements, commentaries, or recommendations on important issues which are published in *Pediatrics* or *AAP News* in a form suitable for saving and filing.

The *AAP Policy Reference Guide* is a comprehensive collection of all Academy policy statements. Current statements are published in their entirety. This handy resource is indexed and cross-referenced for convenience and clarity.

Patient education literature

Public education, hand in hand with professional pediatric care, has dramatically increased the quality of child health. Pediatricians know that educational literature from the Academy contains up-to-date and scientifically accurate information reviewed by experts from Academy committees and sections. The information is practical and easily understood; the topics are important to pediatric-aged patients and their parents.

These brochures, posters, booklets, and videotapes cover such topics as immunization, breast-feeding, developmental milestones, injury prevention, car safety, child care, substance abuse, adolescent depression, health insurance. and sports activities. Some are available in several languages.

Healthy Kids

Healthy Kids, an exciting new publication from *American Baby* and the American Academy of Pediatrics, addresses all the elements that go into raising a healthy, happy child, from basic information on health care to an analysis of a child's developing mental and behavioral patterns. *Healthy Kids* is presented in a comprehensive series of three age-specific publications – starting with birth to 3 years old, children ages 4 to 10 years old, and adolescents.

Academy members receive a supply of free copies of each issue of this magazine to distribute to their patients.

Other benefits

Members receive numerous other benefits and services. They receive considerable discounts on registration at Academy scientific meetings and purchases of Academy publications. They may participate in insurance plans at low group rates (comprehensive major medical, office overhead, hospital indemnity, disability income protection, dental, term life, universal life, and preferred auto insurance). Members enjoy group discounts on long distance telephone services, and car rentals. Through a special program with a national bank, Academy members can apply for a gold or silver credit card and may contract for "professional services," a system that allows members to accept credit card payments. A toll-free telephone number enables members to have quick access to the Academy's staff and resources in Illinois and Washington, DC. Office-based pediatricians interested in research can apply to the Academy's research fund for financial support.

Opportunities for involvement

Chapters

The Academy is a democratic organization, divided into nine regional districts with 59 United States chapters and seven chapters in Canada.

Chapters are the channels of representation and communication for individual members. Academy members voice their concerns at chapter meetings, by sending resolutions to the Annual Chapter Forum, and by electing chapter and district leaders.

Chapters represent the health needs of children and are important players in developing and implementing child health policy at the state level. Each chapter establishes its own legislative priorities and accomplishes them largely through volunteer member efforts. Chapters have a proud history of "Speaking Up For Children."

Members take part in implementing Academy programs by participating in chapter initiatives, serving on chapter committees, and coordinating national and chapter activities. Members working through the network of chapters have passed child passenger safety laws in all 50 states; shortened the statute of limitations for minors; established bioethical review committees at local hospitals; and developed local coordinators for media relations, child health financing, and the tobacco-free society initiative.

Sections

Pediatricians with a special interest, specialty, or a subspecialty may form into sections which, as with the Academy's committees, serve as a resource of expertise for the Academy. Fellows may join one or more sections of their choice. The sections present educational programs during the annual meetings and spring sessions, develop educational projects, and promote pediatrics in other specialty societies. Many of the sections have established separate dues to help them accomplish their mission.

Conclusion

For most pediatricians, membership in the Academy is the hallmark of professionalism and service to children. Membership benefits include continuing education programs, collegial efforts to establish standards for care, authoritative resources, opportunities for involvement in chapters, sections, and committees, an effective advocacy arm for the health needs of children, and fellowship with peers.

Checklist

✓ Have you carefully considered the advantages of membership in the Academy?

✓ Do you periodically review the *Publications Catalog* for pertinent books and pamphlets?

✓ Have you taken advantage of Academy-sponsored CME courses?

✓ Do you effectively use Academy staff and resources?

✓ Do you understand the benefits of the insurance available to Academy members?

✓ Are you involved in your local Academy chapter?

✓ Do you have an interest in joining any of the Academy's sections?

Illustration Credits

Figure 2-1: Location Scorecard. *Medical Practice Management* by Horace Cotton. Medical Economics Company, Inc, Oradell, NJ 1985

Box, pg 39: Telephone Quality of Care Checklist: Katz, HP: *Telephone Triage and Training in Pediatric and Family Practice: A Handbook for Health Care Professionals,* 2nd Edition, Philadelphia, PA, FA Davis, Co, 1990

Figure 8-1: A Four-Step Approach to Improved Telephone Service and Quality. Katz, HP: *Telephone Triage and Training in Pediatric and Family Practice: A Handbook for Health Care Professionals,* 2nd Edition, Philadelphia, PA, FA Davis, Co, 1990

Figure 8-3: Telephone encounter entries. Beaumont Clinic, Green Bay, WI.

Figure 9-1: Sample job description for receptionist. Pediatric Services Incorporated, Parma, OH.

Figure 9-2: Sample job description for insurance clerk. Pediatric Services Incorporated, Parma, OH.

Figure 9-3: Sample job description for office manager. Pediatric Services Incorporated, Parma, OH.

Figure 9-4: Sample job description for day nurse. Pediatric Services Incorporated, Parma, OH.

Figure 9-5: Sample performance review form. Pediatric Services Incorporated, Parma, OH.

Figure 9-6: Sample employee handbook. Pediatric Services Incorporated, Parma, OH.

Figure 10-1: Health questionnaire for a new patient. Pediatric Associates, Hollywood, FL.

Figure 10-3: Well child care check sheet. Dorothy Davies Johnson, MD, and Barbara Jones Deloian, RN, PNP.

Figure 11-1: Newborn information booklet. North Suburban Pediatrics, Evanston, IL.

Figure 11-2: Practice information folders and booklets. Pediatric Associates, Hollywood, FL; Drs Piel, Patton, Aicardi, Gonda & Ernster, San Francisco, CA; Drs Martin Gershman, Mitchell Sollod & Robert Verhoogen, San Francisco, CA.

Figure 12-1: Patient registration form. Pediatric Associates, Hollywood, FL.

Figure 12-2: 1990 standardized insurance form (HCFA-1500). US Department of Health and Human Services, Health Care Financing Administration, Bethesda, MD.

Figure 12-3: Health care information transfer request form. Pediatric Associates, Hollywood, FL.

Figure 12-4: Health care information response form. Pediatric Associates, Hollywood, FL.

Figure 12-5: Sample initial collection letter. Beaumont Clinic, Green Bay, WI.

Figure 12-6: Sample second collection letter. Beaumont Clinic, Green Bay, WI.

Figure 12-7: Sample third collection letter. Beaumont Clinic, Green Bay, WI.

Figure 14-2: Patient charge sheet. Clairemont Pediatric Medical Group, Inc, San Diego, CA.

Figure 14-3: Patient charge sheet. KidsHealth, Inc, Knoxville, TN.

Figure 15-1: Avoid hold harmless clauses. American Society of Internal Medicine. *An A.S.I.M. Guide for Physicians and their Staff: The PPO Perspective.* Washington, DC, 1986.

Figure 16-1: Sample patient satisfaction survey. Ross Laboratories, Columbus, OH.

Figure 16-2: Explanation of educational videocassette library. Pediatric Associates, Hollywood, FL.

Box, pg 120: Suggestions for Pediatricians: William Robertson, MD, and W. Parker, Seattle, WA.

Figure 22-2: Sample parent questionnaire. Donald Moore, MD, Boulder, CO.

Figure 22-3: Unisex adolescent health inventory. Donald Moore, MD, Boulder, CO.

Figure 22-4: Sample adolescent questionnaire. Donald Moore, MD, Boulder, CO.

Figure 26-3: Common problem educational materials. Salt Lake Pediacenter, Salt Lake City, UT.

Figure 26-4: Sample patient education materials. American Academy of Ophthalmology, San Francisco, CA; American Cancer Society, Atlanta, GA; American College of Obstetricians and Gynecologists, Washington, DC.

Figure 28-1: Sample letter for discontinuing professional courtesy to families of physicians. Pediatric Associates, Hollywood, FL.

Box, pg 170: 10 Commandments for Effective Consultations. ©1983, American Medical Association.

Box, pg 177: Investment Advisor Questionnaire. ©1988, American Association of Retired Persons, Washington, DC.

Figure 34-2: Sample brochure. Lucy Osburn, MD, Salt Lake City, UT.

Index

Notes

Notes

Notes

Notes